Thick Film Hybrid
Microcircuit Technology

Thick Film Hybrid Microcircuit Technology

D. W. HAMER

State of the Art, Inc.

J. V. BIGGERS

The Pennsylvania State University

WILEY-INTERSCIENCE, a Division of John Wiley & Sons, Inc.
New York • London • Sydney • Toronto

Library of Congress Cataloging in Publication Data

Hamer, Donald W   1925–
    Thick film hybrid microcircuit technology.

    Includes bibliographical references.
    1. Microelectronics.   I.   Biggers, J. V., 1929–
joint author.   II.   Title.

TK7874.H34   621.381′73   72-3191
ISBN 0-471-34700-0

Printed in the United States of America

10 9 8 7 6 5 4 3 2 1

PREFACE

In 1969 we initiated a series of five-day seminars on thick film, aimed at people who had little or no background in this field.

There was no text to turn to when the seminar series was started. Use of articles reprinted from newspapers and periodicals would have resulted in swings from oversimplified to highly technical presentations. Poor subject balance also would have been a problem. We were thus forced to come up with something of our own that had balanced content and uniform technical depth. After giving these seminars over a period of two years, we have learned what must be amplified, or dropped, or changed in order to produce an effective seminar.

This book is based on the seminar text. It differs in organization from the text used for the seminars only insofar as reading a book is a different learning experience than is attending a seminar.

The technical level of our presentation reflects the fact that many interested people have a limited background in the physics and chemistry of thick film composites. We spend additional time in discussing materials and processing, because these are of great importance in the *manufacture* of thick film circuits. Applications information has been almost eliminated. The book is about the technology of thick film, not its application.

D. W. Hamer
J. V. Biggers

State College, Pennsylvania
March 1972

v

CONTENTS

Chapter 1   *Introduction to Thick Film Microelectronics*   1

Chapter 2   *A First Look at Thick Film Technology*   29

Chapter 3   *The Economic Rationale for Thick Film Hybrids*   56

Chapter 4   *Thick Film Materials*   69

Chapter 5   *Screen Printing*   95

Chapter 6   *Firing Thick Films*   116

Chapter 7   *Properties of Thick Film Components*   131

Chapter 8   *Trimming Thick Film Elements*   159

Chapter 9   *Bonding and Soldering*   193

Chapter 10   *Discrete Devices for Thick Film Circuits*   242

Chapter 11   *Packaging*   277

Chapter 12   *Artwork, Layout, and Design*   303

Chapter 13   *The Economics of Thick Film Hybrid Microcircuit Production*   332

Appendix I   *The Technology of Monolithic Integrated Circuits and Thin Film Integrated Circuits*   357

Appendix II   *Digging Deeper*   392

Index   421

Chapter 1

INTRODUCTION TO THICK FILM MICROELECTRONICS

Before discussing the main topics of this book we examine some introductory matters to gain the proper background knowledge. We examine (1) historical developments—both in electronics in general and in integrated circuits in particular; (2) how integrated circuits (and, specifically, thick film) are affecting the electronics industry; and (3) the basic terminology of microelectronics.

HISTORICAL DEVELOPMENTS—ELECTRONICS IN GENERAL

Figure 1-1 shows forty years of solid growth in electronics. What are the forces behind this growth? Why has it continued for four decades? Few other industries of the same size have been able to maintain such growth.

We know that in recent years computers, industrial instruments, space technology, microelectronics, and integrated circuits have all contributed to the continuation of the well-established, long-term growth of the electronics industry. But how? What is the interrelationship between electronics and microelectronics? A brief look at the technology changes in electronics in the past will help to explain some of these relationships.

1

Electronics and Communication. Electronics is tied closely to the story of communications. Probably the main forward steps that man has made in his ability to communicate are (1) spoken language, (2) written language, (3) printing presses, and (4) electronic communications. Each had the effect of tremendously broadening human communicating skills. Use of language made it possible for primitive man to communicate subtle and

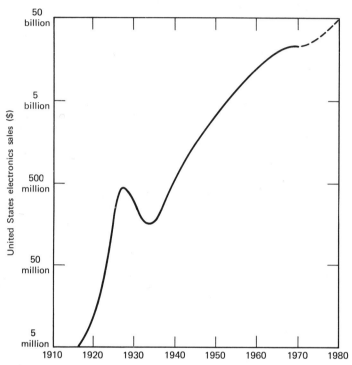

Figure 1-1 Growth patterns in the electronics industry. (*Source. IEEE Spectrum,* December 1969, p. 57.)

complex desires, thoughts, and ideas. One man could enrich the thoughts and knowledge of another man, and the synergistic effect lifted man to true civilization. The concept of putting spoken words in an equivalent written form permitted man to bridge time and distance with his ideas. Mathematical language further developed and enhanced his capability. The printing press extended the advantages of written language to many more people, and man's power of communications became even greater. Each one of these developments, if one were to try to measure the "power" of man's communicating abilities, resulted in an orders-of-magnitude increase in capabilities. Man who makes use of mathematics, music, visual arts, and complex spoken language, all aided by mass distribution via printing presses, is much more effective than man who possesses spoken language only.

Electronics has improved man's communicating capabilities by an order of magnitude equal to that of the printing press. There have been continuing basic technological developments in electronics that have further enhanced this capability, the integrated circuit being the latest.

THE THREE "ERAS" OF ELECTRONICS

The First Era. The "passive components" era, as it may be called, began before 1900 with the invention of the telephone and the telegraph. Together with wireless telegraphy these two inventions are the foundation of today's electronic communications world.

Equipment in this period was made with passive components such as coils of wire, conductors, magnets, capacitors, and resistors and by electromechanical devices such as switches, levers, and relays.

The telecommunications industry that was launched by these developments was the foundation for the still-to-come electronics industry. Some of the names of the original inventors—Bell and Marconi, for example—are familiar names today in communications and electronics.

The Second Era. Fleming's invention at the turn of the century of the first active device—the electron tube—started the second period. (An active device is, put simply, something that allows control of a large amount of voltage or current with a very small electrical input. It permits us to put "in" a small signal and to get "out" a big signal. This cannot be achieved with passive devices.)

The electron tube expanded man's communication capabilities once more. Now it was possible to send voice messages by wire over *long distances;* until then telephone's distance capability had been limited because the signal slowly lost strength over long distances. With an active device a weak signal could be amplified over and over—allowing us to talk over much greater distances.

The active device also lets us send voice messages without wires. Wireless communications, though known before, had been limited to coded pulses of noise, such as those released by a high-voltage spark jumping across a gap. Eventually the active device would allow transmitting not only *voice* over long distances without wires, but other signals, such as music, pictures (television), and other information.

The electron tube—the first "active" device—thus opened still further areas of freedom in communicating. Not only the spoken word could be communicated without connecting wires, but all sorts of aural and visual information, even complex machine-to-machine talk. This invention—with the help of the already existing passive electrical devices—now made available the needed technological resources to start a new industry: electronics.

The rapid growth of the new electronics industry is shown in Figure 1-2, which lists the dollar sales of vacuum tubes from 1920 to the present.

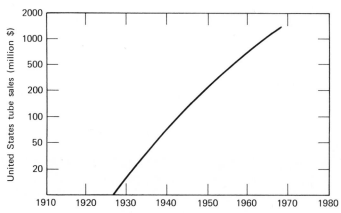

Figure 1-2 The growth of tube sales. (*Source. IEEE Spectrum,* June 1969, p. 26.)

The pattern of continuing growth over a long period is exponential in nature, as indicated by the semilog graph. The tube industry has expanded by an order of magnitude every two decades since the 1920s—an annual growth of 12% compounded every year for forty years or more!

The reason for this growth is that "interesting" things can be done with the tube. At first a new tube could be made to perform only in a limited way or perhaps only in the laboratory. However, as the technology of making tubes (glass forming, glass-to-metal sealing, materials technology, vacuum technology, plastics, automated handling techniques, etc.) improved, new fields opened up to feed electronic industry sales—and, of course, electron tube sales as well.

Sales in the various passive-component industries grew *with* the tube sales during these years. These subindustries, many having their roots in the telephone-telegraph business of the nineteenth century, had their own technologies, which were as varied as the shapes and functions of the components involved. Driven by both opportunity and need, the technologies of component making improved and the passive-component makers were able to keep up with advancing electron tube technology.

Figure 1-1, showing the growth of electronics, is repeated in Figure 1-3, with the contributions of the military market in the forties and later of

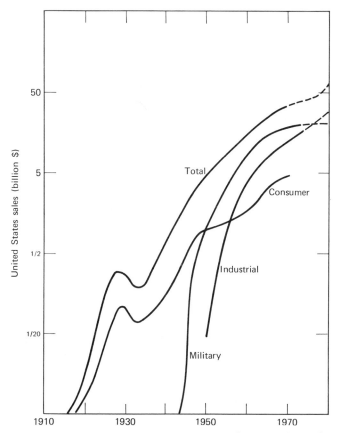

Figure 1-3 The sales history of the United States electronics industry. (*Source. IEEE Spectrum,* December 1969, p. 57.)

the industrial electronics industry added. It illustrates how the industry—built originally on radio and telephonic communications—fed itself with new industries as the various components and electron tube technologies advanced.

Thus the electronics industry was able to grow through the decades of the second era because one technological development after another in the electron tube and passive-components business allowed the industry to tackle more and more complex things. Steady advances in the technologies of the participating industries made one new product after another practical. (Component development, of course, was not *solely* responsible for these products and markets. The designers of equipment and circuits certainly contributed. The development of component art and of equipment design go hand in hand—each unable to survive without the other.)

Radio became big business in the twenties. Military electronics arrived in the forties. Television became generally available in the late forties and early fifties. Industrial electronics—more or less fathered by the military—gained significance in the fifties. This has been the pattern of industry growth for the active-device era: growth of one major product after another, made possible (or practical) by advancing technologies in the various component industries. As one product stopped developing and became a stable industry, another new "industry" started and made continued growth possible.

Consider the variations in technology of the various participants in the electronics industry. The tube makers work with glass/ceramic/metal sealing—exotic materials and complex shapes; the capacitor makers with the many dielectric materials, insulators, electrodes, and assembly techniques; the wire makers with metal drawing technologies and insulation material; the equipment assemblers with the various assembly techniques; and finally the circuit designer who starts it all with his mathematical techniques for circuit synthesis. There is not much overlap in these technologies.

The second era of electronics—the era of the active device thus encompasses fifty years of continuous rapid growth (except for the thirties)—averaging 12% per year. The technologies are component based and differ widely, with very little overlap.

The Transition Period (between the Second and Third Eras). The 1950s mark the ending of the second period of electronics and the beginning of the third period. The transition time extended into the 1960s and 1970s. It was the transistor, of course, that was the start of this transition.

During the transition time old balances in the electronics industry are going to be upset, resulting in tough times for some and good times for others. This is what makes the transition time very exciting, and very frustrating.

By the late 1940s electronics as a growth industry had just about come to an end. If it had not been for the transistor, the growth pattern that we saw earlier in this chapter would have been very different. The electron-tube-oriented technologies—forty years or older—were running out of ways to improve. Performance and reliability of the electron tube were beginning to push theoretical limits. Since tubes were technology limited, new applications for the tube would be unlikely to develop. And without new applications a continued annual growth of 12% would be very hard to achieve.

To cite one example of its technical limitations, the electron tube, even though it can function as a switch, *never* in all the forty years of steady improvements in performance and reliability could compete, in a broad sense, with electromechanical relays. It was for this reason that the telephone company retained electromechanical relays when they began to modernize in the forties and switch to the dial systems. Other limitations had to do with size, cost, strength, and life.

The transistor was invented in 1948 by Shockley, Bardeen, and Bratten at the Bell Laboratories. It was a remarkable invention—backed by some remarkable advances in materials technology. Here was a solid state device that, at least theoretically, could do almost anything a tube could. It was also strong in many areas where the tube was weak; it was *very* small (almost too small, in fact, for the mechanical handling capabilities of those days); it was reliable (at least potentially)—being constructed like it was—just a piece of matter; and it was potentially inexpensive. Thus a brand new technology arrived, completely mysterious to most of the participants in the electronics industry at that time. It threatened to limit tube sales eventually, but at the same time it opened vistas of all kinds of new markets for electronics.

Small size had for some time been desired in the electronics industry because of the need of complex systems to be light and portable. Mini-components of various kinds had begun to come along—small versions of electron tubes, the ceramic capacitor, and so on. Miniaturization of electronics had made a feeble start, but the transistor gave it a start with its great reduction in size. The various passive-components industries now began to miniaturize along with the transistor. These efforts have been successful, and many components makers have participated fully in the transistor revolution. The state of their technology allowed them to make further developments, hence to survive. Tube makers, however, at least in areas where the transistor performed well (not, e.g., in CRTs), had little choice and had to join the revolution by getting into transistors.

We are all familiar with the results of the transistor's appearance on the electronics scene. The switching capabilities of the transistor almost single-handedly opened up the computer business (which forms the basis for the rapid growth of the industrial electronics business, as shown in Figure 1-3). The inexpensive pocket radio so popular today is the result of the transistor, as is the success of the radio broadcasting business (in spite of television). Many space and airborne systems and other complicated electronic marvels, such as modern weapons systems, exist because of the transistor's size and reliability.

The technical limitations of the electron tube were thus circumvented. This allowed one last jump in electronics industry growth through the 1950s and into the 1960s. Without the transistor the long-established growth pattern in electronics might have ended by 1950, converting the industry to one that lives on without major technical innovation, as do other mature, basic industries today (automobile, steel, furniture, etc.).

New firms became leaders by embracing the new technology; old leaders that failed to enter the new field eventually lost their position in the electronics industry.

The basic technology of the transistor meanwhile underwent several almost back-to-back upheavals. The first transistors were point contact devices. These were soon replaced by alloy transistors—almost before the point contact got off the ground. The wide use of the original transistor material—germanium—soon began to be jeopardized by better-performing silicon. Alloy junction technology went down before the onslaught of diffusion. Each of the new developments took down many good men and firms that were too loyal to the old technology. This rapid succession of one technology rolling over the previous one is in good measure responsible for the bloody trail of transistor maker "bodies" (bruised and mauled at least).

As we saw, the greater part of the second era of electronics was characterized by one new market application building on top of the another—all based on various technologies that never really changed (only improved) from the beginning of the era. But the last years of the era—the transition period, so to speak—had a different character. New markets still came along, thus producing continuing growth for the electronics industry, but now technology was no longer stable. The first decade of the transistor's existence witnessed four new technologies—from point contact germanium devices to diffused junction silicon devices. Improvement came from dumping one technology in favor of another rather than from the slow improvement of a single technology. From a business management standpoint, this produced real problems. How is one to pay for all the investments involved if the technology lasts only two or three years before another comes along? In the early days of the second era decades were available to recoup investment; now only a few years are available. This explains why the period has proved to be a painful one for many people involved in semiconductor technology.

By 1960 the industry had come to still another impasse—another technological brick wall, as serious as or perhaps even more serious in its implications that that which the tube's performance limitations had placed on the industry. Some of the new systems had so many components that, no matter how carefully they were connected, a loose wire, a crossed connection, or some other similar mistake was bound to occur, thus preventing the system from functioning. Systems designers could envision all kinds of enticing new products—but, alas, they were too complex to be assembled into a working whole. The problem of unreliable connections seriously limited such plans. If more complex products were to become a reality, the connection difficulty would have to be circumvented.

The 1950s saw the beginning of the resolution of this interconnections impasse. The solutions would lead to today's thick film, thin film, and monolithic technologies. These three technologies all offered "solutions" to the interconnection problem. The technological capabilities of thick film, thin film, and monolithic silicon opened the third era of electronics—the period of the integrated circuit.

The Third Era—the Integrated Circuit Era. In the preceeding section we noted how the advent of the transistor made possible one last surge of growth in the second era—the active device era. This is depicted in Figure 1-4, which is a repeat of Figure 1-2 (showing tube growth over the years),

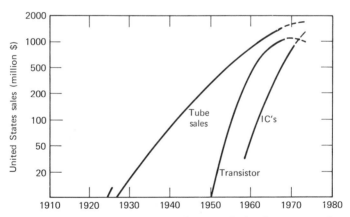

Figure 1-4 The sales growth of integrated circuits (ICs), tubes, and transistors.

but with data on discrete semiconductor sales and integrated circuit sales added. Note the fast growth of the discrete semiconductor; in only a decade the growth topped out, however, nipped, of course, by the integrated circuit (IC).

The IC growth curve in the figure shows a much different rate than did the devices of the second era. This rapid growth, characterized (like the transistor industry) by a rapidly moving technology, has made it a very exciting and perilous time for those in the industry. New industrial giants have arisen by making use of these technologies. Note that the extreme rapid growth is being sustained even on the very broad basis of hundreds of millions of dollars. This reflects some of the pressures of need that were waiting—and were released—when the technology appeared on the scene.

But some of the most significant characteristics of the third era are not reflected in the chart. They were hinted at in the preceding paragraph when it was mentioned that new firms have won major positions (not to mention the hundreds of smaller firms that are also gaining entry).

One of the *really important* characteristics of the third era is that many of the old, well-established industry relationships are altering. The biggest change is in the classic components maker-components assembler relationship. Third-era components (now often part of the IC) are being made by technologies very different from those that are familiar to the older components makers.

Furthermore, the IC maker is taking over a portion of the classic role of the equipment assembler, in that he is in effect doing much of the assembly. And the "assembly" is being done *differently*—via diffusion, vacuum evaporations, and screen printing rather than with soldering iron and nimble-fingered girls.

This situation has not only been a strange and uncomfortable one for the component makers and equipment assembler, but also for the equipment designer. Integrated circuits operate differently, both functionally and economically, and new design rules must be followed. Often the new rules are so changed that the circuit designer no longer even design the equipment—this being the job of the systems designer. The systems designer draws little boxes and labels them. Circuit designers design what is in the little boxes and need not concern themselves about the purpose of the final equipment.

Thus the integrated circuit has brought change for almost everyone in the industry—from the components maker to the circuit designer. The old rules no longer apply, and the established fifty-year-old relationships between the various firms in the electronics industry will no longer exist as we go into the integrated circuit era.

Integrated circuits (IC) produce circuits with the individual component (or elements) already interconnected. Thus the IC maker is taking over a function that has traditionally belonged to the equipment assembler. The IC producer has in effect integrated forward—closer to the end product.

The old electronics industry participants are not usually willing to give up, however; to counter this trend of forward integration on the part of the IC makers, many firms with long-established traditions of assembling and marketing equipment integrate backward by making IC's themselves. They find that they *must* do so if they wish to control their traditional share of the value added. Figure 1-5 shows how the IC, replacing many of the components, has much of the assembly labor costs built into it.

	Total Value Added (%)	
	Discrete Components Used	ICs Used
Labor	21	7
Material	18	11
Components	61	82

Figure 1-5 Comparison in value added of IC-made equipment with component-made equipment. (*Source.* Integrated Circuit Engineering Corporation, *A Management Guide to Integrated Circuits*, 5th ed.)

Another situation that has come with the integrated circuit era is increased overlapping of technologies. In the days of the second era, the technologies of making components, assembling them, and designing the equipment had little to do with one another. People who made components did not need to know how the components worked or what they were used for. The assembler was not concerned with the technology of making components, but; worried only about "having them there on the floor when he needed them." To the designer, the components were abstract symbols. This is completely different when ICs are being made. The user or the maker of ICs must have technological capabilities across the board. It is rare to find all these technological skills developed to an expert level in one person—but they have to be available within the firm. Also, each individual needs *some* expertise in areas outside his specialty. The separation of technologies of the "old days" and the overlap of today's IC era are illustrated in Figure 1-6.

The main result of the start of electronic's third era is that it is allowing the industry to resume its traditional growth pattern.

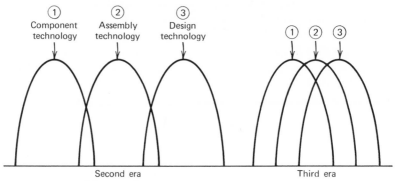

Figure 1-6 Changes in technological overlap.

HISTORICAL DEVELOPMENTS—ICs

According to the *Random House Dictionary of the English Language,* "integrated" means "Combining or coordinating separate elements so as to provide a harmonious, interrelated whole." With such a broad definition, several approaches to integrating electronic circuits should be possible. Our approach in this book is through *silicon monolithic* integration, *thick film* integration, *thin film* integration, and finally *hybrid* integration. We try to clear up some of the conflicting terms that often confuse people when discussing ICs. We also continue the tale of how today's electronics industry is forced to undergo a basic change.

According to the dictionary definition, printed circuits are a simple form of integrated circuit. They manage to combine all the separate wires of a device into one piece. There is little or no miniaturization (which is also usually associated with integration), and the only kind of component that is integrated is the conductors. Even with these limitations, we are all aware of how the printed circuit has managed to fill a very basic and important need by improving reliability of interconnections. The printed circuit accomplishes some of the basic goals of integration of electronic circuits. As said before, the restriction of the type of component to be integrated to *conductors only* limits the printed circuit's scope, as does the fact that it is not miniaturized.

If one does not care to call the printed circuit board an early IC, it can at least serve as an example of one of the relatively rare new technologies in passive components that developed in the second era. Without the integrated conductors of the printed circuit board, the computer of today would be a hopeless tangle of wires. The thing that keeps the printed circuit from becoming a true IC in the sense usually thought of today is that its technology will not allow production of other types of components.

Silicon Monolithic Integrated Circuits. The most significant of the various developments that led to the main IC technologies of today has to do with the diffused silicon device.

The term *diffused* refers to a method of introducing one material into another. The phenomena of diffusion are used in making silicon semiconductor devices to introduce small amounts of materials into the basic silicon material.

Diffusion techniques for the first planar transistors were used in the mid-fifties, eventually displacing the alloy junction types. Figure 1-7 is a

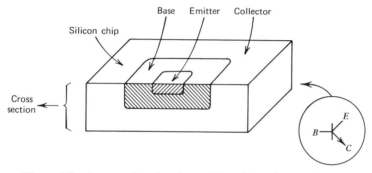

Figure 1-7 Construction of a planar diffused-junction transistor.

cross section of the construction of a planar diffused transistor. The sketch shows all the main parts of a transistor chip, the base, emitter, and collector—on a single plane. All the necessary IC technologies are used in making this planar diffused-junction transistor.

In 1956 Ross at Bell Laboratories developed an integrated silicon binary counter using planar *pnpn* structures, starting a string of developments that in a few years would result in the IC as we know it today. In 1958 Texas Instruments (Kilby) developed a silicon circuit containing diodes, transistors, and resistors separated by mesa techniques. The various components were interconnected with wire jumpers as indicated in Figure 1-8.

The Texas Instruments development was the first real silicon IC. It used a monolithic structure and managed to get more than one kind of component into the monolith. Of great significance was the combination of active *and* passive components, operating side by side, produced with the same basic technology. If one had to pick any one single development (it is not really fair to do this) and say "it started here," this invention would be where the third era started. If not here, certainly with the next development from Fairchild.

Very shortly after Kilby's invention, a major improvement in technique was introduced by Noyce and his co-workers at Fairchild. Instead of using

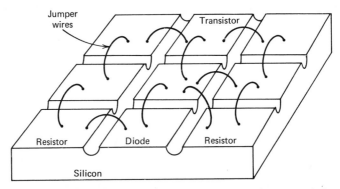

Figure 1-8 The Kilby/Texas Instruments IC, with mesa isolation and jumper connections.

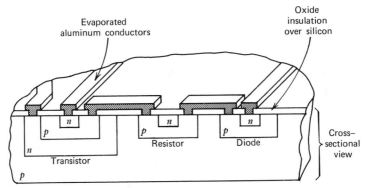

Figure 1-9 The Noyce/Fairchild IC, with evaporated interconnections.

wire jumpers to interconnect the various components, separated by mesas, Noyce used diffused junctions for isolation and vacuum evaporated metal to make the connections (Figure 1-9). There is controversy about which of the two—Noyce or Kilby—was the actual inventor of the IC. The matter is in the courts where decisions have been made and reversed, with appeals continuing.

With the Fairchild development, the basic form of the silicon monolithic IC was set. Diffused silicon technology along with vacuum evaporation technology presented a true integrated approach, which allowed transistors, diodes, capacitors, and resistors to be *interconnected* with conductors. This approach solved much of the interconnect problem.

Another very important series of developments were being made meanwhile at Bell Laboratories that would in time make large-scale manufacture of ICs economically practical—the process of epitaxy, by which one kind of silicon can be grown on a slice of another type of silicon.

It should be noted that the silicon IC was a "triple barrelled" development. Not only was a way around the *interconnection difficulties* at hand, but the small size and the batch-process nature of the processing gave promise of *extreme miniaturization* and *very low cost* as various processing difficulties were overcome.

There are limitations in silicon monolithic ICs, however. The range of components possible and the quality of these components are somewhat limited. IC versions of some circuits do not work because of the individual components' poor performance. Integration for some types of circuits is not possible with this technique.

Thick Film ICs. In the late forties and early fifties the makers of ceramic capacitors were pursuing another approach to the integration of electronic circuits that would eventually evolve into what we now refer to as the *thick film IC*. This approach is based on screen printing and uses "fired-on" materials for making components.

Ceramic capacitors have electrodes made from "fired-on silver." These electrodes are screen printed. They are made from a mixture of silver, glass, and organics. The ceramic capacitor, with its high dielectric constant, had won wide acceptance by the early fifties because of its low cost and small size. Capacitor engineers, fighting to improve size and cost, soon hit upon the idea of putting two capacitors on a single dielectric with a common electrode on one side. Since this resulted in two capacitors with only three leads, it amounted to a very small beginning in another approach to solving the intercorrection problem.

Next in the evolution of thick film ICs came several capacitors on a single piece of dielectric instead of only two. Screen-printed carbon composition resistors were added to make resistor-capacitor combinations. Now, with both capacitors and resistors (as well as the interconnecting conductors) it is possible to get a fair degree of integration of passive devices. This resulted in elimination of many interconnections. These thick film circuits were *also* true ICs—although at the time they were developed they were not called ICs. (The term "integrated circuit" was first applied to the monolithic silicon devices and for some time applied only to this type. Inclusion of thick and thin film as ICs came later.)

Centralab Division of Globe Union pioneered these thick film devices and deserves a large share of the credit for starting technologies that eventually developed into today's thick film hybrid IC technology.

One of the problems that Centralab encountered as did the firms that took up the manufacture of these all-passive-component ICs, was that the baked-on carbon resistor was not very good. Certainly not good enough for many of the resistor-capacitor circuits that were used. The carbon resistor was noisy, it had a rather high temperature coefficient, its value was difficult to control closely, and it did not perform well under rugged operating conditions. The development of the fired-on resistor cleared up many of these problems and released the thick film IC from a very limited to a much broader range of usefulness.

DuPont, the major supplier of the fired-on silver compositions used by the makers of the capacitors and of resistor/capacitor combinations, had a naturally strong technical base for developing a replacement for the carbon resistor. They pioneered in the development of new fired-on resistor materials that could replace carbon. Other firms that were making screen-printed *R-C* circuits also had been working on the problem, and such companies as Sprague and CTS, too, developed (for their internal use) resistor systems that were great improvements over the baked-on carbon. All of these compositions were of the fired-on type.

There are many applications where resistors only are needed. Alumina is used as the substrate for these applications instead of titanate materials (more difficult to handle and process) to produce a better resistor. One may think that the limitation of the thick film IC to resistors and capacitors is serious. The lack of active device capability would seem to cripple the process. However, today's market for this type of circuit is quite large—over $40 million—and is growing nicely.

Early in the game, recognizing the limitations of not having active devices as part of their circuits, Centralab and others attached tubes or transistors—much in the same way as these items were attached to conventional circuits. This then might be called the advent of the *hybrid* integrated circuit—it was a pioneering effort to get around some of the limitations of thick film having only passive device capability.

Centralab, along with Onandaga China (now a part of Air Reduction Co.—the Airco Speer Electronics Division) produced a thick film hybrid IC used in a fusing device during the Korean War. This is probably the first thick film hybrid circuit—and perhaps could take credit for being the first *integrated circuit* also—since it was produced in the early 1950s, with development models going back to the late 1940s—long before silicon monolithics came along. See Figure 1-10.

It was IBM that finally placed thick film into the "big-time" category. Because of its inherent "producibility," they decided to use the thick film

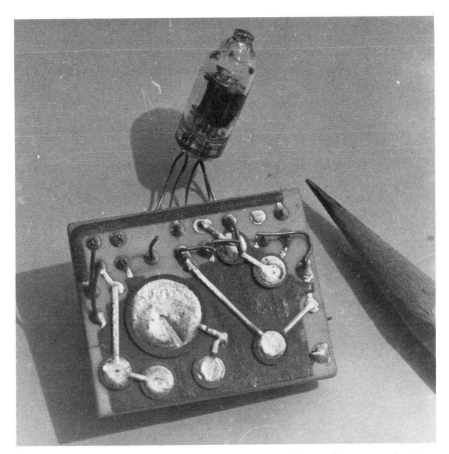

Figure 1-10 An early thick film device. The composition resistors are printed on titanate substrates. Capacitor chips and small vacuum tubes are attached with solder. (*Source.* H. Simon, Airco Speer; photograph by State of the Art, Inc.)

in making the circuitry for their 360 series computer. Conductors and resistors were of thick film. Capacitors, diodes, and transistors were attached as separate units. A highly animated process was developed that has produced billions of thick film circuits. See Figures 1-11 and 1-12.

Thus the thick film IC, pioneered by such firms as Centralab, CTS,

Sprague, DuPont, and IBM, achieved much the same result as did the developers of the silicon monolithic circuit. They created a compatible technology for making more than one kind of component in which the interconnection problem was solved to some degree.

It should be emphasized that the limitation of not being able to include active devices (except by attachment as discrete additions) is a disadvantage that restricts usefulness and to some extent leaves the field wide open to the silicon monolithic—which has no such limitation. What saves thick

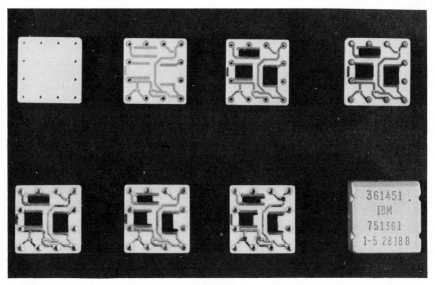

Figure 1-11 The assembly sequence of IBM's "SLT" thick film circuit. (Courtesy IBM.)

film is that with added active devices (hybrid ICs, i.e.) it can offer such advantages as high performance, quality, precision, low parasitics, and a wide range of component values. Since silicon monolithics cannot offer this performance, the usefulness of the thick film IC is thus firmly established.

Thin Film ICs. A third approach to integration has been that of thin film. Here the technology is that of vacuum deposition of the passive elements—as compared to screen printing and firing for thick film.

It is possible to deposit conductors on a smooth-surfaced insulating substrate (glass or glazed alumina, e.g.) by placing the substrate in a vacuum chamber and evaporating a thin layer of a conductor material such as gold on the surface of the substrate. The pattern of the conductors can be delineated by placing a mask over the areas that need no gold or by depositing the conductor over the entire surface and later selectively etching

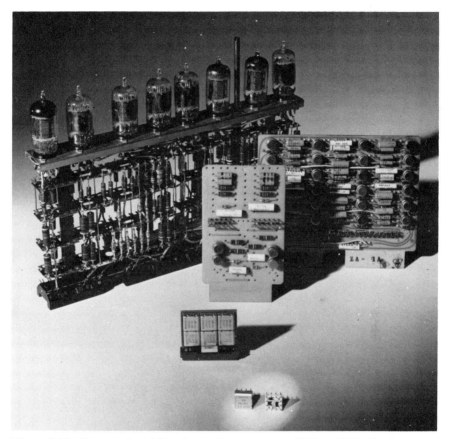

Figure 1-12 Progress in miniaturization in computers, 1950 to 1964, the last step in miniaturization being the result of thick film IC's (Courtesy IBM.)

away the areas that are not needed. The latter method is accomplished by photolithographic means.

Capacitors can be made by sputtering an insulating dielectric over a conductor, and later another conductor layer over the top of the insulating dielectric. Resistors can also be sputtered or evaporated.

Thus thin film has about the same capabilities as does thick film—conductors, capacitors, and resistors can be made. Also, the same disadvantage exists—no active device capability is in the process.

Minicomponents. Playing a fairly important role in the area of micro-electronics and closely associated with hybrids—at least for the time being—are minicomponents. Many discrete components added to thick or thin film ICs are conventional versions of miniaturized components, ranging from transistors in plastic packages to miniature conductors, small capacitors, and variable components. The use of these components sometimes represents a hangover from the old thinking of discrete componentry of the second era. It is true that in many instances the use of minicomponents broadens the scope of circuit capabilities. Many components are available in no other form. In time, use of these discrete add-ons in the shape of minicomponents will fade away, as the various components become part of compatible IC technology, or as they are "undressed" and adapted specifically for attachment as discrete add-ons for hybrid circuits. (The multilayer ceramic capacitor chip is a prime example of adapting a minicomponent for use as a hybrid add-on.)

Miniaturization. So far in this chapter we have emphasized that ICs are used primarily to eliminate interconnections. This no doubt is the most important factor—or it will be in the end—but something that cannot be ignored is the small size of the integrated circuit. For a very complex circuit, small size is advantageous because it cuts down on space and weight. We mentioned the big push for miniaturization that got off the ground in the fifties with the development of the transistor, helped along with the miniaturization efforts of all the various other component makers. These developments allowed production of such diverse products as pocket radios, computers (that did not require warehouses to fit them into) and compact airborne equipment.

Integrated circuits (especially the silicon monolithic) have capabilities of carrying miniaturization much further than was possible in the era of discrete components. Elimination of individual leads and separate packages alone saves lots of space and weight. The IC has created new markets where small size is important. Extreme miniaturization is a most important secondary benefit of the IC era.

Reliability. The interconnection difficulties of discrete components were essentially a reliability problem, and in eliminating connections, the IC has cleared up a crippling reliability problem. In addition, the basic nature of the construction of the three different types of ICs naturally lends itself to enhanced reliability—over and above the interconnection improvement.

They are all essentially one solid chunk of material. Higher reliability leads to a situation where all sorts of markets can be (and have been) opened that are based on the inherent reliability of the integrated circuit.

Cost. Another advantage of the IC that cannot be ignored is lowering of the basic costs of electronic circuits. It should be obvious that in making several resistors at one pass of a screen printer or making many transistors at once on a silicon chip is less expensive than the same part made one at a time. The advantages of lower cost are just now coming into being because in the early years of the IC technologies, processes were "rough" and yields were low. Costs were much higher, and many applications had to wait until the price was right. The innate low cost of the IC approach to "assembling" electronic circuits would make possible many new electronic products even without the ICs other advantages of size and reliability.

THE IC INDUSTRY TODAY

The electronics industry has been in a ferment for twenty years because of the transistor and the IC. We now look at the effects these technological innovations have had, both on the electronics industry itself and on the newly established "IC industry."

As noted earlier, electronics has been growing by a factor of 10 every twenty or twenty-five years for half a century. We are now just getting started in what we have called the third era of electronics—the IC era. In the past few years there has been some slowing of the well established growth rates of the electronics industry; this is probably not indicative of a long-term trend, however, but is rather a slowing brought about by the limitations of the technology of the second era. The old growth rate of 10% per year will not reappear for a while, several years being needed to reestablish the growth that will result from future new applications of ICs.

Electronics Industry Sales. Figure 1–13 shows recent sales figures in the United States electronics industry. The breakdown is into the traditional electronics market segments: consumer, government, and industrial.

We see that the only really dynamic sector of today's electronics industry is the industrial sector. With all the other changes taking place in the electronics industry (many of them caused by the industry moving into the third era) having only a portion of the industry "healthy" adds still another set of problems.

Microelectronics Sales. It should be noted, however, that the sales of ICs are not necessarily following the overall industry trends. As an industry shifts from second era discrete component designs to IC designs, increasing IC sales are possible even in a shrinking industry. The growth of IC sales through the recent years is to a considerable extent due to the conversion from discrete to IC rather than to an overall electronics industry growth. The added capabilities of IC-built devices will be largely responsible for continuing electronics equipment growth in the 1970s. Conversion will play a less important part in future growth of the IC industry.

	1968	1969	1970	1971	1974
Government	10.7	10.7	10.6	10.0	12.5
Consumer	4.2	4.6	3.9	4.2	5.3
Industrial	8.3	9.5	10.1	10.2	13.7
Total	23.2	24.8	24.6	24.4	31.5

Figure 1-13 United States electronics sales (billion $). The figures for 1971 and 1974 are estimates made by *Electronics*, in its annual forecast issue, January 4, 1971.

	Monolithic ICs			Hybrid ICs			
Year	Factory Sales	In-House Production	Total	Factory Sales	In-House Production	Total	Grand Total
1965	70	10	80	30	280	310	390
1969	400	100	500	80	330	410	910
1973	730	320	1050	220	390	610	1660
1979	1050	490	1540	360	520	880	2420

Figure 1-14 ICE estimates of IC production (million $). (*Source.* Integrated Circuit Engineering Corporation, *Status of Integrated Circuits—1970.*)

Figure 1-14 shows IC sales trends. The projected IC industry growth between 1969 and 1973 is 82%, whereas the McGraw-Hill estimate (Figure 1-3) of growth between 1969 and 1974 for the entire electronics industry (one additional year) is only 31%. This growth differential between the IC industry and the overall electronics industry exists because (1) conventional components are being replaced by ICs, (2) IC elements are furnished "assembled," with ICs thus replacing assembly labor (see Figure 1-5), and

(3) ICs are allowing new kinds of electronic equipment to be produced that cannot be produced conventionally.

Figure 1-15 indicates how some of the more vulnerable components industries are being affected by the increased use of the IC.

	Industry Sales (Million $)			
	1969	1970	1971	1974
Transistors	396	364	353	291
Receiving tubes	191	187	173	136
Resistors	418	349	359	415

Figure 1-15   The slowest growing components industries in the United States. (*Source. Electronics*, January 4, 1971.)

Returning for a moment to Figure 1-14, we see that one of the most important aspects of the hybrid IC industry is the extent to which it is "captive." About 80% of today's business in hybrid ICs is captive. ICE predicts more emphasis in years to come on factory sales for hybrids, as opposed to captive, although other sources of opinion (including the author) do not agree that the present 80:20 ratio will change significantly.

The ICE figures indicate an increasing shift to captive monolithic IC production—away from outside purchasing. The reason is that now it is much easier to go into monolithic production than it was in the past and that pressures for backward integration are increasing.

Hybrid ICs. The hybrid industry today is dominated by thick film (75 to 80% of the total production is thick film, not including IBM). Total hybrid industry output is also dominated by IBM's immense thick film output (probably over $250 million per year).

There are about 400 firms today (1971) producing hybrid ICs. Eighty of them are firms that sell custom hybrid circuits. Of the remaining, many are no more than in-house prototype laboratories, but some sizable captive operations are either on stream or heavily committed to large production levels.

Some of the biggest captive thick film operations are at IBM, Delco Radio, RCA (Consumer Products Division), and Zenith. Examples of large custom houses are Centralab Division of Globe Union, CTS, and Sprague.

Europe's development of hybrid ICs is every bit as dynamic as the hybrid growth in the United States, but the structure of the industry is (today, at least) much different. Thick film in Europe is being produced almost exclusively by noncaptive operations. This is because the basic structure of the electronics industry is not changing in Europe as it is in the United States. Backward integration is not yet nearly so strong a trend.

TRENDS IN THE HYBRID INDUSTRY—SUMMARY

The present domination of thick film over thin (80:20 ratio) is not expected to change significantly in the near future, but with all the major in-house commitments (except Western Electric) opting for thick film, the ratio will have to eventually shift toward even more thick film as these heavy producers (e.g., Delco, RCA, and Zenith) come fully on stream.

Monolithic IC production is now dominated by noncaptive vendors, but the trend toward captive operations will accelerate. Hybrid production now is and will continue to be primarily a captive industry.

Integrated circuits are the most dynamic portion of an electronics industry that contains very dynamic sectors (such as industrial and commercial electronics) and "sick" sectors (such as the military). The IC has been taking a larger portion of the total electronics dollar and will continue to do so in the seventies.

The IC is responsible for a shift in value added in electronics equipment *away* from the final assembly operation toward the IC maker. Trends are now quite visible that the equipment maker is not going to put up with such a threatening trend—thus captive operations are assuming a major importance in the overall IC industry.

The IC, hybrid *and* monolithic, is the driving force behind most projected electronics industry growth, and is responsible to a great extent for starting one of the most significant changes in the electronics industry structure in decades—the altering of the classic raw materials/component maker/equipment manufacturer relationship.

In being responsible for this basic altering of industry structure, decisions to participate in ICs or not to participate can be extremely important long-term decisions for a company. This is eloquently brought out by Figure 1-16. The leader's survival in a market is not assured—especially in a field whose technology is rapidly changing. The 1970 leaders in the newer MOS technology hint that by 1980, when MOS may be the prime IC technology, a new set of leaders will be on hand.

The IC industry cannot be expected to be either static or peaceful. Today's participants are not guaranteed a future role. Today's nonparticipants

Vacuum Tubes 1950	Transistors 1960	Bipolar ICs 1970	MOS ICs 1970
RCA	Texas Instruments	Texas Instruments	American Micro-Systems
Sylvania	Transitron	Motorola	North American Rock-well Microelectronics
General Electric	Philco	Fairchild	General Instrument
Raytheon	General Electric	Signetics	Texas Instruments
Tung-Sol	RCA	National Semi.	National Semiconductor

Figure 1-16 Leaders, at various times, in the active device industry. (*Source. Electronic News*, September 7, 1970.)

can still get on board—but they should expect an exciting time of it if they do decide to participate.

WHAT IS COMING

The impact of the third, electronics, era of modern communication technology—the IC era—is just beginning to be felt. The sales of the old era production are still significant, although the growth is gone.

Compared with the electronic components business as a whole, the IC industry is still small. Designers are just beginning to take advantage of the new horizons being opened because of the new freedoms of integration.

Eugene Fabini states (*IEEE Spectrum,* July 1969, p. 30) that "Major technologies have three stages: stage 1 when you do what you need to, only you do it better; stage 2 when you do new things you never did before; and stage 3, and this is the important one, when you change your lives to match the new capability that the technology gives you." Using the internal engine as an example—we have "progressed" to stage three of this technology, with such institutions as the supermarket, suburbs, and ghettos representing the ways in which we have changed our lives to match this technology.

Some developments in electronics would have us in stage three—such as television and radio—but generally we are in stage two of electronics technology—doing things with electronics we never did before: automotive electronics, computer control, going to the moon. Stage three is yet to come—but we hear talk of it with developments leading to the elimination of money, and to wide-band two-way communication networks connecting residences. Obviously, integrated electronics is heavily involved in activity having to do with Fubini's second technological stage, and it is the amazing capabilities of IC's that will propel us, ready or not, into the third stage.

DEFINITIONS

The terms used in IC technology are often confusing and have been often misused or misunderstood. To aid in sorting out the various definitions, Section 3 of Mil STD-1313A, (December 8, 1967) is repeated here, being one source of authoritative definitions.

3. DEFINITIONS

3.1 *Terms for equipment divisions.* The definitions of part, subassembly, assembly, unit, group, set and system, as well as the ancillary terms accessory and attachment are contained in MIL-STD-280.

3.2 *Microelectronics.* That area of electronic technology associated with or applied to the realization of electronic systems from extremely small electronic parts or elements.

3.3 *Element (of a microcircuit or integrated circuit).* A constituent of the microcircuit or integrated circuit that contributes directly to its operation. (A discrete part incorporated into a microcircuit becomes an element of the microcircuit.)

3.4 *Substrate (of a microcircuit or integrated circuit).* The supporting material upon or within which the elements of a microcircuit or integrated circuit are fabricated or attached.

3.5 *Microcircuit.* A small circuit having a high equivalent circuit element density, which is considered as a single part composed of interconnected elements on or within a single substrate to perform an electronic circuit function. (This excludes printed wiring board, circuit card assemblies, and modules composed exclusively of discrete electronic parts.)

3.5.1 *Multichip microcircuit.* A microcircuit consisting of elements formed on or within two or more semiconductor chips which are separately attached to a substrate.

3.5.2 *Hybrid microcircuit.* A microcircuit consisting of elements which are a combination of the firm circuit type (see 3.6.2) and the semiconductor types (see 3.5.1 and 3.6.1) or a combination of one or both of the types with discrete parts.

3.6 *Integrated circuit.* A microcircuit consisting of interconnected elements inseparably associated and formed in situ on or within a single substrate to perform an electronic circuit function.

3.6.1 *Monolithic integrated circuit.* An integrated circuit consisting of elements formed in situ on or with a semiconductor substrate with at least one of the elements formed with the substrate.

3.6.2 *Film integrated circuit.* An integrated circuit consisting of elements which are films formed in situ upon an insulating substrate.

3.7 *Microcircuit module.* An assembly of microcircuits or an assembly of microcircuits and discrete parts, designed to perform one or more electronic circuit functions, and constructed such that for the purposes of specification testing, commerce and maintenance, it is considered indivisible.

Note: To further define a particular type of circuit, additional modifiers may be prefixed. This is particularly desirable in the case of the hybrid circuit.

The microelectronics tree shown in Figure 1-17 will also help to understand the interrelationship between the various technologies of microelectronics.

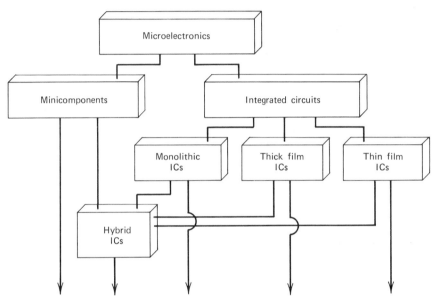

Figure 1-17 The microelectronics tree.

SUMMARY AND REVIEW

We are now seeing the end of the second era of electronics—the era of the active device in discrete form—and are moving into the third era—that of IC. Using Fubini's divisions, we have passed the first-stage technology where we did things we had been doing, only better (smaller, more reliable computers, communications gear, etc.) and are well into the second stage where we are doing things never done before.

The primary accomplishment of the integrated circuit has been the removal of the interconnection barrier, although its small size and low cost must not be ignored either.

The three separate technologies of ICs—silicon monolithic, thick film, and thin film—all have advantages and disadvantages and all are firmly established as contributing and participating technologies. The use of combinations—hybrid ICs—expands the capabilities of all three technologies.

The effects of these new technologies on the electronics industry have been far reaching. Fundamental changes have taken place. To continue to survive as healthy participants, it is often necessary for the old second-era participants to change. Components makers must find new markets. The equipment and systems assemblers must find new ways of obtaining added value for their portion of the work.

ACKNOWLEDGMENTS

We are much indebted to a fine article in the June 1969 issue of *IEEE Spectrum* by the late Jack A. Morton of Bell Laboratories, entitled "Strategy and Tactics for Integrated Circuits." The author here develops the concept of the eras of electronics and focuses on the interconnection impasse of discrete components.

Chapter 2

A FIRST LOOK AT THICK FILM TECHNOLOGY

We now introduce—briefly here, and in much greater detail later in the book—the subject of *thick film integrated circuits.*

The basic thick film processes are *screen printing* and *ceramic firing* (as compared to diffusion, photolithography, etc., for silicon monolithic, ICs and vacuum deposition for thin film ICs; for a brief introduction to monolithic and thin film technology, see Appendix I).

Passive components in thick film integrated circuits consist of metal-oxide-glass systems. They are chemically bonded to a ceramic substrate by high temperature firing. A comparatively heavy amount of thick film material must be deposited on a substrate in order to make good conductors, resistors, and capacitors. Printing methods capable of depositing heavier amounts of ink must be used. A very old process for printing thick ink applications is *screen printing.* Screen printing is used to put coloring into fabric, to apply decorations to glassware, and for many other applications. It is also employed in making printed circuits for applying etching resist or plating resist. In each of these applications there is a need for a "heavy" coating of material. Screen printing is thus ideal for thick film ICs.

The thick film process is (on the surface at least) very straightforward and easy to grasp. For instance, to make a resistor, simply screen-print it on a ceramic substrate, and then fire it to fuze it to the substrate and

29

to develop the final resistance characteristics. This simplicity promises economic advantages and easy technological control. The technology of assembling circuits in this manner is neither so demanding nor so difficult as competing IC processes such as vacuum deposition, epitaxy, or diffusion. The basic simplicity of the process is one of the major attractions of thick film. (However, as with all simple-seeming things, there *are* complications.)

THE MATERIALS OF THICK FILM INTEGRATED CIRCUITS

Substrates. Alumina-based ceramics are the most common substrate material, accounting for over 95% of all thick film applications. Alumina has the needed strength, electrical, and thermal properties and is widely available at attractive price.

Almost all alumina ceramic used for thick films is the 94 to 96% purity alumina material. The other 4 to 6% is a mixture of calcia, magnesia, and silica which helps to give the alumina substrate enough reactivity so that the thick films will bond strongly. The 99% grade alumina is used for thin film ICs because of its superior high-frequency characteristics and its smoother surface. (Figure 2-1.)

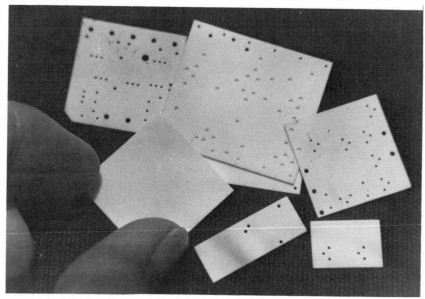

Figure 2-1   Alumina substrates. (Photograph by State of the Art, Inc.)

For thick film ICs a very smooth surface (such as that obtained with 99% alumina) is undesirable because better adhesion can be had with rougher surfaces. Alumina substrates for thick films normally have an as-fired surface finish of 20 to 30 μin., five to ten times the roughness of thin film substrates. The influence of surface roughness is not nearly so great with thick film as with thin film. The thicknesses of screen-printed filmst usually range from $\frac{1}{2}$ to 1 mil (500 to 1000 μin. A 25-μin. substrate surface "looks" relatively smooth to a 1000-μin. thick film, whereas a 1-μin. surface "looks" very rough to a 200-Å thin film. (See Appendix I, Figure A-27.)

Conductors. Conductors are applied as a pastelike organic-metal-glass mixture called inks or pastes.

The organic materials are added to give prefiring strength to the mixture and to control the fluid characteristics. The organics consist of a plastic base and a thinner. The thinner gives the proper viscosity and is driven off after screen printing by drying at relatively low temperatures. The solid organic base, in which the metal/glass system is suspended, holds the dried film to the ceramic substrate until it is fired. The solid organic materials must be chosen so that they will burn off without undue disruption of the film. (Figure 2-2.)

The glass is chosen partly for its melting point, although other characteristics are also of considerable importance. Most paste systems must fire at temperatures ranging between 500° and 1000°C. A variety of glasses with different melting points is needed to cover this range. Lead borosilicate glasses are commonly used.

The metals used for thick film conductors must withstand the high temperatures needed for "attaching themselves" to the substrate without oxidizing or entering into reactions with other materials. Noble metals such as platinum, palladium, gold, and silver and the various combinations and alloys of these metals are common conductor materials.

To control adhesion, solderability, and chemical stability, the glass/metal ratio, the particle size and shape of the metal components, and various mixtures and alloys of different metals are all important variables. Organic/inorganic ratios and the materials of the organic portion of the conductor formulation are manipulated to control the fluid properties.

Being heavily loaded with precious metals, thick film conductor inks are not inexpensive. Prices range from a low of $2 per troy ounce for silver to $100 or more per troy ounce for platinum-rich compositions. But each ounce will cover from 2 to 3 ft^2, which allows approximately 3000 feet of a 10-mil-wide conductor; the cost in a circuit thus is not so bad as it might seem from the per ounce price.

Resistors. Resistor compositions could be made of a great variety of materials. For good stability (of resistance) with temperature, however, very few satisfactory systems are available. Like the metal conductor pastes, these inks have organic additives that control the fluid properties.

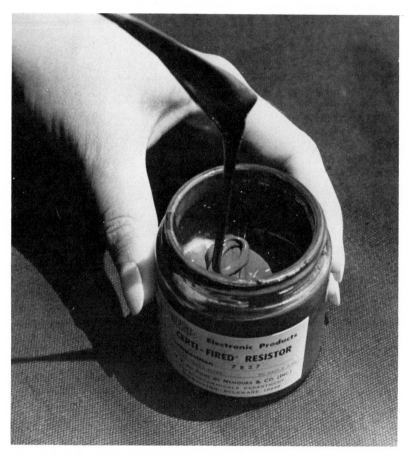

Figure 2-2 A thick film resistor paste (ink composition). (Photograph by State of the Art, Inc.)

The firing treatment is much more critical for thick film resistor compositions than it is for thick film conductors. The final value of the resistance depends almost as much on the firing treatment as it does on the basic composition. Other resistor performance characteristics are also strongly influenced by the firing treatment. (Figure 2-3.)

The conduction mechanism in thick film resistors is not well understood. Resistor systems such as the palladium-palladium oxide-silver system depend largely on physical contact of the individual conducting particles (in the glassy matrix) for conductivity. As the conductor/insulator ratio changes the number of contacts changes; hence the resistance changes. Other thick film resistor systems apparently depend more on the resistivity of a continuous phase, which is heavily influenced by the peak temperature and

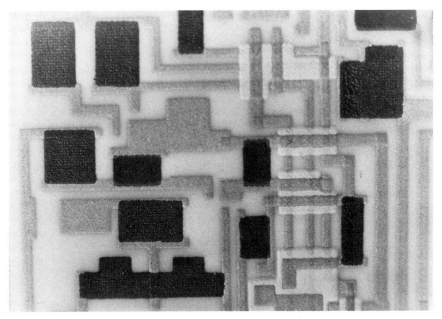

Figure 2-3 Thick film resistors. The pattern of screen is still showing in resistors. Note also the crossovers at the right (lighter color). (Circuit by JW Microelectronics, Inc.; photograph by State of the Art, Inc.)

dwell at the peak temperature, increasing amounts of the continuously conducting compound being created as the firing temperature goes higher or the time at temperature is extended.

Systems other than the palladium-palladium oxide-silver-glass system that have been used are thallium oxide, platinum group oxide mixtures, ruthenium oxide based systems, and various other proprietary concoctions.

The costs of resistor pastes are similar to those of thick film conductors, since they also contain rather expensive materials.

Capacitor Dielectrics. Increasingly useful capacitor compositions are becoming available for thick film users. Most of the push is toward systems with higher dielectric constants. The most common approach is to produce mixtures of high dielectric constant materials (titanates) held in a matrix of glass.

With high-K crystal/glass mixtures the capacitance (or the dielectric constant) is little different from that of the low dielectric constant glass component until the amount of glass is reduced to very low percentages. Even with very small amounts of glass, the dielectric constant of the film can be drastically reduced from the high dielectric constant value of the crystalline additive. In spite of this situation, dielectric constants well past 1000 are now available. (Figure 2-4.)

Simple glasses and recrystallized glasses are used for low value capacitors.

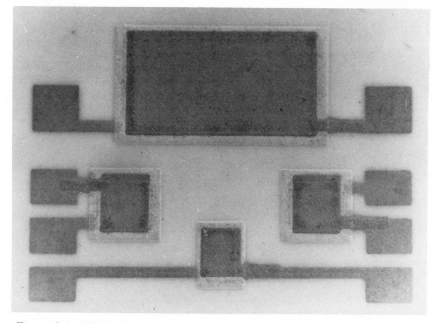

Figure 2-4 Thick film capacitors (a test circuit). (Pattern by DuPont; photograph by State of the Art, Inc.)

Crossover Materials. There is often a need in complex, high-density circuits for one conductor to cross another. To do this, an insulating layer must be placed between the two conductors. Although this can be accomplished with monolithics and thin film ICs, it is *particularly* easy to do with thick film. The materials used for crossovers are very similar to the low dielectric constant compositions used for building low-value capacitors.

In the simplest possible system one could use the same glass as in the resistor or conductor pastes, but without the metal or ceramic additives. There are serious problems here though. The conductors will tend to react with such a glass, in that they will move, shift, or sink, thus causing a short. Because of this problem, another type of crossover material is more useful: glasses that recrystallize on cooling. With recrystallizable glasses, the fired crossover is converted during firing from a glass to a solid mass of polycrystalline ceramic which will not allow sinking or shifting of the top conductor when refired (because the melting point of the crystalline ceramic is high). (Figure 2-5.)

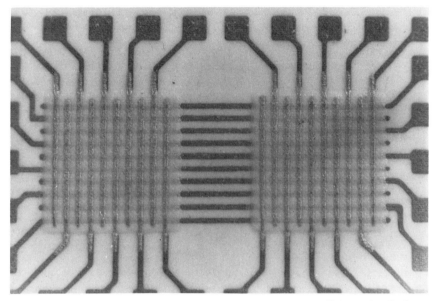

Figure 2-5 Thick film crossover construction—a test array. (Pattern by DuPont; photograph by State of the Art, Inc.)

If the circuit consists of a single complex chip, it is usually possible to get from the chip to the outside leads without a crossover; but if the circuit consists of many chips, it is next to impossible to get from one chip to the other or from one chip to the outside without conductor crossovers. The availability of crossover pastes, plus good progress in development of fine-line printing capabilities (fine for thick film, that is; approximately 10-mil lines on 20-mil- centers or less is considered fine-line thick film printing) has helped considerably in making very complex ICs available. Thick film is thus playing a major supporting role in LSI and MSI.

The capability that thick film has for easily producing crossovers, when looked at in a somewhat broader sense, permits the thick film IC producer to make miniature multilayer circuit boards by a very simple and economic process. Most IC manufacturers involved in LSI, MSI, and other multichip ICs use thick film for their interconnects.

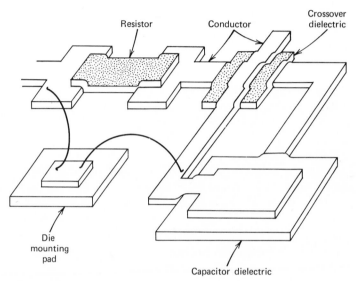

Figure 2-6 Use of thick film materials for making conductors, resistors, capacitors, mounting pads, and crossover insulators.

Protective Coatings. Resistors, capacitors, and conductors sometimes need to be covered with an insulator. Resistors and capacitors are subject to attack by humidity, for example. They would operate more reliably if sealed with an impervious material. Some thick film resistor compositions containing easily reducible oxides need protection from the reducing atmospheres that are used in silicon die bonding. Conductors also need to be insulated at times (for instance, when a wire jumper is to pass over the conductor).

These protective coatings are usually lower melting point glasses that are screened on as a last step in the thick film manufacturing process.

THICK FILM EQUIPMENT

Screen Printers. A screen printer is a device that holds the screen stencil and the substrate to be screened in proper relationship while the ink or paste is pushed through the screen onto the substrate. There are many different ways of doing this. The method chosen depends on the circuit complexity and resolution needed and the rate at which it is to be done.

A screen printer must have a platform on which to hold the substrate in place accurately. This is done by placing the substrate on a flat metal pedestal against the stops (for accurate positioning). It is common practice to use vacuum to hold down the substrate and keep it from slipping and from sticking to the screen after the printing stroke.

Once the substrate is positioned and held down, the screen printer must bring the screen stencil into proper position over the substrate. If the screen stencil is movable, it is generally kept out of the way above the substrate pedestal during loading. For printing it is moved down over the pedestal and held in place, just over, but not touching the substrate. If the screen stencil is stationary, the pedestal is generally loaded in front of the screen and moved under the screen for printing.

After the substrate has been brought into proper position with relation to the screen, a charge of paste, stored on the top side of the screen, is pushed before a squeegee (a blade of slightly resilient material) which is brought across the screen with a steady forward motion plus some downward force. As the squeegee blade advances, its downward force forces the screen into contact with the substrate just at the point where the squeegee is over the substrate. In the mesh of the screen where no emulsion exists, the paste is forced down through the screen mesh and into contact with the substrate. After the squeegee passes, the tension on the screen causes the screen to snap back, separating from the substrate, and ink that came in contact with the substrate adheres to the substrate. The amount of ink that sticks to the substrate is a function of the thickness of the screen and emulsion, the ink rheology, the width of the line, the surface of the substrate and a host of other conditions. Although subject to many variables, the amount that is laid down on successive passes is quite constant. (Figure 2-7.)

The screen printing steps just described can be made in a variety of ways, and with considerable automation if desired. Precision-built machinery is needed for good control of the positioning of the pattern and the amount of ink to be deposited. (Figure 2-8.)

Screens. Screen printing is accomplished by forcing a paste through a pattern of open meshes, as described above. To delineate the areas where paste is to be forced through the screen, the screen cloth is coated with a photosensitive emulsion. Upon exposure to light through a mask, portions of the emulsion are made insoluble (Figure 2-9). The soluble (unexposed) portion of the emulsion can then be washed away. The holes that are

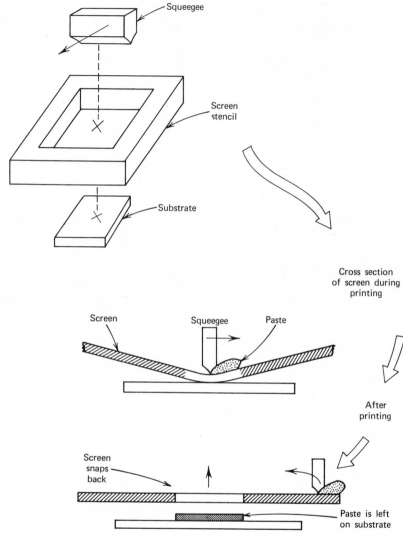

Figure 2-7 Schematic representation of screen printing.

plugged with emulsion will not allow paste to pass through. The emulsion-less areas are where printing will take place.

The amount of material that goes through the screen onto the substrate depends on the size of the wire, the size of the holes, and the thickness of the emulsion. Resolution is limited to approximately the finest mesh size that can be used. The finest size used for thick film screen printing

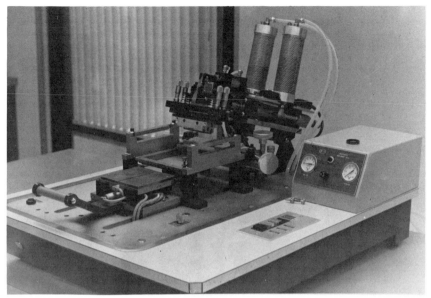

Figure 2-8 A laboratory or low-production screen printer. (Printer by Affiliated Manufacturers, Inc.; photograph by State of the Art, Inc.)

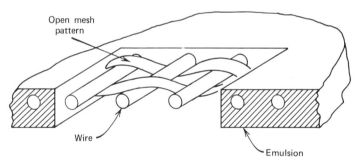

Figure 2-9 A portion of a screen stencil pattern showing details of the screen and its emulsion. Mesh size and emulsion thickness control, print thickness.

is 400 mesh (400 openings/in.). Two hundred mesh is used for most applications. At 200 mesh/in., the average opening would be 5 mils (less wire diameter); thus about 5 mils is the smallest dimension that can be held (unless finer mesh screen is used).

Mesh size is a major limitation on dimensional geometry of thick film. For larger patterns—over 25 mils—this has little effect, but for smaller dimensions the mesh will exert considerable influence. Using smaller mesh helps, but then the amount of material that will be laid down becomes a limiting factor. Progress is being made in getting around these limitations by using *metal masks*. Metal masks allow resolution down to 2-mil lines with 2-mil separations. (It is common to refer to screen printing resolution capability by saying "2 by 2" instead of "2 mil lines on 4 mil centers" or "two mil lines separated by two mil spaces.")

Screens are tightly stretched on stiff frames (cast aluminum is common). It is important to use a screen with the mesh stretched to proper tension. As a screen wears, however, it stretches, and some of this tension is lost. When this happens, snap-back capability (among other things) begins to degrade. Stretching with use can be counteracted to some extent by increasing screen/substrate separation. (Figure 2-10.)

Screen stencils are mounted on the screen printer by clamping or bolting.

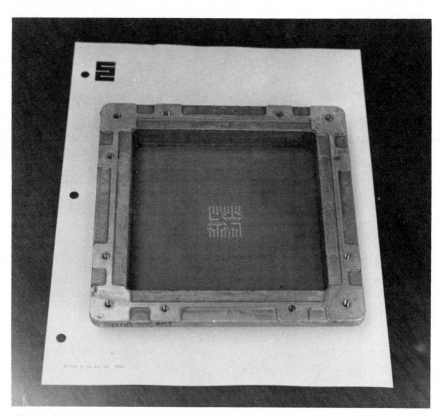

Figure 2-10 A screen stencil. (Screen by Industrial Reproductions, Inc.; photograph by State of the Art, Inc.)

The need for rigidity and parallelism is great. The screen is located over the substrate in its proper position by adjustments on the screen printer that allow "back and forth" and rotational movement, in precise amounts. Once properly located, the adjustments are "locked in" so that the screen printer prints on the substrate in *exactly* the same place each time it is cycled.

Squeegees. Squeegees are made of such materials as neoprene or polyurethane. Solvents used in thick film pastes attack the squeegee, causing wear, swelling, flaking, and so on. (Polyurethane is replacing neoprene, because of improved solvent resistance.) The screening edge of the squeegee blade is beveled. During travel of the squeegee across a screen the beveled (angled) edge creates a situation where paste is forced forward and downward. The downward force is a function of this "angle of attack." Squeegee design, amount of wear, softness, holding angle, and similar factors all have an effect of the way paste is metered into the open holes of the screen.

Kilns. The most common kiln used in firing thick film is a muffled moving metal belt furnace. Printed substrates are loaded into the metal belt at the entrance end of the kiln. The belt moves the substrates through the furnace. As a part starts its trip through the furnace (kiln) it is first heated enough for the organic additives (vehicle) to start volatilizing and burning out. This part of the process must be orderly—neither too fast nor too slow. At too fast a pace the burnout is disruptive, resulting in blisters in the film, separation of the composition from the substrate, and so on. If burnout is too slow, the parts may retain carbon when they go into the hot zone where glass melting and other reactions take place. Carbon sets up undesirable reactions resulting in bubbles in the glass or reduction of some of the oxides in the composition. The kilns are vented to remove the products of combustion. (Figure 2-11.)

The *hot zone* of the kiln is a region where the substrates are brought up to the peak temperature and held for a period of time. The length of the hot zone is usually about the length of the *preheat zone*. The *cooling zone* is an unelemented section where the parts cool off before being discharged. (Figure 2-12.)

Thick film kilns are usually muffled in order to better control ventilation, to keep vaporized products of the thick film firing reactions away from the elements, to act as a heat radiator, avoiding hot spots, and to keep products of the furnace such as element flakes and brick dust off the thick film circuits. Quartz is the most common muffle material although inconel and mullite are also used.

The maximum temperature needed is about 1000°C (1800°F) although having kilns capable of 1100°C is a good idea, because these higher temperatures are likely to be advantageous for firing capacitors.

The most sophisticated feature of thick film kilns is the temperature controls. The need for the close temperature control takes thick film furnaces out of the "simple" class. Some of the best resistor systems—that is, those that make the most stable resistors—are systems in which the resistance varies as much as 3%/°C firing difference. Control capability of 1°C or more therefore is needed for maximizing yields.

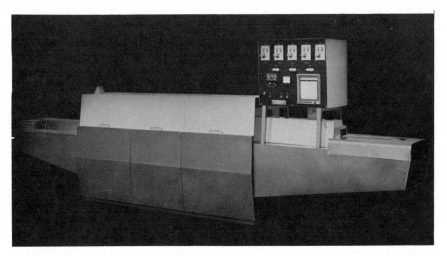

Figure 2-11 A thick film kiln (furnace). (Courtesy of W. P. Keith Company.)

Trimmers. Without the ability to adjust thick film resistors (and more recently capacitors) thick film elements would be limited in their usefulness because it is impossible to screen-print and fire to a precise value.

Machines are available that can very capably and economically trim thick film resistors and capacitors. Of the many different approaches to trimming that have been tried *air-abrasive* trimmers were able to capture the overwhelming majority of the trimming market, but in the recent past *laser* trimmers have proved capable enough so that the day of sole rule by the air-abrasive trimmer is over.

Air-abrasive trimmers abrade the resistor (or capacitor) material away by bombarding the resistor body (or capacitor electrode) with a stream of compressed gas loaded with abrasive particles. The size of the stream is controlled by use of very small nozzles. The position and direction of

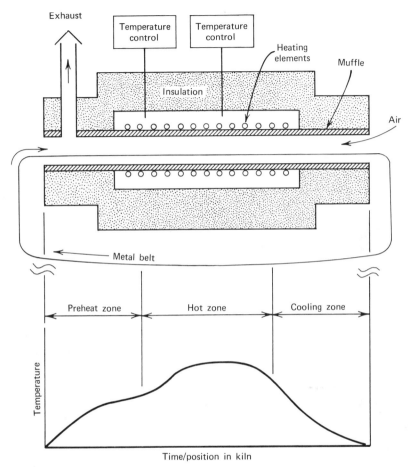

Figure 2-12   A cross section of a thick film furnace (kiln) and its temperature profile.

the nozzle is precisely controlled by the mechanics of the equipment. Air-abrasive trimmers can trim to less than 1% tolerance for less than 1¢ per resistor.

Laser trimmers are inherently faster than air-abrasive ones, and can do the trimming without damage to nearby components. The laser trimmer is better for *dynamic trimming* (trimming not to a specific value, but to a circuit performance level), because the laser trimming action will not harm delicate components such as transistors. Laser trimmers function by directing a focused high energy beam on the material to be removed. The

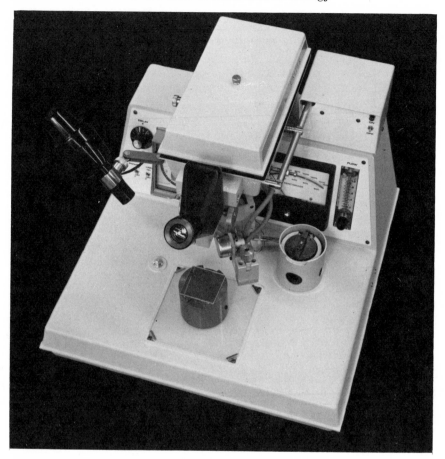

Figure 2-13 A die bonder. (Courtesy of Unitek, Inc.)

high-energy concentration of the beam vaporizes the material without disturbing (very much) nearby material.

Assembly and Packaging Equipment. This equipment is employed in thin film and monolithic fabrication as well as in thick film operations.

Die bonders are used to attach transistors, diodes, or monolithic IC chips to metallized substrates. Die bonders are machines that allow one to pick up the tiny die (or chip), move it into proper position over a heated substrate, and then lower it into position, doing some rubbing and scrubbing to remove dirt and oxide as the chip is brought into contact. As the chip heats up, it begins to alloy with the gold substrate pad. (Alloy "preforms" are sometimes added to ensure good bonds.) This work is usually done by hand, with the operator viewing the bonding operation under a stereomicroscope. Micromanipulators that reduce movements of the hand to extremely small motions are often used to locate the tools and position the chips. (Figure 2-13.)

Methods other than eutectic bonding are also popular. They include plastic bonding, soldering (or brazing), and use of miniature special packages (such as LIDs).

Wire Bonding. There are two important methods of wire bonding. In *thermocompression bonding* a combination of heat and pressure is used to attach a very fine gold or aluminum wire first to the pad on top of the semiconductor chip and thence to the thick film, or thin film, pad on the substrate. Miniature tooling moved around with micromanipulators

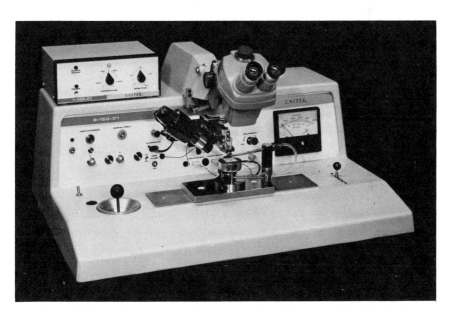

Figure 2-14   A thermocompression wire bonder. (Courtesy of Unitek, Inc.)

is again featured, with the work progress being viewed through a microscope. A microscope is essential, since one is bonding 1-mil wires to pads of only a few thousands of an inch square. (Figure 2-14.) A thermocompression bond is made by bringing a wire in a heated holder down over the bonding pad of a heated chip, applying pressure to make a bond, then moving the holder over to the next stitching spot. Wire is pulled through the capillary as the movement is made. The second bond is made and the wire is then cut off or broken (by pulling).

In *ultrasonic bonding* the silicon chip need not be heated. The wire is brought down into contact with the chip much in the same way as in the thermocompression bonders, and ultrasonic energy is applied to make the bond. This process is somewhat more difficult to control than thermocompression, but it has an important advantage in not using heat, which can damage a silicon chip. Ultrasonic bonding is especially helpful in avoiding the long heating periods needed for wiring multichip ICs. Chips attached to substrates with plastic materials or soft solders cannot withstand thermocompression bonding and thus require ultrasonic bonding. The combination of plastic die bonding and ultrasonic wire bonding is attractive because it avoids high temperatures. (Figure 2-15.)

Face Bonding. The high cost of making wire bonds and their relatively low reliability created pressure for better methods. Several methods of eliminating leads exist, most of them involving placing the chips upside down on the substrate. The two main methods for leadless bonding are *flip chip* bonding and *beam lead* bonding.

Flip chips have small balls or bumps of metal resting in (protruding from) "windows" in the insulated surface of the monolithic chip. Electrical contact is made to the chip through the metal bumps in these windows. The chip is turned upside down and bonded to matching pads on the substrate by ultrasonic energy, soldering, and so on.

The other approach—beam leads—uses very small leads that extend out over the edge of the silicon die. The beam lead chip is attached to the substrate by thermocompression methods. Its main advantage is that the leads and the bonds are visible—considered to be important for high-reliability bonds. A disadvantage of beam leads is that they use extra silicon area.

The two face bonding methods have many limitations, but the pressure for adaption of these approaches (or something similar) to replace the wire bonded devices is intense. Both are being used more and more.

Several large manufacturers of ICs have developed their own versions of leadless bonding. Motorola, GE, Fairchild, and Signetics have all announced special automated systems. Most of these systems involve a tiny stamped metal lead frame, held in strip carriers, automatically bonded to the chips—all connections made simultaneously.

Bonding Other Devices. All kinds of passive devices can be bonded to thick film—soldering being the most popular method of attachment. Multilayer ceramic chip and tantalum chip capacitors give great versatility and make high-capacitance values available to hybrid ICs. Development of these components for use in hybrids has been an important factor in improving and expanding hybrid IC capabilities. Resistors also can be added in chip form, although they are not used as much as capacitor chips. Other components such as small inductors can also be added.

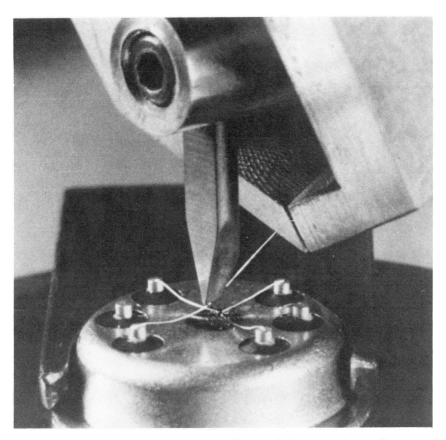

Figure 2-15 Close-up of an ultrasonic bonding head during a wire bonding operation—about to make a bond on the silicon chip. (photograph courtesy of Tempress Division, Sola Basic, Inc.)

Packaging. There are so many approaches to packaging that it is difficult to say much here except that thick film adapts to all kinds of packaging, from expensive flat packs to inexpensive dip-coated plastic packages. Since thick film hybrids are rugged, requirements for packaging them are not as demanding as those for thin film or monolithics. Packaging is thus often much less expensive for thick film than for other types of ICs.

THE PROCESS STEPS IN MAKING A THICK FILM CIRCUIT

The same simple amplifier that is used in the appendix for illustrating monolithic and thin film processing is "built" here using thick film techniques. The circuit layout is changed to allow illustration of crossovers. (Figure 2-16.)

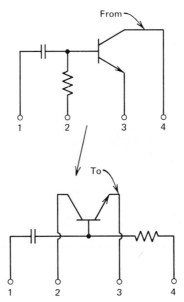

Figure 2-16 The schematic of a sample circuit to be "built" in Figure 2-17.

Screen-Print Capacitor Electrode (Figure 2-17a). The first step is to screen print the bottom capacitor electrode. This is done (in our example) with a palladium-silver conductor paste and fired at 1000°C.

Print Capacitor Dielectric (Figure 2-17b). Next, the capacitor dielectric is screened-on *over* the bottom electrode. To avoid shorts created by bubbles, the dielectric thickness is built up by making *two* passes of the screen. A fairly coarse mesh screen (160 mesh) is used so that the final buildup of film will be over 1-mil thick. (The dielectric laid down on the first print is dried before printing the second layer.)

Print and Fire Top Electrode and Other Conductor Patterns (**Figure 2-17***b*). Before firing, the top electrode and other conductor patterns can also be printed. After printing and before firing the parts are subjected to a 15-min drying at 125°C. The same drying is used between successive printings if more than one is made per firing. This firing step is also at about 1000°C (1800°F). The capacitance value obtained is strongly dependent on temperatrue, so great care must be used in controlling temperature.

Print and Fire Crossovers (**Figure 2-17***c*). Next the crossover composition is double-printed (to ensure dielectric integrity). The conductor composition is printed over the unfired crossover. After drying they are cofired at 900°C. This firing temperature is sufficiently below the previous capacitor dielectric firing to avoid changing the capacitance of the capacitor. (The need for crossovers in a simple circuit such as this is obviously unnecessary, but is done here for purposes of illustration.)

Print and Fire Resistors (**Figure 2-17***d*). The resistor paste is screened-on and fired between 700 and 850°C depending. on the resistor system that is used.

Adjust Resistor (**Figure 2-17***e*). The resistor is then adjusted. Air-abrasive sand blasting is used for adjustment. This can be automatic, the resistance being monitored as adjustment proceeds; the flow of abrasive will stop when the proper value is reached. Laser trimming would be a suitable alternate method.

Protective Coating (**Not Illustrated**). After the resistor is adjusted, the resistor and the capacitor are coated with a low-temperature glass fired at 500 to 600°C. The capacitor will need protection from humidity. Certain resistor compositions can change resistance if exposed to reducing situations (as in the case of the upcoming die bonding step).

Final Steps (**Figure 2-17***e, f*). The next step is to mount the transistor. This is done by eutectically bonding the chip to the gold pad and then wire bonding to the substrate from the chip (thermocompression or ultrasonic). Gold is often chosen for wire bonding pads, but other thick film conductor types will also accept wire bonding.

Tinned copper leads flattened at the ends can be soldered to the edge of the substrate where the four thick film conductor paths terminate.

To get a stronger connection it is common in thick film to use substrates with holes in them. The wire can be bent into the holes and swaged or staked into place prior to soldering. To protect the circuit from physical

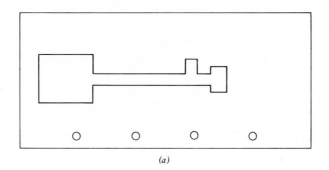

(a)

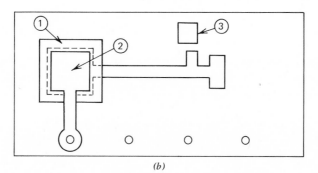

(b)

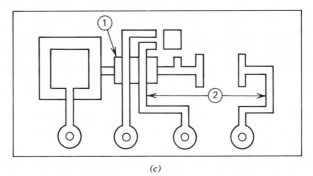

(c)

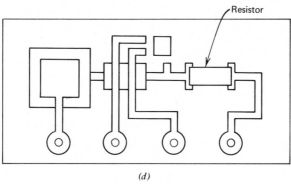

(d)

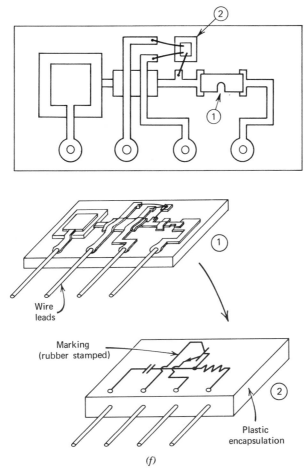

Wire
leads

Marking
(rubber stamped)

Plastic
encapsulation

(f)

Figure 2-17 The fabrication steps in making a thick film hybrid circuit. (a) Print and fire capacitor bottom electrode (palladium-silver, 200-mesh screen, 1000°C). (b) 1, Double print capacitor dielectric (160 mesh). 2, Print top electrode (200 mesh, palladium-silver). 3, Print gold mounting pad. 4, Fire at 950° to 1000°C (to proper capacitance). (c) 1, Print crossover dielectric (double pass, 160 mesh). 2, Print remainder of conductor patterns (palladium-silver, 200 mesh). 3, Fire at 900°C. (d) Print and fire resistor (160-mesh screen, 750° to 850°C). (e) 1, Trim resistor (air abrasive or laser). 2, Mount transistor (eutectic die bond-thermocompression wire bond-gold). (f) 1, Attach leads. 2, Encapsulate and mark.

damage, humidity, and so on, a variety of packages and encapsulation can be used ranging from expensive high performance hermetic packages (not for the package with leads as described here, though) to simple dipping or potting in epoxy or silicone.

COMPARISON OF THE CAPABILITIES OF THE THREE TYPES OF INTEGRATED CIRCUITS

We have described briefly the steps in processing the three types of ICs: monolithic and thin film hybrid (discussed in Appendix I) and thick film hybrid. It should not be difficult to guess at this point which type is best

Table 2-1   Comparison Chart of Silicon Monolithic, of Thin Film, and Thick Film ICs

Category to be Compared	Monolithic	Thin Film	Thick Film
Setup cost	3	2	1
Maintain-capability cost	3	2	1
High-volume runs, cost	1	3	2
Low-volume runs, cost	3	2	1
Resistance range	3	2	1
Resistor tolerance	3	1	2
Resistance stability	3	1	2
Other resistance characteristics	3	1	2
Capacitance range	3	1	1
Capacitance tolerance	3	1	1
Capacitance stability	3	1	1
High-voltage	3	1	1
High-power	3	2	1
High-frequency	3	1	2
Linear circuits	3	1	1
Digital circuits	1	3	3
Volume efficiency	1	2	3
Reliability	1	1	1

for various applications. Table 2-1 ranks the three types from 1 for "best" to 3 for "worst" in various categories. If two of the types are fairly close, they are given the same rating. Keep in mind that the "worst" rating is not necessarily bad—just not so good as the other types.

Setup Costs. Original equipment is obviously expensive for monolithic and less expensive for thick film. A very rough estimate of funds needed for minimum (prototype only) facilities might be $50,000 for thick film, $80,000 for thin film, and $250,000 for monolithic (for equipment only).

The people needed for setting up and operating an IC facility and the expenses arising because of these "people costs" are usually more significant than raw equipment costs. The skill inventory and time needed for monolithic is rather high compared with either of the film technologies. One or two years are required to put a monolithic facility on line, but only a half year or so for thick film. Thin film takes a bit longer than thick film. (These estimates assume availability of knowledgeable people.) Equipment cost is only a *part* of getting started—the total cost might be closer to $75,000, $150,000, and $500,000 when "people" and "time" costs are included. These costs are much lower today than a few years ago.

Maintain Capability Costs. Maintaining a prototype facility at a state-of-the-art-level can be very expensive for monolithic, but is nominal for thick film. Glenn Madland reported in *Electronic Products Magazine* ("Prototyping Microcircuits," December 1967) that to keep on top of things in monolithic could cost $500,000 per year. This is high for today, but nevertheless the point is well made that it is expensive to keep up. Maintaining thick film capability would run no more than $50,000 per year. Thin film is somewhat more expensive than thick film. (Table 2-2.)

Table 2-2 Comparison of Costs of Setting Up and Running IC Facilities

	Cost to Set Up Laboratory Facilities		Cost to Maintain Facilities ($/year)
	Equipment Only	Equipment, People, and Time	
Monolithic	$250,000	$500,000 (2 years)	200,000
Thin film	80,000	150,000 (1 year)	75,000
Thick film	50,000	75,000 (½ year)	50,000

Low-Volume Production Costs. The simple setups for thick film give this technology the easy "victory" for short production runs where prorated setup and design costs loom large. Tooling that could cost $5000 in monolithic would cost only a few hundred dollars in thick film. Turnaround time can also be fast. As circuits increase in complexity, thick film's advantage declines. Thin film again is in-between, but is closer to thick film than to monolithic in cost.

High-Volume Production Costs. The monolithic resistor has the advantage here. If the circuit can be done in silicon monolithic, and volume will support it, *nothing* can touch the costs of monolithic. Cost per component can be only a fraction of a cent in a monolithic IC. It is *this* advantage that is primarily responsible for the success of silicon monolithics, and which will keep them in the leading position in the years to come.

Resistor Tolerance Capability. The closest tolerance capability is that of thin film, followed by thick film. Both can be trimmed to fractions of 1%. Five percent is an outside limit with monolithic, and this is hard to maintain, whereas the close tolerances of trimmed film are easily obtained.

Resistor Temperature Stability Capability. Thin film ICs result in the most stable resistors, but thick film can do almost as well. Thin film can produce a 50-ppm TC with relative ease, whereas thick film has to "struggle." Monolithic resistors are very unstable. Coming thick film advances will probably make it capable of producing the most temperature-stable resistors.

Resistor Range. Thick film can commercially produce the widest range of values. Thick film resistor materials are available through five or six orders of magnitude—up to several megohms per square.

Thin film is limited to about 1000 $\Omega/\square$, but with meandering fine lines can overcome much of the limitation. Silicon is limited to about 400 $\Omega/\square$ (unless buried resistor techniques are used, going to about 10,000 $\Omega/\square$). There is little room to produce long meanders because of the high substrate cost.

Other Resistor Characteristics. The biggest advantage is low noise in thin film, and the worst disadvantage is parasitics in silicon monolithics. Time stability of thin films is excellent.

Capacitor Range. Thick and thin film, through ability to "piggyback" discretes, have an extremely wide range available.

Capacitor Characteristics. Use of discrete chips in either thick or thin film ICs gives them superior performance in almost any category. Screen-printed or vacuum-deposited capacitors are also good.

High-Voltage and High-Power Capability. The small size of silicon mono-lithics argues against high-voltage capability. Both thick and thin film have excellent high-voltage capabilities, including the ability to add high-voltage or high-power solid state devices as hybrids. There is considerable hope for eventual success of monolithics in the 200- or 300-V range, but not much higher.

High-Frequency Performance. Since microwave uses components whose characteristics depend on exact geometry and on very low loss substrates, this field turns to thin film almost extensively. Thick film can compete very effectively with thin film from UHF up to 1 or 2 GHz. Monolithic is a poor third.

Linear Circuits. Thick and thin film are excellent. Monolithic is not so good, but is rapidly gaining in capabilities. In time monolithics will have a good portion of the less demanding linear circuits.

Digital Circuits. All silicon monolithic. The technology is a natural for this type of circuit. Monolithic's capabilities here, as well as in low cost and small size, allow almost no competition.

Reliability. All are very good. Thin film has a good reputation with extensive documentation, but it is not *inherently* more reliable to any extent than the other types. All three are very reliable when compared to conventional circuits.

Volume Efficiency. Silicon monolithic by a wide margin. Thin film is some-what more compact than thick film.

Summary. In its size, low cost in high volume, and adaptability to digital circuits, silicon monolithic is clearly "the best." For specialized circuits where a large variety of quality components are needed, the film types are clearly superior. In small production runs the film types cost less, with thick film being clearly ahead of thin film.

There is a definite place for all three. Some circuit types that can efficiently be done in only one way, but the overlap of the three is such that almost anything can be handled by one of the approaches. Combined, they make a powerful trio.

Chapter 3

THE ECONOMIC RATIONALE
FOR THICK FILM HYBRIDS

In this chapter we consider the economics of ICs. We show the driving forces behind their increasingly widespread use. To be sure, they have advantages other than economic—such as their small size and high reliability—but even these advantages can often be dollarized. *Low cost* thus is a major reason for the wide use of ICs today. What used to be commercially impractical is now possible. Most of the many new business opportunities enjoyed by ICs exist because of the basic economy of integrated circuits. Much of the rationale behind the present and future success and popularity of integrated circuits is primarily economic.

There are two ways in which thick film hybrid circuits justify their existence and use: (1) they bring silicon monolithic IC advantages and economies to more applications than could silicon monolithic alone and (2) they (sometimes) have certain economic advantages of their own.

THE LOW ELEMENT COST IN MONOLITHIC
INTEGRATED CIRCUITS

Circuit elements (the individual transistors, diodes, resistors, etc.) of the monolithic silicon IC are *very* inexpensive.

Cost-Yield Relationships—An Example. This amazingly low element cost can best be examined by reviewing manufacturing costs of a typical monolithic IC. As a specific example, let us look at the manufacturing costs of a 40 × 40 mil chip containing 20 circuit elements. This example represents a typical bipolar linear circuit today. Our example does not represent state-of-the-art element density. MOS ICs, and many digital ICs, can be even *more* dense—that is, a 40 × 40 mil chip could have many more than 20 elements.

If a 2-in. silicon wafer were used, there would be about 2000 chips per wafer. With 20 elements per chip there are 40,000 elements on each wafer that are processed. To take this 2-in.-diameter wafer through all

Table 3-1   Chip Costs at Various Yields

Process Yield (%)	Good Parts	Cost ($)	
		Per 20-Component Chip	Per Assembled Element
100	2000	0.02	0.001
50	1000	0.04	0.002
25	500	0.08	0.004
10	200	0.20	0.01
5	100	0.40	0.02
1	20	2.00	0.10

the process steps—epitaxy, diffusions, metallization, testing, scribing, *up to* packaging (not including packaging)—would cost (at the factory level) about $40.

Table 3-1 shows the costs allocated to each completed IC chip and to each element on the chip for a variety of yields. It is easy to see that even at very low yields a silicon IC could compete favorably with conventional discrete component circuits. Our 20-element chip could be a low-power amplifier circuit, for instance. Even with a 1% yield and a factory cost of $2, it could complete against conventional construction costs (especially since the individual elements are all connected, so that final assembly costs for the IC will also be reduced.

Even with the cost of packaging included, the IC amplifier would be quite inexpensive. The way in which packaging affects overall costs is shown in Table 3-2. A high-volume IC operation could package (including test) the 20-element chip for approximately 40¢ (40¢ in *this* example—packaging costs can vary widely from this figure as the package type ranges from plastic to mil-standard hermetic).

Competitive Problems Having to Do with Yield. Chip yields have always varied widely. The average yield in a well-run firm for a circuit of the complexity used in our example might today be 40%. This means the chip can cost about 5¢ and the packaged unit about 45¢. Some firms have higher yields, however, and some, unfortunately, must struggle along on much lower yields. It is not hard to understand the profit problems that a firm experiencing 10% yields would be facing in a market whose leaders are realizing 50% yields and basing prices on yields of 30 to 90%.

Table 3-2   Packaged IC Costs—Various Yields

Yield (%)	Cost ($)		
	Chip Cost	Package Cost	Total Factory Cost
100	0.02	0.40	0.42
50	0.04	0.40	0.44
25	0.08	0.40	0.48
10	0.20	0.40	0.60
5	0.40	0.40	0.80
1	2.00	0.40	2.40

This yield range is typical of today's IC industry. It shows that the yield leaders can be involved with very profitable operations, and the yield "laggers" can lose heavily.

Differences in costs due to different yields are smaller as we enter the 1970s. Average yields are approaching or passing the 50% level (with packages thus becoming a relatively large part of the overall cost). Only a few years ago the average yield was 10%, the leaders getting 25% yields and the beginners and the technologically weak firms experiencing 1%. Reference to Table 3-1 or 3-2 should convince the reader that these were indeed perilous times. The penalties for being a technological follower were severe, and the rewards for being a leader could be great. In the newer IC technologies (such as MOS) this is still the case.

Cost Trends Today. In spite of what seems to be the rock-bottom cost of silicon ICs, costs *continue* to trend downward. There are three reasons for this trend:

1. Costs go down as yields go up (see Tables 3-1 and 3-2).

2. Final costs go down as the number of elements per chip increases. Consider that a package cost for a chip with 40 elements is not much different from that for a chip with 20 elements. As yields go up, more elements per chip become practical. (See Figure 3-1.)

3. Costs go down as new technologies or techniques are introduced—as with LSI or with MOS ICs.

Typical yields over the years for a 20-element chip such as that used in our example would be as shown in Table 3-3. Thus because of yield improvement chip costs have been coming down for a long time and are likely to continue downward in the future. This is verified by the reduction

Table 3-3   IC Yield Improvement

Year	Yield
1960	Less than 1%
1965	10%
1970	40%
1975	80%

in average unit prices for digital ICs over the past years reported by EIA in 1968, and by Integrated Circuit Engineering (ICE), in 1970 (*Status of Integrated Circuits, 1970*). Table 3-4 lists these data. Note how EIA underestimated the rate at which costs would decrease. The ICE data were published before drastic recession-induced price reductions in 1970, so that their 1971 estimate is probably also high.

IC costs are declining also because the number of elements per chip, hence element density, is increasing. Today, in MOS memory devices, chips with over 5000 elements are on the market, and 100,000 to 1,000,000 element chips are in "sight" (see the next subsection). The effect of the number of elements per chip on cost is shown in Figure 3-1. It shows how increasing yields, increasing number of elements per chip, and increasing element density have brought IC costs down over a period of years. The cost per element at any one time has been a function of the sum of (1) chip packaging costs (which decreases with more elements per chip) and of (2) chip cost (which increases with the number of elements per chip, because of lower yields). Until recently chip yield problems kept monolithic IC makers from taking advantage of packaging economics. Now

Table 3-4   History of IC Costs

Year	Unit Cost ($)	
	EIA	ICE
1962	65.00	
1963	39.26	
1964	16.93	
1965	7.25	
1966	4.33	
1967	3.00	3.32
1968	2.15	2.33
1969	1.65	1.63
1970	1.25*	1.15
1971	1.07*	0.70*
1973	0.85*	
1975	0.75*	

* Forecast

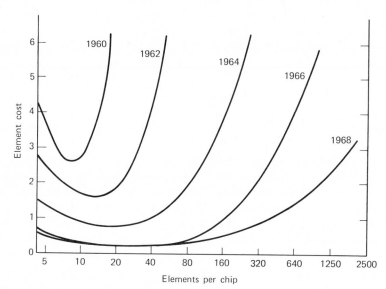

Figure 3-1 IC economics over the years. (*Source.* Integrated Circuit Engineering Company, *Integrated Circuit Engineering—Basic Technology,* 1966.)

(1971) the most economical combination is approaching 1000 elements. Devices with several thousands of elements are becoming commonplace because the penalty in increased element cost is not severe.

What is Coming in the 1970s? At the 1970 IEEE Convention in New York City, Robert Noyce, President of Intel (and the "coinventor" of the IC), was a member of a panel that devoted an afternoon to prognostications of what is going to happen in the coming decade. His predictions were as follows:

IC complexity: up to 100 fold from today.
IC costs: down 100 fold.
1980 MOS selling price: 1/20¢ per gate.

The reduced cost history of ICs has been impressive. We are all aware of many things that have become technologically possible and economically practical because of IC technology. But with cost reductions and increased chip complexity still coming, such as Dr. Noyce predicted, new application possibilities are truly mind boggling. Not only will today's products be available at lower cost, but products that previously could never be considered practical will become possible. New design rules will have to be evolved—partly because ICs work differently, but also because of different economic rules having to do with the new cost structure.

One of the best examples of how IC economics allow things to be done electronically that were not economically practical in the past is in the rapidly burgeoning area of semiconductor memories. A semiconductor memory "bit" requires several transistors and resistors—one version being essentially a "flip-flop" circuit. The cost of flip-flops in complex chips is now so low that they can compete (in some applications) with memory systems using magnetic cores. Other similar opportunities will open up as IC technology advances—such as Noyce's 1/20¢ gate. These low costs will allow all sorts of applications that are not practical today.

The *low element cost* is a major reason why ICs are being used today, and will *continue* to be used in increasing amounts in the future. This low cost is based on processing many parts or elements at the same time on a single wafer. It is one of the factors that underly predictions of a $50 billion United States electronics market within the next decade. Without ICs, the prospect for electronics would not be nearly as bright.

THICK FILM COSTS

As already mentioned a major reason for use of thick film hybrids is that they allow the low element cost possible with silicon monolithics to be expanded into new areas where monolithic ICs cannot go by themselves. Many types of circuits require precision elements, high-performance components, or more than one type of active device. Thick film hybrid technology is often the only way that the needs of the circuit can be met.

In addition, thick film has its *own* economic "punch," though less strong and dramatic than that of monolithics.

Thick Film Tooling. Tooling for thick film is inexpensive and available on a fast-delivery cycle. This allows thick film to be extremely competitive in short-run situations, and is of course, helpful on longer runs. Of the three types of IC, thick film is usually the least expensive. (See Table 3-5 and Figure 3-2) in short production runs.

Thick Film Conductors. Conductors of thick film offer good isolation, low conductivity, and they are inexpensive to lay down. All the conductors needed for an entire circuit can be "manufactured" with a single pass of a screen printer. The economics of thick film conductors are very similar to those of printed circuits. In fact, pitted economically against printed circuits, thick film is very cost effective. Substrate costs are lower than high-quality PC board costs when one takes into account that what would require several square inches on a PC board can take only 1 in.^{2} on a substrate. Even if all technological capabilities of thick film were to be ignored except for its conductor capability, there might be a place for thick film as a kind of compact, low-cost PC board.

Multilevel Circuit Capabilities. This will be another major justification for thick film. In multichip circuits, getting from one chip to another or from one chip to the outside world is often impossible without many crossovers. Thick film offers one of the most attractive approaches to multilevel circuits—being reliable and inexpensive and having relatively low parasitics. The most common interconnect approach today with complex arrays is multilayer thick film.

Resistors. Thick film resistors offer a very wide range of resistivity with capabilities of producing close tolerances and excellent resistor characteristics. Since several can be screened at the same time, the thick film resistor can be quite economical. The ability to print resistors, several at a time, added to the low-cost conductor capability, gives to thick film an advantage that is very potent. Thick film resistor costs are low enough to be highly competitive with the least expensive carbon composition resistors.

Capacitors. Thick film capacitors also offer considerable economy when several can be printed at the same time. The costs of thick film capacitors are not so low as resistors, but under the right conditions costs can be competitive with the least costly discrete capacitors.

Discrete Add-Ons. Discrete add-ons offer little in the way of economy, but they serve to broaden the capabilities of thick film hybrid circuits. In this way they not only allow the economic advantages of monolithic ICs into more areas, but also allow those economies peculiar to thick film processing to be expanded into more areas.

Functional Testing. This aspect of thick film capabilities is getting increasing attention and, along with multilevel conductor capabilities, is a very important advantage and justification for thick film hybrids.

A large part of the cost of a hybrid circuit can be in the cost of the purchased semiconductor chips (see Chapter 13). Any cost reductions here could be very significant. A highly effective approach to reducing these costs is to take advantage of the *adjustability* of thick film resistors (and capacitors). The circuits are designed so that less expensive semiconductor chips can be used. The final circuit performance depends on use of "sloppy" (inexpensive) active devices "peaked" into desired performance by use of resistor trimming. This often requires complex test equipment and redesign of the circuit to add the proper resistors, but it can result in significant savings.

Another example: where a discrete device circuit would use potentiometer, a thick film circuit will use a screen-printed resistor—trimmed to value. This substitution invariably results in significant savings.

Another much more simple example of functional testing is illustrated by a timed RC circuit. Done the "old way," it would consist of a resistor and a capacitor, each with about half the tolerance of the final time interval desired (time is proportional to the product of the resistance and the capacitance). For timing to within 2%, 1% tolerance is required of each of the discrete components. With thick film, however, an inexpensive loose-tolerance discrete capacitor can be used, and the resistor trimmed to whatever value the capacitance of the capacitor demands.

Effective functional trimming depends on the easy, accurate and economic trimming capabilities of thick film resistors. Major cost reductions have been reported when this technique is used. Indeed, the trimmability of thick film resistors (and lately of thick film capacitors) is such that one gets precision resistors with thick film ICs whether they are needed or not. Trimming equipment has advanced to the point where trimming to 1% tolerance is very easy and inexpensive.

SYSTEMS LEVEL COST CONSIDERATIONS

General Cost Comparisons between Conventional Circuits and the Various Types of ICs. Table 3-5 shows how the various IC types compete with one another (and with conventional circuits) at different production levels. Note the extreme low cost of silicon monolithics; monolithics should be used if the tooling cost can be justified. This information comes from a paper given in S. Stulberg of Raytheon at Wescon's Symposium on Hybrids in 1968. The cost data are thus now (1971) at least three years old. Tooling costs for monolithic ICs are somewhat less expensive now—and the costs

Table 3-5   Cost Comparisons between ICs and Conventional Circuits

Type of Circuit	Tooling Costs (in dollars)	Size of Production Run				
		1 to 25	100 to 1000	1000 to 10	10 to 100	100 and Up
Conventional PC board	1,200	50	30	25	18	15
Thick film	1,800	50	30	25	15	12
Thin film	2,000	75	45	30	20	15
Monolithic	20,000	30	15	8	6	4

of monolithic IC production have also come down more than have either thick film or thin film costs. Conventional circuit costs have moved upward slightly.

Figure 3-2, in a similar comparison, draws almost the same conclusions. Conventional circuitry is the least expensive for very low production, then thick film takes over, and finally monolithic is the least expensive. Use of thin film at any level or of thick film in high-volume production runs must be based on a need for performance not available in the less expensive approaches.

Conventional versus Monolithic—"Specific" Comparison. Table 3-6 shows how ICs can be used to reduce costs of similar equipment built with discrete components. The data are from the 1966 edition of ICE's *IC Engineering—Basic Technology*, originally taken from an EDN magazine article published in the mid-sixties, hence are badly out of date. (IC costs

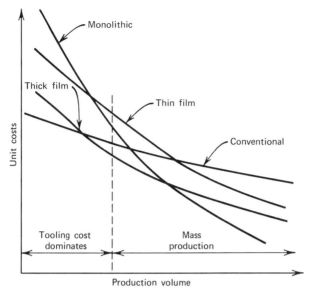

Figure 3-2 Comparison of circuit costs at various production levels. The costs of manufacturing different kinds of IC are compared to those of manufacturing conventional circuits. (*Source.* Integrated Circuit Engineering Company, *The Status of ICs—1971, 1970.*)

today are probably one-tenth of those in 1966.) The example has been retained for illustration here because comparisons of this nature simply are not made any more. The mid-sixties were about the time that it was first possible to reduce costs by using ICs, and a comparison such as this was of considerable interest. One would not bother to make such a comparison today because the savings are taken for granted. Note that not

Table 3-6 Conventional (Discrete) versus IC Costs

Discrete Version		IC Version	
3696 discrete components on		182 ICs on 7 printed circuit	
28 printed circuit boards	$1051	boards	$748
Assembly labor	87	Assembly labor	21
Back panel wiring	150	Back panel wiring	30
Testing	43	Testing	10
Total	$1331	Total	$809

only the individual component costs are reduced, but also the assembly labor.

Cost Comparisons—LSI versus Simple ICs; The Schneider/Honeywell "Digitest" Multimeter. In 1969 France's Schneider bought out a new model of a multimeter. The redesign involved use of one LSI module which cost $8 (plus $30,000 for tooling from the United States General Instrument Corporation with a guarantee of buying 10,000 circuits). The combined cost of the module and tooling amortization was $11. The new model also used 50 discrete transistors. This redesign replaced an older model that used 12 standard ICs which cost a total of $35, plus 180 transistors costing heaven only knows how much. The old model retailed (in France) for $400, the new model for $250. This illustrates the use of newer, more advanced monolithic technology as a way to further reduce costs (over reductions made possible by a shift from discretes to ICs).

Cost Comparisons—Overall, Rather Than Initial, Cost. The popular "systems" approach to costs examines *other* cost items than initial cost. The cost of using, cost of repairing, and finally the cost of enduring loss of service must also be considered. ICs are useful as reducers of these other costs. This was the prime reason for use of ICs in their early years when their initial cost was usually much higher than for the same item constructed with conventional components.

Cost of Using. Costs such as those of power consumption can be significant. Savings from weight reduction are sometimes important. Power consumption savings might not seem much—but consider their importance in a battery-powered circuit on a moon mission. The weight of airborne equipment influences the operating costs of commercial airlines. One pound of extra airborne electronic equipment on a commercial cargo jet costs over $1/year in fuel, and also results in lost revenue of more than $1/year. The cost of extra weight, considered over the 20 years or so of the airplane's life, make weight reduction important.

Table 3-7 shows some old (and therefore interesting) data on the premium that can be paid for weight reductions. The progress that has been made—some of it because of ICs (which were not used much in those days)—is most obvious in the first item: "deep space." The $20,000/lb premium made space experiments very expensive in those days. NASA's space shuttle, being designed in the late 1970s to serve orbiting space laboratories, has a target cost of under $100 for putting 1 lb of material into orbit. This puts the weight premium for deep space *below* that of present-

Table 3-7 Premiums That
Can Be Paid in Weight
Reduction

Application	Premium
Seep space	$20,000/lb
Nonorbit	$2,000/lb
Portable	$800/lb
Airborne	$300/lb
Vehicular	$7/lb
Stationary	5¢/lb

Source. Wallmark, *Microelectronics*,
McGraw-Hill, New York, 1963.

day weight reduction premiums for airborne equipment, which run around
$200/lb.

The Cost of Repairing. ICs are much more reliable than are conventional
circuits. They do not break down as much, and when they do, repair
costs tend to be lower because of modular replacement. Maintenance and
repair costs of many IC systems approach zero.

The Cost of Being out of Service. This is somewhat harder to measure in
dollars, but is nevertheless a very important item. The cost in lost profits
to a computer service firm because their computer is broken can be very
serious—lost profits, lost customers, and so on. The cost of an out-of-service
piece of electronic equipment intended for entertainment is usually limited
to personal frustration; the cost is incalculable for life support systems
in a spacecraft. In life support applications redundant systems are needed,
so the cost of insuring against out-of-service time can be very high. In
many instances ICs are the only approach that is reliable enough to even
consider.

Other Cost Reduction Possibilities. The hybrid IC can often reduce costs
of the nonelectronic parts of a device. An example of this would be placing
a thick film hybrid voltage regulator on (or inside) an automobile's alternator. Part of the overall comparison between the thick film hybrid
version and the older electromechanical regulator would be the savings
made by eliminating the wiring between the old style bulkhead-mounted
regulator and the alternator (including the cost of *installing* the wiring).

Overall Cost Comparisons. Table 3-8 shows how one might look at all costs rather than first cost only when making a decision about which system should be purchased. System A turns out to be less expensive in the end than system B in spite of the fact that it is 50% more expensive originally. Higher first costs, but lower overall costs was a common situation in systems built with integrated circuits in the early 1960s. Now not only are the "other" costs less, but original costs are also less.

Table 3-8　An Overall Cost Comparison

	A	B
Original cost	$3000	$2000
Use cost	100	1000
Maintenance cost	200	1500
Out-of-service cost	400	2000
	$3700	$6500

SUMMARY

The impact of monolithic ICs on the cost of electronic equipment and systems—both in initial cost and in overall cost—is significant. In years to come this impact will be felt even more strongly.

An important role played by thick film (and thin film) hybrids is to bring these cost and performance improvements to more areas than monolithics ICs alone could do. In addition, thick film hybrids offer economically attractive approaches to low-cost resistors, capacitors, and complex conductor interconnect systems. Functional trimming of resistors allows major reductions in costs of discrete active devices are variable passive components.

Chapter 4

THICK FILM MATERIALS

The switch from conventional circuit construction techniques to a thick film hybrid process entails for many a drastic change in outlook concerning the materials used. Assembly of a printed circuit board requires little materials knowledge. The components are purchased in final form and can be treated as "black boxes," the only concern being that of not altering the device's property during assembly.

In thick film circuit techniques the situation is definitely reversed. The circuit assembler has now become a producer of components who must be concerned with the effect of his processes on the properties of the circuit elements.

It would certainly be possible to produce a thick film circuit without an understanding of the nature of the materials used and their possible chemical and physical interactions during the different steps of the thick film process. It is the authors' opinion, however, that any successful thick film operation must be based on a materials awareness on the part of the engineers who design and produce the circuits. The aim of the next four chapters is to provide this understanding or "materials philosophy."

The diversity of backgrounds of the people involved in the design and production of thick film circuits makes preparation of these chapters somewhat difficult. We have assumed only a basic knowledge of physics and chemistry in this presentation. We hope to parlay this knowledge into the desired "materials philosophy."

In this chapter we examine the "raw materials" most important in producing the thick film components—the inks and substrates. Chapter 5 will cover the screen printing process, including printer design and important aspects of fluid flow. In Chapter 6 the chemical reactions between the ink and substrates that take place during firing are described. The design and operation of the thick film kiln are discussed. Chapter 7 concludes the materials presentation with a description of typical physical and electrical properties of the different components.

The remaining chapters are devoted to discussions of nonthick film subjects—and to driving home the basic "materials philosophy" introduced in Chapters 4 to 7.

THICK FILM INKS

There is a similarity between the process of screen printing and conventional lithographic techniques. Because of the similarity, screen printing mixtures are often referred to as inks. The term "paste" is also used to describe these materials because of their pasty consistency. These terms are used interchangeably throughout this book along with the somewhat more "sophisticated" or "dignified" term "composition."

The basic purpose of the thick film ink is to produce a fired composite that will control the electrical conduction process. In conductors we want unhindered conduction or low resistivity; in resistors, modulated conduction over a range of resistances; and in dielectrics, low conductivity.

Before beginning our discussion of the inks, it might be wise to review briefly some facts about electrical conduction in solids. If we prepare a rectangular sample of material and electrode the ends as shown in Figure 4-1, we can cause current to flow by application of an electric field.

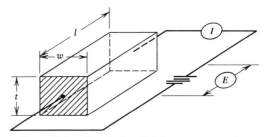

Figure 4-1   Electrical resistivity measurement.

The magnitude of the current will depend on the sample dimensions, the voltage applied, and the material. We can relate these quantities with the equation.

$$V = RI \qquad (4\text{-}1)$$

where V = applied voltage
R = resistance (Ω)
I = current (A)

The resistance, R, is the proportionality factor between current and voltage. The defining equation for R, in terms of a specific material, is

$$R = \rho \frac{l}{tw} \qquad (4\text{-}2)$$

where R = resistance
ρ = resistivity
l = length of sample
t = thickness of sample
w = width of sample

It is sometimes convenient to rearrange this equation and define a property called sheet resistivity.

$$R = \frac{p}{t} \frac{l}{w} \qquad (4\text{-}3)$$

where R = resistance

$\dfrac{p}{t} \equiv p_s \equiv$ sheet resistivity

$\dfrac{l}{w} =$ aspect ratio = N

In a rectangular resistor, the aspect ratio can be considered to be the number of squares N, of dimension W $\times$ W (Figure 4-2).

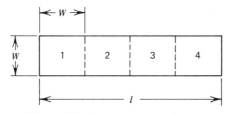

Figure 4-2   A four-square resistor.

In the example above, $N = 4$. The resistance in terms of these quantities is

$$R = p_s N$$

It is important to note that this resistance is based on a unit thickness.

We usually make three broad classifications of a material based on the value of the resistivity: conductors with low resistivity, insulators with high resistivity, and semiconductors in which the resistivity is not constant but varies with applied voltage at a fixed temperature (with resistivity between conductors and insulators).

The value of the resistivity determines the current flow in a particular material. This current flow is the result of a movement of charged carriers. Several types of carriers are possible, but in the materials of interest to us we shall consider only electrons as the moving species.

The magnitude of the current flow for a fixed sample configuration and applied voltage is determined by the number of mobile electrons and their drift velocity. At absolute zero the number of mobile electrons is related to the specific material, and their velocity depends on the atomic arrangement in the solid. The number of free or mobile electrons increases with temperature and their mobility decreases.

At any particular temperature the conductivity is a combination of these two factors. In a conductor (with large numbers of free electrons) the increase in atom-electron interactions (decreased mobility) outweights the contribution of the added conduction electrons. As a result, its conductivity decreases with increasing temperature.

In theory an insulator has no mobile electrons and would be a nonconductor. All real dielectrics have impurities that contribute mobile electrons so that insulators have a low but measurable conductivity.

In a real insulator with a small number of conduction electrons, the percentage gain in mobile electrons outweighs their decreased mobility, and the conductivity increases with temperature. In the third class of materials, the semiconductors, there is a delicate balance between the mobility and number of mobile electrons. Applied voltages can also increase the number of electrons so that these materials behave as conductors or insulators depending on temperature and voltage levels.

THICK FILM CONDUCTOR INKS

Three types of materials are used in producing a thick film conductor: the metal or functional material, a glassy phase or permanent binder, and a mixture of several organic liquids. Examination of a micrograph of the surface of a thick film conductor would show a predominance of exposed metal particles.

Each of these components plays a specific role in the development of the properties of the finished composite. The functional material provides a conductive path, the glass binder holds the functional materials in point contact during firing and "glues" the conductor to the substrate, and the organic liquids make possible the screen printing of these solids.

Resistance measurements would show that the fired composite was a good conductor with a resistivity on the order of 10^{-3} Ω-cm. This value is considerably lower than a homogeneous sample of the functional material, i.e., a palladium silver alloy would have a resistivity of about 10^{-6} Ω-cm. Examination of a micrograph will show that the actual conduction path through the composite is a system of metal particles in contact. The nature of these contacts will determine the conductor resistance.

While the uses of a conductor in the thick film hybrid circuit may seem obvious, they are worth listing if only to serve as the starting point for this section in which we examine the composition of conductor inks.

The conductor serves at least one of the following functions in the hybrid circuit:

1. Interconnection between circuit elements (Figure 4-3).

2. Mounting pads for discrete components and other types of interconnections (Figure 4-4).

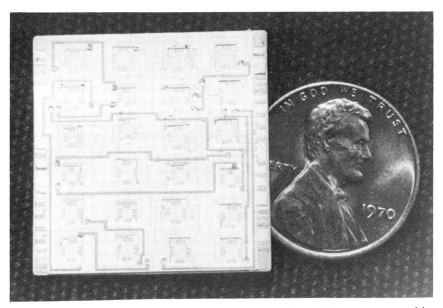

Figure 4-3 Thick film conductors used as interconnections; these are on a multi-layer circuit. Note buried conductor runs (faint shadows). (Photograph by State of the Art, Inc.; circuit from *J W Microelectronics.*)

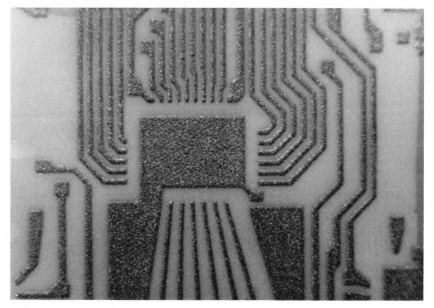

Figure. 4-4 Thick film conductor composition serving as a mounting pad (for a complex IC chip). (State of the Art Photo.)

3. Resistor terminations (Figure 4-5).
4. Electrodes for screen-on capacitors (Figure 4-6).

The conductor inks should produce a composite with the following properties:

1. Conductivity must be high to minimize voltage drops and heating.
2. Adhesion must be good because leads and discrete devices are attached directly to the conductor.
3. Bonding of leads and devices to the conductor surface must be possible.
4. The composite must be stable during processing and use. Ideally, the conductor properties would show no change with time, temperature of operation or storage, environment, and thermal cycling.

The composition of the three components of the ink as it relates to these functions is now described.

Functional Materials. The purpose of the functional material is to provide a conductive path through the composite. For conductor inks the functional materials are metals or alloys.

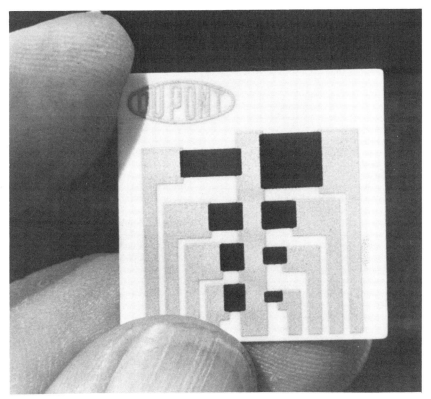

Figure 4-5 Thick film conductor composition serving as thick film resistor terminations. (Test circuit by DuPont; photograph by State of the Art, Inc.)

Many factors must be considered in choosing the proper materials. There are economic considerations, processing behavior, stability, and factors relating specifically to the function, that is, conductor functional materials, resistor functional materials, and so on. Many of these factors are universal and they apply to all of the materials under consideration. Cost, for instance, should always be as low as possible and the materials should be stable after processing to avoid physical and electrical changes. We shall not deal with these in any more detail.

We will concern ourselves with the specific materials properties that enable the component to fulfill its particular functions.

For the functional phase of the conductor ink, the important materials considerations are surface characteristics of the powders, chemical reactivity, ease of preparation, and process compatibility.

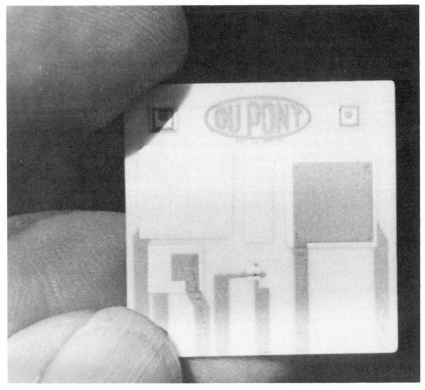

Figure 4-6 Thick film conductor composition serving as a thick film capacitor electrode. (Test circuit by DuPont; photograph by State of the Art, Inc.)

We have already observed that the overall resistivity of the composite is determined by the contact resistance of the individual metal particles.

There are two limiting types of contacts in the conductor. Inks fired at low temperatures would produce composites with point contacts only. There would be essentially no reaction between the metal particles, and the contact resistance would be a complicated function of the contact pressure and composition of the metal surfaces.

In composites fired at high temperatures there would be considerable diffusion and possibly melting of the metal particles to form a more or less homogeneous junction. The contact resistance in this case would be a function of the degree of sintering and composition of the metal surfaces.

The composition of the metals surface is dependent primarily on contaminants. The most harmful would be oxide or nitride surface layers formed during firing by reaction of the metal with the glass or furnace atmosphere. As an example, copper cannot be used as the functional material in a conductor composite fired in air. After firing, all the copper particles would be coated with an oxide layer. This surface layer would lead to high contact resistance and poor sintering behavior.

The bonding behavior of the composite will also be influenced by the formation of surface contamination. All of the bonding techniques used to attach leads and discrete devices depend on a clean metal surface to produce good bonds. Any surface contamination will make bonding more difficult. The formation of an oxide or nitride layer that is not removed by the flux makes soldering impossible.

Since the surface properties are so important in determining both the resistance and the bonding characteristics of the composite, it is clear that the functional metal or alloy must be extremely nonreactive. The relatively high firing temperatures and oxidizing atmosphere in the thick film furnaces, coupled with the use of reactive glasses as permanent binders, eliminate many metals and alloys from consideration as functional materials. Reactions during soldering and bonding must also be considered. Of particular importance is solder resistance. Metals that are soluble in molten solders present many difficulties. In practice, only precious metals such as gold, silver, palladium, and platinum can be used.

The functional materials are incorporated in the ink as small particles, usually less than 5 μM in maximum diameter. The size distribution and shape of these particles will influence many of the important electrical and physical properties. In a conductor, the screening behavior of the ink, the bonding characteristics of the composite, and its electrical resistivity will all be influenced by these factors. Production of metal powders of controlled size and shape is not an easy matter. Very desirable metals or alloys may be eliminated from consideration because it is not possible to form powders from them economically.

The reasons for the requirement that the functional material must be compatible with the process will become clear as we proceed with the description of the chemical interactions possible during the production of a thick film circuit.

A good example of this requirement is the use of conductor inks with silver as a functional material for resistor terminations. Under certain conditions the silver from the conductor can diffuse into the resistor, completely changing its resistance value. The use of the silver conductor is not compatible with the process in this case.

Because of the conflicting materials requirements for any component of the ink, it should be evident that the ink manufacturers and the user will be required to make many property tradeoffs in ink formulation and processing. For instance, compositional changes to maximize conductivity in a particular ink might lead to poor bonding performance, high cost, or difficult processing. The thick film engineer should be constantly alert to the possible tradeoffs necessary in his particular application.

Permanent Binders. The permanent binders are all low-melting glasses. They serve two functions in the conductor composite: (1) they hold the metal particles in contact and (2) they bond the composite to the substrate.

Before discussing the desirable properties of the permanent binders, let us take a closer look at glasses. Solids are usually classified as crystalline or amorphous depending on the arrangement of the atoms. If there is a regular and repeated order extending over distances that are large compared to the atomic dimensions, we call the material a crystalline solid. If there is considerable atomic disorder in the material, it is classified as amorphous.

Glass is a good example of an amorphous material. There may be some identifiable groups of atoms in glass, but they are small, extending only a few atomic diameters. These groups are distributed in a random fashion throughout the glass. We say that the glass has "short range" order only. Because of the atomic arrangement, glasses behave physically more like liquids than solids. For instance, most crystalline solids possess a definite melting point where they change from a solid to a liquid of low viscosity. Glasses, on the other hand, have no sharp transition from a solid to a liquid. The viscosity of a glass decreases steadily with increasing temperature until a point is reached where there is detectable flow. When the glass reaches a viscosity of approximately 500 poise, it is considered to have melted.

The properties most important when selecting a permanent binder are the temperature-viscosity relationship, surface tension properties, chemical reactivity, and coefficient of thermal expansion.

The temperature-viscosity behavior of the glass will determine the firing range of the composite. While it is impossible to establish absolute values, it is generally observed that the necessary flow of the glass to coat the metal particles and substrate can take place only at viscosities lower than 500 poise. With increasing temperature, the viscosity continues to decrease, and there is a point at which the glass becomes too fluid and flows out on the surface of the substrate leaving a porous, poorly structured composite.

The surface tension and wetting properties of the glass in contact with the metal particles will determine the mechanical properties of the metal-metal contacts of the functional materials. If the glass formed a *complete* layer around each particle, the composite would have high resistivity because there would be no metal-metal contacts. What is needed then is a partial wetting of the metal particles so that they can be held in place but still remain in direct contact. The surface tension of the glass at the glass-ceramic interface will help to determine the amount of reaction that can take place between the permanent binder and the substrate.

The reactivity of the glass is also important in determining this bond. The structure of the substrate is discussed later in the chapter. For now, it is important to know only that the substrate has a glassy phase that must react with the permanent binder if a good bond between the composite and substrate is to be formed.

The reactivity of the glass and metal must also be considered. Because of the effect of surface contamination on electrical resistivity and bonding behavior, it should be evident that little or no reaction can be tolerated.

The last criterion is the thermal expansion of the glass. The normal firing range of the thick film circuits is 500 to 1000°C, and they may operate from −55°C or lower to 125°C. The thermal expansion of the glass should match that of the substrate over this range; otherwise cracking and peeling of the thick film composite could result. Even if cracking did not occur, the stresses set up in the composite due to thermal mismatch could affect its electrical properties because of their point contact nature.

The choice of a specific glass involves the tradeoffs discussed for functional materials. Many different proprietary glass systems are in use. They are based on bismuth oxide, cadmium oxide, or lead borosilicates.

Organic Additives. The purpose of the organic additives is to impart fluid properties to the mixture of solid functional and as a permanent binder material so that the ink can be screen printed.

Aside from the fluid characteristics, which will be covered in Chapter 5 (Screen Printing), the only materials properties of interest to us are related to the removal of the organics during firing.

The organic additives contain large amounts of carbon. If the organics are not eliminated from the ink before maximum firing temperatures are reached, they will decompose and carbonize. There are several undesirable consequences of this decomposition. The carbon could react with either the metal or glass phases. The reactions with the glass would produce a gas causing pinholes and other discontinuities in the composite. The point contact properties of the metals could also be altered by reaction. In dielectric composites the carbon could increase the conductivity to unacceptable levels.

There are an almost unlimited number of organic liquids meeting the necessary requirements. They include water, organic solvents, terpenes, and liquid resins. Specific examples are methyl, ethyl, butyl, propyl and higher alcohols, the corresponding esters of these alcohols, pine oil, alpha terpineol, and beta terpineol. Several organic additives will normally be required to produce the optimum fluid characteristics for a screen printing ink.

Conductor Ink Compositions. To complete the coverage of conductor inks a brief summary of the most popular compositions is given. The inks are classified according to the functional materials—either single component or alloy systems.

One-Component Systems. 1. Silver. The silver powder-glass-frit systems were the first developed and still find some use today in thick film hybrids. They are the lowest in cost and have several other good points—ease of processing, high adhesion, and ease of bonding and soldering. They can also be cofired with many resistor and dielectric formulations. It is unfortunate that the silver tends to migrate under high field and high humidity ambients. This "migration" leads to interactions, primarily with resistors and dielectrics, which can affect the electrical properties of the other thick film components. In the case of resistors, the effect is to lower the resistance of the areas in which the silver has diffused. This, in turn, lowers the total resistance of the screened-on element. In screened-on capacitors, silver migration leads to increased conductivity as well as a decreased effective thickness of the dielectric. This thickness decrease raises the capacity and makes the capacitor more prone to short circuits. The migration problem is so widespread that test specifications covering metal migration rate have been written. In one test, a water drop is placed between a pair of electrodes under test. A DC field of 600 V/in. is impressed, and the time to short circuit is measured. In a test cell with 5 mil electrode spacing times of $\frac{1}{2}$ sec or less to short circuit are common for pure silver compositions. Silver alloys have somewhat longer times to failure. Detracting from another attractive characteristic (ease of soldering) is a strong tendency of silver to dissolve (leach) rapidly in molten solder. Migration and leaching problems keep silver from wide use as a thick film conductor.

2. Gold. Usually used where silicon devices are attached by gold-silicon eutectic bonding or where ultrasonic gold or aluminum wire lead bonding is employed. The high cost and poor solderability of gold systems are a disadvantage. Special indium-bismuth solders can be used, but the solder bonds are still very weak.

3. Others. It is safe to say that almost all metals have been tested for possible use in conductive inks. Commercial inks are available using platinum, palladium, iridium, rhodium, ruthenium, and osmium, to name a few.

Alloy Systems. In order to produce superior formulations and reduce the cost, alloys of different noble metals have been developed for thick film applications. An almost unlimited variety of multicomponent alloy systems are available. In each system there are many metal/metal and glass/metal ratios that produce a variety of properties.

1. Platinum-Gold Systems. Combines desirable electrical and physical characteristics of both platinum and gold. Drawbacks include the need for precise firing control to develop maximum substrate adhesion.

2. Palladium-Silver Systems. Developed as a lower cost substitute for platinum-gold. Films have high adhesion and good solderability. As with any silver-containing alloy, there is evidence (not serious) of silver migration under certain conditions. Loss of adhesion in high temprature storage can be a problem. Solder leach resistance is much improved over silver, but is not as good as in platinum gold.

3. Palladium-Gold. Used as a cheaper substitute for platinum-gold.

4. Other Systems. There are many other conductive inks on the market that contain alloys with several components. As in the case of single-component systems, it is safe to say that untold thousands of combinations have been tested.

RESISTOR INKS

The resistor inks are in many ways similar to conductor inks. The functional materials are chosen in part from the same metals and alloys and the permanent binders and organic additives are basically the same. The surface is composed mostly of glass with only a few particles of the functional materials exposed. This contrasts sharply to the surface of the conductor which was mostly metal particles.

The conductor ink used only a metal phase to promote good conductivity. The functional materials in resistor inks are combinations of the three basic types of electrical conductors previously described—conductors, insulators, and semiconductors. In the conductor, the resistance of the composite was primarily determined by the contact properties of the metal particles. While the actual mechanisms of conduction in a resistor composite are unknown, it can be inferred from the resistance levels, the voltage sensitivity, and the temperature-resistance behavior that the contacts are semiconducting in nature.

In theory this should be the case. By decreasing the metal content of a typical thick film conductor ink, a point will be reached where all of the metal particles in the fired composite are separated by a layer of glass. Because of interactions between the glass and metal phase and the impurity level of the glass, these layers are likely to be semiconducting. Depending on the glass/metal ratio, these glass layers could be extremely thin. Since the voltage drop in the ink system would be essentially across the glass layers, high fields would result with only moderate applied voltages. With the glass layers functioning as semiconductors, we could expect resistances intermediate between conductors and insulators.

In practice this approach to making a resistor ink does not work well because of the rapid increase in resistivity as a function of glass layer thickness. This leads to a situation where changes in resistance can only be observed over a narrow composition range. Too little glass and the composite has metal-metal contacts and is a good conductor. Too much glass and the glass layer is thick and of high resistance. This behavior is shown graphically in Figure 4-7.

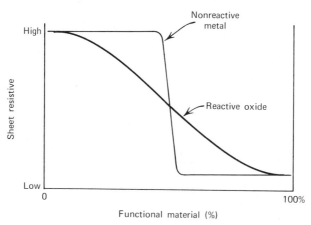

Figure 4-7 Relationships between functional material content and sheet resistance, showing limited useful range for a "nonreactive" system.

One solution to this problem is a functional material that reacts with the glass phase to form thicker semiconducting layers. Mixtures of glass and thallium oxide are an example of this approach. The thicker semiconducting layer permits the composite to function as a semiconductor over a wider range of glass to functional materials ratios.

The use of functional materials that contain combinations of metals, oxides, and semiconductors would also tend to extend the range of glass to functional materials ratios over which the composite would behave as a resistor. In these systems it is almost impossible to determine the actual conduction mechanism because there are so many possibilities.

While the resistor serves only one function in the circuit, the many performance demands placed on it make selection of the functional materials and permanent binders difficult. The electrical parameters of the resistor include sheet resistivity, resistance change with temperature, resistance change with voltage and noise. Typical values of these properties and measurement methods are presented in Chapter 7.

Functional Materials. Many of the criterion for selection of the conductor functional materials are directly applicable. These include surface characteristics, chemical reactivity, and ease of preparation.

The surface characteristics and reactivity of the functional materials will determine the kinds of particle-particle contacts that exist in the composite. These contacts will be responsible for the electrical behavior of the composite. The many possible reactions between the functional materials, permanent binders, and furnace atmosphere are discussed in Chapter 6.

There are an infinite number of precious metal and metal-oxide combinations suitable for resistor applications. Because of the complexity and proprietary nature of the functional materials, it is possible to give only a very limited description of the different systems. For classification purposes, these systems are divided into single- and multicomponent categories.

Single-Component System. *1. Thallium Oxide.* Mixtures of fine particles of thallium oxide and a lead borosilicate glass produce thick film resistors with sheet resistivities varying from about 50 $\Omega/\square$ to 10^7 $\Omega/\square$. This range of resistivities is obtained by varying the thallium oxide content from 85 to 25 wt %. Airco Speer (the Electronics Division of Air Reduction Company) who markets this system, claims that the resistor characteristics are insensitive to changes in furnace atmosphere. (The same cannot be said of some of the multicomponent systems described later.) The firing temperatures are about 550°C, which is much lower than most of the precious metal in multicomponent systems. The cost of thallium oxide based inks is also considerably less than inks based on precious metals.

2. Other Systems. Silver, gold, palladium, platinum, rhenium, palladium oxide, and rhenium oxide have been used as the functional material in conjunction with appropriate glasses. The major drawback to most of these systems is their sensitivity to composition. Glass frit-silver powder mixtures have sheet resistivities of less than 1 $\Omega/\square$/mil at 48% silver and 10^5 $\Omega/\square$/mil at 46% silver. Palladium-glass systems on the other hand have a useful range from 33 to 70% palladium.

Multicomponent Systems. *1. Pd-PdO-Ag.* This pioneer system of DuPont is still in use today. Sheet resisistivities from 1 $\Omega/\square$ to 10^6 $\Omega/\square$ are available. The firing of these inks requires careful control, since the resistance values are extremely sensitive to furnace atmosphere and firing profile. This behavior is due to the complicated chemistry of the system—oxidation of Pd and Ag, reduction of PdO and AgO, alloying of Pd and Ag, and doping of the oxide and metal phases by the glass can all occur. The extent of the reactions depends on furnace temperature and atmosphere as well as base composition.

2. Pd-Ag. These formulations were developed as an improvement on the original Pd-PdO-Ag compositions. The composites produced by this system are somewhat more stable with temperature than the Pd-PdO-Ag mixtures. Firing control is critical, as these inks are much more sensitive to temperature and furnace atmosphere than the Pd-PdO-Ag systems.

3. Other Systems. There are commercially available systems using a whole host of precious metal and oxide combinations. Compositions containing ruthenium and rhenium are becoming popular because of their better resistance stability.

Permanent Binders. The glass systems used in conductor composites are modified for use in the resistor systems. The lead borosilicates are sometimes replaced by cadmium or zinc borosilicates. The role of the glass in fixing the electrical properties of the resistor make its composition more critical. Bond strength requirements are not an important aspect of the thick film resistor, and this function of the glass may be deemphasized.

Organic Additives. In most instances the organic systems are identical with the conductor inks. Some modifications may be necessary because of the different ratio of functional material to glass.

DIELECTRIC INKS

Dielectric materials have two main applications in thick film circuits—crossover insulators and capacitor dielectrics. A third application is as protective seals. The electrical conduction process in these materials has already been described. Because of the small number of conduction electrons, they are good insulators with resistivities exceeding 10^{13} Ω-cm.

The main difference in the materials for the two applications is the magnitude of the relative dielectric constant, K.

A capacitor is essentially an electrical charge storage device. If we construct a parallel plate capacitor, as shown in Figure 4-8, we can store

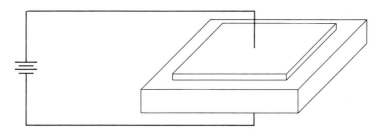

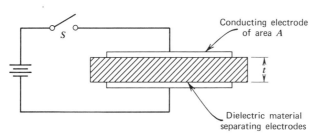

Figure 4-8 Capacitor construction.

a certain amount of charge on the plates by first applying a voltage and then disconnecting the voltage source. The amount of charge is related to the applied voltage, the geometry of the capacitor, and the material between the electrodes.

The equation

$$Q = CV$$

where Q = charge
C = capacitance
V = voltage

relates the Q and V.

The capacitance, C, is defined for the parallel plate capacitor as

$$C = K\epsilon_0 \frac{A}{t}$$

where K = relative dielectric constant
A = area of electrodes
t = electrode spacing
ϵ_0 = constant

The relative dielectric constant used in this equation is determined by the material between the electrodes. Typical values of K are air 1, plastics 2 to 20, glasses 4 to 40, and polycrystalline ceramic materials 6 to 10,000.

Simply stated, a capacitor filled with a $K = 10,000$ ceramic material has a storage capacity 10,000 times that of an air capacitor.

Crossover Dielectrics. It is extremely difficult to design any but the simplest thick film circuit without the use of conductor crossovers. The crossover material acts as an insulating layer between the crossing conductors. A complex crossover pattern is shown in Figure 4-9. Several electrical param-

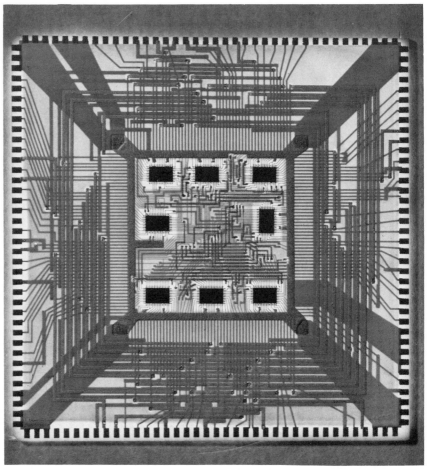

Figure 4-9 Complex crossovers. The buried conductors are made more visible with backlighting. (Circuit and photograph courtesy Raytheon Company.)

eters must be considered for crossover materials. These include breakdown strength, insulation resistance, dissipation factor, and relative dielectric constant. Typical values of these properties are listed in Chapter 7.

Functional Materials. In some cases the functional materials for crossovers are simple glasses. There are many compositions with the proper electrical properties. The choice of composition is usually dictated by other properties of the glass. The most important are temperature-viscosity characteristics, compatibility with conductor formulations, and thermal expansion.

Compatibility requirements are easily stated. The crossover dielectric must not react with the conductor composite in any way that would cause deterioration of its electrical properties or those of the conductor.

As for the temperature-viscosity characteristics of the glass, we must consider two factors—the structure of the dielectric layer and the problem of relative movement of the top electrode either laterally or vertically.

The structure of the dielectric film is of importance because it relates to the electrical properties. If the film is not dense and continuous, there are likely to be shorts between the top and bottom electrode. To produce a flaw-free film, it is desirable to use a glass that has a low viscosity at firing temperatures. The low viscosity allows for considerable flow during processing.

To prevent relative movement of the top electrode—sinking or swimming—a glass with a high viscosity at firing temperatures is dersirable.

These opposing requirements place severe limits on the use of conventional glasses as crossover dielectrics. For most applications it is possible to separate only two conductors. The attempt to build multilayer crossovers would result in short circuits and poor lateral registration.

To overcome the problem of sink and swim, modifications to the glass compositions must be made. It is possible to formulate a glass that will partly recrystallize with proper thermal treatment. The formation of the crystalline phase drastically alters the temperature-viscosity relationship of the glass. At a particular temperature the glass on initial firing may have a viscosity of 100 poise. After recrystallization, the viscosity at the same temperature may be 1000 poise or greater. With systems of this type, it is possible to construct complicated multilayer structures without fear of conductor movement.

Thermal expansion characteristics must be matched to the conductor composites and the substrate to prevent flaw formation and subsequent shorting.

Permanent Binders. Since the functional material is a glass, no additional permanent binders are required.

Organic Additives. The same basic systems used for the other inks are sufficient for crossover applications. It is important to have the best possible flow characteristics so that a flaw-free film can be printed. It is also mandatory that binder removal be complete; otherwise carbon may be trapped in the dielectric leading to higher conductives than desired.

Capacitor Dielectrics. The capacitor dielectrics are more complex than crossover materials. They are similar to resistor systems with separate functional and permanent binders.

Functional Materials. The essential difference between the crossover dielectric and the capacitor dielectric is the magnitude of the relative dielectric constant. In addition to the electrical properties listed for crossover, the capacitor dielectric must have a high K.

There are many ceramic materials, based primarily on $BaTiO_3$, which have high values of relative dielectric constant. By mixing small particles of these materials with glass, it is possible to produce a composites with K's approaching 1000.

The important property of these functional materials is their reactivity. The K's of the ceramic are very sensitive to composition. The glass permanent binders used in the inks contain elements which can significantly lower the K. For this reason it is desirable to limit the reaction between the ceramic and the glass or at least control it so that the K's are reproducible after processing.

Permanent Binders. The permanent binders are chosen from the same glass systems used in conductor and resistor inks. There are two overriding considerations for capacitor dielectrics—reactivity of the glass with the ceramic functional materials and the requirement that the composite must be completely flaw-free after firing.

The reactivity problem has already been touched upon. The requirement of a flaw-free dielectric cannot be compromised. Any flaws in the dielectric layer that short circuit the top and bottom electrodes will render the capacitor useless. To produce these flaw-free dielectrics, extreme care must be taken in selection of the glass system and in processing.

Organic Additives. The same systems used for the other inks find application in the capacitor dielectrics. It is extremely important that the ink have the best possible rheological properties so that a flaw-free film can be printed. It is also mandatory that binder removal be complete at low temperature or carbon will be incorporated in the dielectric layer—this will lead to excessively high conductivities.

INK MANUFACTURE

Ink manufacture is essentially a two-step process. The functional materials and permanent binders must be formulated and the components of the organic additives mixed together. The second step of the process is a thorough mixing of the three components to produce the homogeneous ink. A simplified flow chart of the process is shown in Figure 4-10.

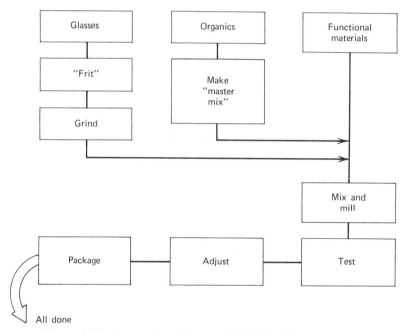

Figure 4-10 Process flow diagram of thick film ink manufacture.

Functional Materials. The important considerations in preparation of the metal functional powders are composition and particle size distribution and shape. It is possible to purchase refined precious metals and alloy powders that can be used directly in the ink formulations. In many cases, however, the ink manufacturer must prepare his own alloys and reduce them to the proper size and shape particles. The preparation of the powders is not as straightforward as it might seem, and in many cases elaborate chemical techniques of precipitation from solutions must be used to get proper sized powders.

The oxide constituents used in resistors and capacitor dielectrics are much simpler to prepare. It is possible to purchase directly many of the oxides. In the case of the capacitor dielectrics, it may be necessary to prereact the components to produce a ceramic which is then milled to produce the proper particle size and shape.

Permanent Binders. The glass systems for use as binders may be purchased with the desired composition and particle size distribution. Because of the specialized applications, it is more likely that the desired composition will be prepared and melted by the ink producer. After melting, the glass is "fritted" to proper size. The fritting process consists of pouring the molten glass into water. The resultant particles are milled to final size.

Organic Additives. The different constituents of the organic system are purchased in bulk and mixed using conventional paint mixing techniques. The high viscosity of many of the organics makes good mixing difficult. The resultant mixture of the organics is called the master mix.

Final Mixing. The final mixing step is carried out using paint mixing equipment, normally a three-roll mill. This step is critical because it must produce a very homogeneous blend of the three ink constituents, but without significantly changing the particle size and shape of the solid components.

CERAMIC SUBSTRATES

The last "raw material" that will be discussed is the substrate. The classification as a raw material is based on the fact that the substrate is a significant participant in some of the chemical reactions that take place during the processing of the thick film inks.

The substrate must serve many functions. The most important are the following:

1. Support the circuit and provide a means for mounting.
2. Protect the circuit from mechanical damage and possibly from the environment.
3. Dissipate heat.
4. Provide electrical isolation.

The materials properties of most interest for substrate applications are resistivity, relative dielectric constant, refractoriness, strength, surface characteristics, chemical reactivity, thermal conductivity, thermal expansion, and dimensional stability.

High surface and bulk resistivity are necessary if the substrate is to provide adequate isolation of the circuit elements.

A low relative dielectric constant is desirable to minimize parasitic capacitance.

Thick film firing temperatures range as high as 1000°C. The substrate must withstand these temperatures without changing dimensions or unduly reacting with the thick film inks. Firing temperatures alone rule out plastics and glasses as practical substrate materials.

There is considerable handling involved in thick film processing so that the substrate must be strong and abrasion resistant.

The surface characteristics will play a significant role in determining the bond strengths of conductor composites. Very little is known about how the substrate surface affects other properties of the composites.

The chemical reactivity of the substrate will also influence the bond strength and possibly other properties of resistors and dielectrics.

Thick films are finding many applications in high power circuits. For this reason it is important that the substrate is a good thermal conductor.

The thermal expansion of the substrate and the mismatch in thermal expansion between the substrate and the composite will influence many of the electrical properties. The overall stability of the thick film device is in part related to this mismatch.

For best performance, it is important that substrate be produced to close tolerances and that these tolerances be maintained during processing and operation of the circuit.

The many competing properties listed eliminate most materials as possible substrates. There is only one group that can be seriously considered—polycrystalline ceramics. A ceramic is a material that depends on some form of high temperature processing to convert the constituents, normally inorganic oxides, into a usable shape. Polycrystalline refers to the many small particles or grains that are held together by a sort of glue called grain boundary material.

For substrate applications three ceramics are popular, beryllium oxide, barium titanate and aluminum oxide.

The beryllium oxide ceramics have high thermal conductivities and are used in high power applications.

Barium titanate ceramics have a high relative dielectric constant and it is possible to make high capacity devices using the substrate as a dielectric.

The aluminum oxide ceramics combine to give the best overall performance and are by far the most popular for substrates. Figure 4-11 is a scanning electron micrograph of the surface of an alumina substrate. The grains of alumina are clearly visible. Their average size is about 3 to 5 μ. Not visible in this micrograph is the grain boundary material which

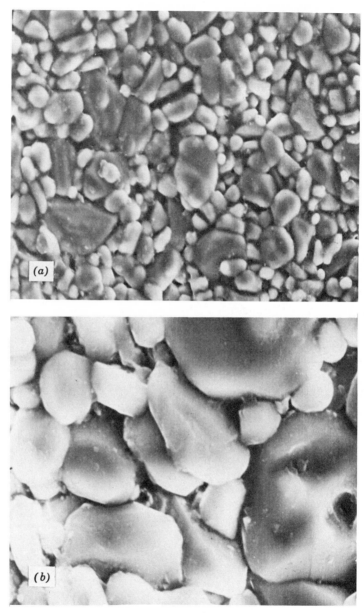

Figure 4-11 Scanning electron micrograph of an alumina substrate's surface. (*a*) 1000×; (*b*) 3000×. (Photographs by J. V. Biggers, Pennsylvania State University.)

is glassy in character. It is the grain boundary glass that reacts with the thick film permanent binders to bond the composite to the substrate.

Substrate Manufacture. The production of the alumina substrates is a typical ceramic processing operation in which fine powders of alumina and other additives are sintered at high temperatures to form a dense, fine-grained polycrystalline structure—in other words, a ceramic. The additives, mainly magnesium oxide, calcium oxide, and silicon dioxide, serve as fluxes, lowering the sintering temperature to a reasonable value. Pure alumina would be difficult to sinter even at temperatures of 2000°C—the addition of 4 to 6% of other oxides permits sintering at temperatures of 1700°C or less without modifying the desirable electrical properties of the alumina.

Very fine powders of the various oxides are mixed together in a ball or rod mill. All the powders are in the micron or submicron range. Water is sometimes added to the powders during milling to aid in the mixing process. Some further size reduction is accomplished, but normally the chief aim of the milling process is to produce a homogeneous mixture. After appropriate milling, the mixture is spray dried. The powder from the spray drier is then pressed in the desired shape on a hydraulically or mechanically actuated press. The pressing operation can be carried out with single or multistation presses using carbide tooling. Production rates of 3600 pieces/hour for a single station press are possible. This operation for multiple station pressing is extremely economical if the tooling costs are spread over a very large number of pieces.

For short runs, temporary designs, a substrate with many holes, or in large area substrates, a tape process is used. The oxide powders are then combined with an organic system that can be cast into a dense, flexible film loaded with alumina and the other oxide additives. The casting process used to produce the tape can be of the batch type or continuous. In the batch operation a movable hopper containing a slurry of the oxides and a suitable organic system is drawn across a glass or smooth plastic surface plate. Material flows from the hopper and is leveled by a blade attached to the hopper. After casting the film is allowed to dry and then stripped from the glass. If the casting is done on organic film, it can either be stripped, or left in place, and burned-off in the kiln.

For the continuous process, a moving stainless steel belt is substituted for the glass sheet. The fixed hopper (which holds the slurry) and the knife blade assembly (which determines film thickness) are similar to those used in the batch operation. The film deposited on the belt travels through a drying section and is then stripped from the belt as a continuous tape. Paper or plastic carriers are used here also.

Substrates are punched from the tape before it is fired. The tooling for the punching operation is much cheaper and easier to modify than the press tooling.

The thermal treatment referred to as sintering that converts the oxide constituents into the dense ceramic substrate is essentially the same for either pressed or tape process parts. Firing is done at temperatures up to 1700°C.

The processing of barium titanate and beryllium oxide substrates is very similar to that of the alumina parts.

Chapter 5

SCREEN PRINTING

The process of stenciling or screen printing patterns is an ancient one. The Egyptians used this technique thousands of years ago to decorate pottery and the walls of buildings and tombs. The concept was simple. A mask with open and closed areas defining the pattern was brought in contact with the surface to be decorated. A fluid ink was forced through the openings in the mask using a rag, fingers, or piece of wood. When the mask was removed, the ink pattern remained.

This is basically the same process used today for production of thick film circuits. A typical screen printer, shown in Figure 5-1, is considerably more complicated but performs the same function—that of forcing the ink through the screen—as did the equipment used by the Egyptians.

In this chapter we look first at some of the rheological properties of the inks. With this as a background, the screen printer and screen printing theory can be examined.

RHEOLOGY

The science of rheology is concerned with the flow of fluids. As far as screen printing behavior is concerned, there are two important fluid prop-

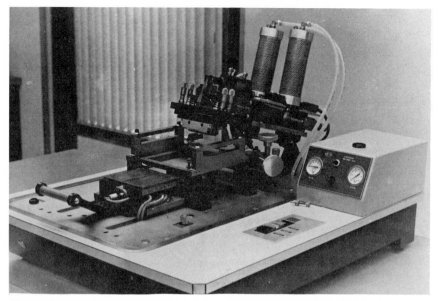

Figure 5-1 A thick film screen printer. (Printer by AMI; photograph by State of the Art, Inc.)

erties that we must consider—viscosity and surface tension. Both properties arise from intermolecular forces within the liquid. Viscosity can be defined as the resistance to motion of one layer of fluid past another layer. Surface tension is related to the imbalance of forces that exists at an interface between two fluids, a fluid and a solid, or a fluid and a gas.

Viscosity. If we imagine that our fluid is stratified in layers as shown in Figure 5-2, then the force required to move one layer past another layer is

$$F = \frac{\mu A v}{y} \tag{5-1}$$

where F = force
μ = coefficient of viscosity
A = area of layers
v = relative velocity between layers
y = distance between layers

In many liquids μ varies only with temperature. These are the so-called *ideal* or *Newtonian* fluids. The temperature variation can be described

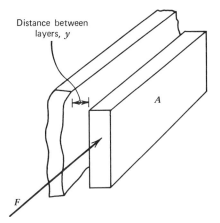

Figure 5-2 Viscosity relationships.

by the relation

$$\log \mu = \frac{A}{T} + B \tag{5-2}$$

where A, B = constants

T = absolute temperature

In many other liquids μ is not only a function of temperature, but will also depend on other factors including rate of force application, magnitude of the force, the direction of the force, and the duration of force. These fluids are called non-Newtonian.

Figure 5-3 illustrates the stress-shear rate behavior of four types of fluids. Curve A shows the behavior of an ideal liquid. The slope of the curve which is the viscosity coefficient is constant for different stress rates.

The other curves represent variations from ideal behavior. Curve B is the stress-shear relation exhibited by a "Bingham Body." This material has a *yield point*—that is, a certain force must be applied before flow will start. In this type of liquid the viscosity coefficient is constant after flow has started. Curves C and D represent different variations of viscosity coefficient with shear rate. The behavior of these nonideal systems is related to the kinds of chemical bonds between the molecules of the liquid.

Viscosity Measurement. Because of the complicated flow behavior of the inks normally used, determination of viscosity coefficients for these systems is not a simple matter. The equipment for measuring shear rate as a function of stress is expensive and difficult to operate.

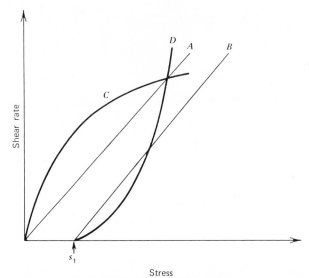

Figure 5-3 Different rheological behaviors—stress-shear relationships. A = Newtonian; B = Bingham Body (yield point = s_1); C = dilatent; D = Pseudo plastic*

Most thick film operators are aware of the importance of ink viscosity on the printing behavior. Thus measurements are often made, but because of the high cost of "complete" viscosity measurement, viscosity checks using simpler (though not inexpensive) measuring techniques have become standard. The authors feel that the use of a Brookfield-type viscosimeter is of limited use in a precision screen-printing operation. This particular technique consists of immersing a rotating spindle in the ink and measuring the force required to produce a fixed number of revolutions per minute (Figure 5-4). It is virtually impossible to relate this measurement to shear rate or the actual printing behavior of the ink. Our main reason for urging caution in using this popular viscosity measuring approach is that people often let the viscosity reading overrule other good performance measurements. Some feel that just because an instrument puts out a definite reading, the number is absolute and meaningful. The instrument is quite useful in bringing a paste to a general viscosity level, but should not be used to change a paste unless production experience has shown a *need* to adjust viscosity. Different lots of material adjusted to a uniform Brookfield viscosity reading will not always have the same printing characteristics.

* Pseudoplastic is often confused with *thixotropic,* a fluid whose viscosity decreases with *time* at a *constant* clear rate.

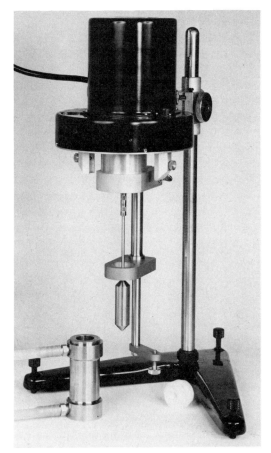

Figure 5-4 A viscosimeter, with water-cooled sample holder for small samples. (Photograph courtesy Brookfield Engineering Laboratories, Inc.)

Surface Tension. Another important property of the ink, which will combine with viscosity to determine its behavior during screen printing, is surface tension. The surface tension is related to the strength of the bond between molecules in the liquid. Most molecules in the bulk of the liquid are surrounded by other similar molecules and the forces are fairly well balanced. The molecules at the interface between another liquid, solid, or gas phase are in a different environment in that they are not surrounded by similar molecules. The relative strength of bonds formed at this interface determines the behavior of the liquid at the interface. Let us consider two hypothetical liquids A and B in contract with an alumina substrate in a vacuum (Figure 5-5). We assume that the A-A bonds in liquid A are much stronger than the A-alumina bonds and that the B-B bonds are weaker than the B-alumina bonds.

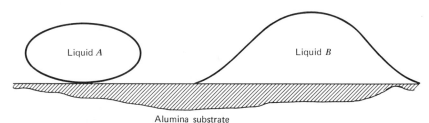

Alumina substrate

Figure 5-5 Relationship between surface tension and wettability. In liquid A the liquid-liquid bonds are stronger than the liquid-alumina bonds. Surface tension predominates. No wetting takes place. In liquid B the liquid-alumina bonds are stronger than the liquid-liquid bonds. Wetting takes place. The liquid spreads until the wetting-surface tension forces are in equilibrium.

If a drop of liquid A is placed on the alumina, the surface molecules will experience an inward-directed force that will tend to minimize the area of liquid A in contact with the alumina. We say that liquid A has a high surface tension.

In the case of liquid B, however, the molecules at the surface of a drop in contact with alumina will experience outward force which will tend to maximize the area of contact. We would say that liquid B has low surface tension or that it wets the alumina.

THE SCREEN PRINTER

The basic elements of screen printer are the screens, screen holder, substrate holder, squeegee, and squeegee mount.

Screens. The screens are woven from stainless steel wire. The diameter of the wire and the size of the opening can be varied depending on process requirements. In general, the larger the opening the more material deposited on the substrate. The opening size is usually given in terms of a standard mesh number. Mesh sizes from 100 to 325 are in use—the most common is 200 mesh. Table 5-1 gives typical dimensions of wire screens.

Table 5-1 Relationship between Screen Mesh Number,
Wire Diameter, and Deposited Thickness

Mesh Number (meshes/in.)	Wire Diameter (mils)	Deposited Thickness* (wet, in mills)
105	3.0	4.44
120	2.6	3.85
145	2.2	3.25
165	2.0	2.92
165	1.9	2.82
200	2.1	2.20
200	1.6	2.35
250	1.6	2.12
250	1.4	1.99
270	1.6	2.02
270	1.4	1.91
325	1.4	1.75
325	1.1	1.55
400	1.1	1.37
400	1.0	1.32

* Assuming a 100% transfer to substrate from screen (transfer is not 100% in real life). An emulsion buildup beyond thickness of screen would result in increase of deposit by amount equal to emulsion thickness (calculations from D. Reimer, "The Direct Emulsion Screen as a Tool for High Resultion Thick Film Printing," *Proceedings ECC*, 1971, p. 963).

The wire mesh is mounted on a rigid cast aluminum alloy frame. The frame is used to keep the screen under uniform tension. Frame size ranges from 5×5 in. to 12×12 in. or larger. The maximum frame size that can be used depends on the particular printer (Figure 5-6).

Screen Pattern. The screens have patterns applied using photolithographic techniques similar to those used in mask making for monolithic and thin film work. After the screen is mounted in the frame, it is coated with a photo-sensitive emulsion which polymerizes on exposure to light. A negative is made of the desired pattern with the opaque areas on the negative corresponding to open areas on the screen. After exposure to light, the unexposed areas are dissolved by the developer and the screen is opened up (Figure 5-7).

Until your thick film operation becomes large enough to justify the ex-

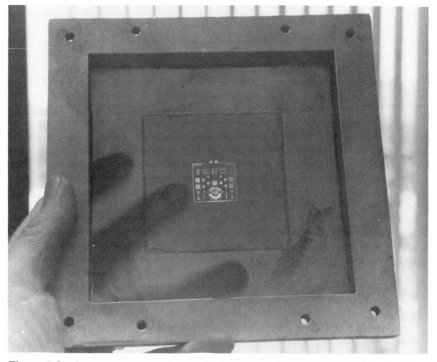

Figure 5-6 A screen stencil. (Screen by Microcircuit Engineering; photograph by State of the Art, Inc.)

pense of a screen making facility, you will have to obtain your patterns from one of the several companies specializing in this work. If fast turn-arounds are demanded by a particular operation, in-house screen making facilities are mandatory. This subject is discussed in detail in Chapter 12.

Screen Holder. The screen and frame assembly is mounted on a holder whose function is to position the screen pattern in relation to the substrate. (Figure 5-8). This positioning must be accurate and reproducible; other-wise, the quality of the thick film circuits will be affected. There are at least two choices in the operation of the screen printer. The substrate can be positioned on a holder that remains fixed during the operation. After the substrate is in place, the screen is brought into proper registration and locked in printing position. Alternatively, the substrate holder may move the substrate into position in relation to a fixed position screen. In either case, the screen holder must have height and leveling adjustments. Good printing practice requires close control of the spacing between the screen and the substrate.

Substrate Holder. The substrate is usually held by vacuum on top of or in a recess in the fixture. The X, Y, and rotational adjustments are provided so that the substrate can be accurately positioned with respect to the screen. There is ample evidence that the more sophisticated printing techniques require recessed holders with the substrate protruding no more than 5 mils above the holder surface. This configuration causes less distortion of the screen and ink flow pattern during the printing cycle (Figure 5-9).

The Squeegee. The squeegee brings the ink supply to the screen openings, depresses the screen so that it is in contact with the substrate, and pushes the ink through the screen openings. The blades are made of neoprene, urethane, or polyurethane. The materials of construction and edge shape of the blade are important factors in the printing process. The squeegee blade must form a good seal with the screen during the printing stroke and maintain a constant angle of attack so that the force exerted on the ink is constant. The blade material must resist wear and attack by the organic liquids used in the inks (Figure 5-10).

Squeegee Holder. The squeegee holder positions the squeegee and provides the proper motions during the various steps of the printing cycle. Motion is usually provided by hydraulic cylinders. Downward pressure is maintained by adjustable springs, air pressure, tortion bars, dead weight, or rigid positioning. There must be no chattering of the squeegee during the printing stroke. Adjustments are normally present for varying the stroke velocity and pressure on the squeegee.

Screen Printer in Operation. There are many different screen printers on the market. They range in complexity from simple hand-operated to completely automated machines. The printing cycle is essentially the same regardless of the degree of automation. The substrate is positioned on the holder, which has been aligned for proper screen-substrate registration. The screen is moved into printing position and locked. (Alternatively, the screen may be fixed and the substrate holder moved into printing position.) Squeegee motion is started with the blade in contact with the screen at some distance from the pattern openings. A supply of ink is pushed along by the squeegee. When the ink reaches the pattern openings, it is forced through by the squeegee blade. This force also pushes the screen into contact with the substrate. When the blade moves on, the screen snaps back due to its tension and leaves the ink adhering to the substrate.

When the squeegee reaches the end of the stroke, it is either stopped and another substrate is loaded so that the printing operation can be carried

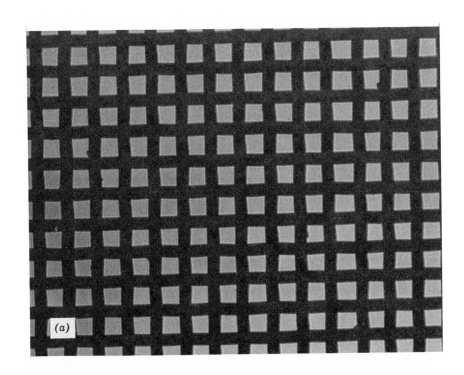

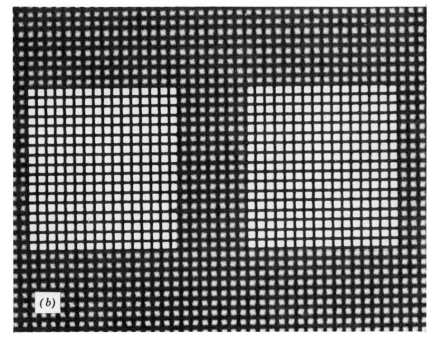

104

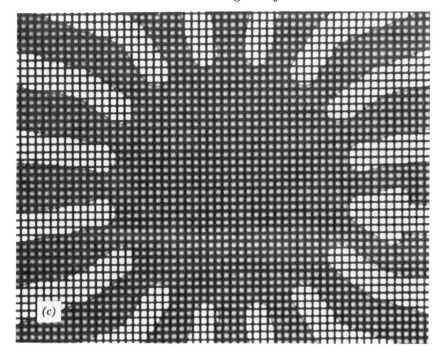

Figure 5-7 Screen patterns. (*a*) Open mesh (325 mesh; 100×). (*b*) A direct emulsion screen showing a pattern purposely designed to conform exactly to the screen mesh (200 mesh; 20×). (*c*) A pattern that cannot conform exactly to the screen mesh. Note that some mesh are partially filled (200 mesh; 20×). (Photographs courtesy Industrial Reproductions, Inc.)

out in the reverse direction, or it is lifted from the screen and returned to its original starting position.

SCREEN PRINTING THEORY

For a process as complicated as screen printing, it would be an extremely ambitious (if not impossible) undertaking to develop a unified theory of printing. We should now be familiar enough with the components of the printer and the fluid properties of the ink to understand in a general way what is happening during printing.

As we can see, screen printing is a process for controlling fluid flow. During screen printing the ink is acted on by an extremely complicated system of forces. The forces include gravity, the squeegee blade, and surface

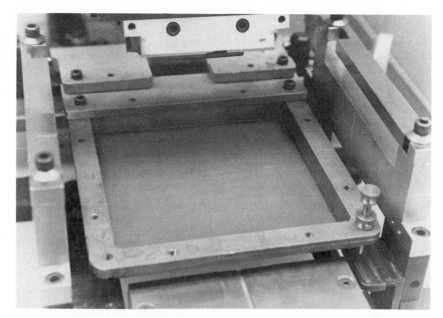

Figure 5-8 The screen held in place in a screen printer. (Printer by AMI; photograph by State of the Art, Inc.)

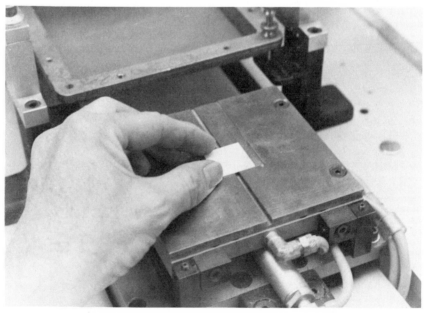

Figure 5-9 The substrate holder. (Printer by AMI; photograph by State of the Art, Inc.)

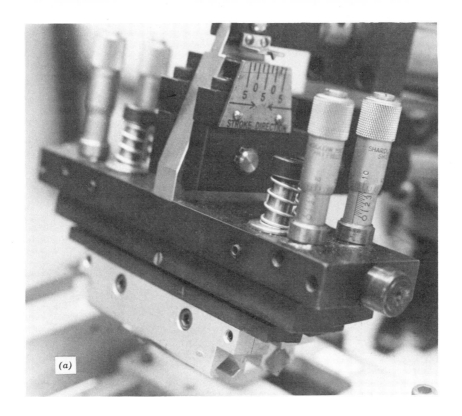

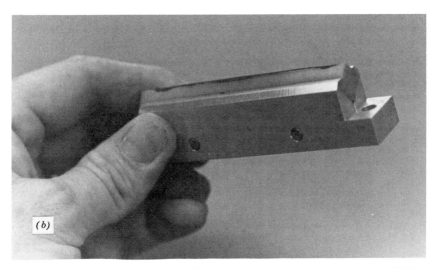

Figure 5-10 (*a*) The squeegee holder, showing adjustments for pressure. (This is a double-squeegee printer—one squeegee for printing forward, another for printing on the backstroke or to act as flood bar. (*b*) The squeegee itself—a square blade held rigidly. The four edges of the blade can be used in succession, rotating as the squeegee wears. (Printer by AMI; photographs by State of the Art, Inc.)

tension forces at the screen wire and substrate interface. The interplay of these forces during the printing cycle is shown in Figure 5-11.

In operation, the squeegee pushes a supply of ink ahead of the blade until the ink reaches an opening. Depending on the mesh size of the screen and surface tension of the ink, it may flow through the screen openings or stay on the upper surface of the screen.

As the squeegee nears the opening, the screen is deflected and contact is made between the underside of the screen (which has the pattern) and the substrate.

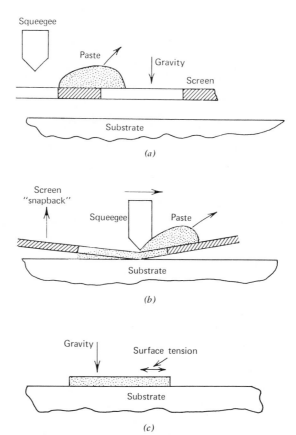

Figure 5-11 The ink transfer process. (*a*) Before printing, paste is on the screen. It will not flow through open mesh because of rheological properties. (*b*) During printing, screen mesh fills with ink. Ink transfers to substrate as screen snaps back. (*c*) After printing, gravity and ink rheology control predrying spreading.

Because of deformation of the flexible squeegee blade, there is a considerable downward force on the ink causing it to flow through the screen openings (if gravity had not already filled them) and onto the substrate.

After the squeegee blade has moved past the opening in the screen, the tension of the screen wires causes the screen to return to its original position above the substrate. The viscosity of the ink and its wetting behavior in contact with the screen wires and substrate determine how much of the ink remains on the substrate and how much returns with the screen.

After the passing of the squeegee and the snap-off of the screen, the printed pattern is free standing. The forces acting on the ink are gravity and the surface forces between ink and substrate. The final dry but not fired shape of the pattern is dependent on a balance between these forces and the inks viscosity, yield point, and so on.

If the ink wets the substrate and has a low viscosity, then the forces of gravity and surface tension would combine to produce outflow from the original pattern outlines. If the ink does not wet the substrate and has a low viscosity, then it is likely that contraction of the pattern will take place. Both of these processes are slowed by an ink with high viscosity. With a very high viscosity ink, we could reach the point where there was little or no movement of the pattern.

Clearly, the best possible dry pattern will be produced with a balanced ink system of intermediate viscosity. Flow could take place to a limited extent to level the pattern and fill in voids left by printing through the screen, but it would not be rapid enough to cause large changes in print dimensions before drying.

PRINTING VARIABLES

Screen printing is easily the most complicated of the thick film processes. Development of inks with better fluid properties and equipment of improved design has made printing a semiscience instead of a black art, as it was originally in the early days of thick film work.

There are still, however, a multitude of variables related to the ink and process equipment that must be controlled if reproducible results are to be obtained. It is not possible to list all or even a large number of these variables in this chapter. A few of the major variables will be described.

Ink Rheology. From the brief description of printing theory and rheology, it should be apparent that the viscosity requirements for an ink are quite complex. During the actual printing step, it is desirable to have a fairly fluid system. After printing, a certain amount of flow is necessary to level the print, but the flow must be limited so that pattern spread is negligible.

The forces on the ink during printing are much greater than after printing. This suggests that an ideal ink system would behave as some combination of a thixotropic and pseudoplastic fluid described in the section on rheology.

During screening, when the forces are large the viscosity would be low, leading to easy flow through the screen openings onto the substrate. After screening, during the drying stage the forces of gravity and surface tension acting on the ink would be much lower; and because of its thixotropic behavior, the viscosity would be higher and flow more difficult. Pseudoplastic behavior could be used to completely limit movement after screening. Some of the many variables that affect the viscosity of the inks have already been listed and they must be included in any list of screen printing variables.

Substrates. The substrate material, its warpage, camber, parallelism, dimensional tolerance, and surface finish will all affect the printing process.

We have already pointed out that almost all thick film circuits use alumina as the substrate material. The alumina manufacturers have the surface finish problem well in control. However, warpage, camber, parallelism, and dimensional tolerance cause serious problems in printing. The difficulties are principally related to variations in screen-substrate spacing. The importance of this is described later in this section.

Screen Openings. The actual amount of open area in the pattern, that is the area of the screen not closed off by the emulsion, is dependent on the number of wires in a unit area and their diameter. The mesh number of the screen gives some indication of the number of openings and their size.

In general, the open area decreases with increasing mesh number, but it is not a linear relation. A screen with a Tyler Mesh of 200 does not have twice the open area of a 400-mesh screen.

We could presume that the amount of ink passing through the screen with all other screening variables held constant would decrease as the open area decreased. This behavior is observed, however, when there is not a linear relation between the two variables. Increases in open area past a certain point will not lead to increased throughput and there is a lower limit of open area below which no ink will flow. Mesh size of thick film screens usually varies betteen 100 and 400, with 200 mesh the most popular.

Pattern Geometry. Patterns of the same mesh size, but with different geometries and orientations to the squeegee motion direction, will have different printing characteristics. The differences are related to screen deformations in the region of the pattern, squeegee force and deformation variations, and basic rheological considerations. A moment's reflection on the process should convince you that a large square pattern will have different printing characteristics compared to a small thin rectangle. It should also not be surprising that different printing behavior would be observed with long thin rectangles oriented with their long axes parallel and at right angles to the direction of squeegee motion. Figure 8-3 shows how size of the pattern can affect deposited thickness.

Emulsion Thickness. The thickness of the emulsion can influence printing in at least two ways. Since the emulsion is generally on the bottom, it is in direct contact with the substrate. A thick emulsion will form a larger pocket and more throughput of ink would be expected. This is true to a certain extent; however, there is an upper limit to emulsion thickness above which there will be no increase in the amount of ink deposited.

The emulsion thickness will also influence the screen deformation in the area of the pattern, which could affect the printing.

Snap-Off Rate. This is one of the most important variables of screen printing. For a given ink system and pattern geometry, the snap-off rate will determine the ratio of ink left in the screen to that on the substrate.

The snap-off rate is primarily controlled by the tension of the screen and the screen-substrate spacing.

The tension is an easily measured variable and should be checked regularly because the screen will lose tension with repeated use.

The screen-substrate spacing is a major consideration in set up of the printer. It may be necessary to control the spacing to ± 0.001 in. for critical printing operations. Holding this tolerance can be extremely difficult because variations in substrate thickness are usually in this range.

Squeegee Material. The roles of squeegee pressure and deformation during printing have already been emphasized. The squeegee material will help to determine these parameters.

Synthetics or natural rubber are used for the blades. The most popular material today is polyurethane. The important characteristics of the squeegee are its hardness, wear resistance, and resistance to attack by the solvents of the ink.

The hardness range normally employed is 50 to 90 measured with a Shore Type A Durometer. This is a simple instrument and should be standard equipment for any thick film operation because regular squeegee checks are a necessity.

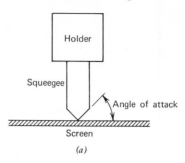

(a)

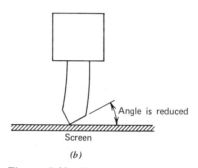

(b)

Figure 5-12 The angle of attack
of a squeegee. (a) Defined. (b)
Changed by squeegee deformation
or wear.

Squeegee Configuration. The squeegee shape and method of mounting are
also important in determining squeegee pressure and deformation.

The shape of the blade can be varied by grinding. The squeegee approach
angle is measured between the surface of the undeformed squeegee and
substrate as shown in Figure 5-12a. The angle of attack will include
squeegee deformation as shown in Figure 5-12b. For a squeegee of given
thickness, the flexibility and deformation will decrease as the approach
angle decreases.

Mounting methods will also play an important role in squeegee deformation. The larger the unclamped height, shown in Figure 5-12b, the more
deformation. The coupling of the squeegee holder to the drive mechanism
is also important. Some printers mount the squeegee rigidly while others
have a "floating" mount. Provisions are sometimes made for varying the
angle of the mount relative to the screen surface.

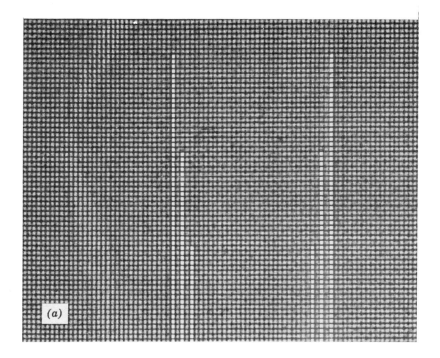

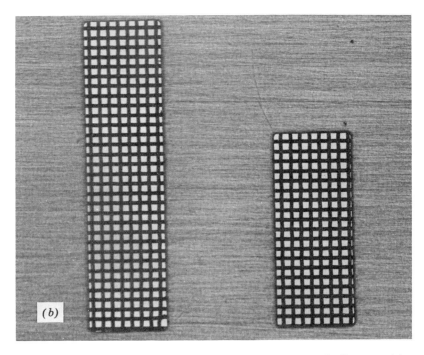

Figure 5-13 Newer types of screens. (a) 2-mil lines, 400-mesh direct emulsion screen (20×). (b) Indirect metal mask with 1-mil foil mesh (20×). (c) Direct metal mesh using an etched square grid structure (20×). (Photographs courtesy Industrial Reproductions, Inc.)

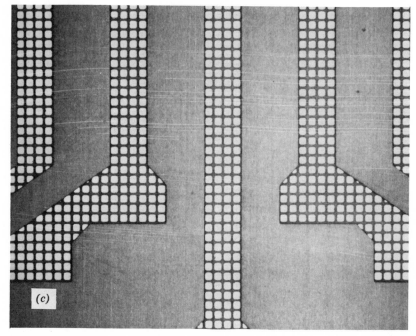

Figure 5-13 (Continued).

Squeegee Motion. Most printers have adjustments that permit changes in squeegee velocity. Experimental data show that the ink throughput remains relatively constant at lower velocities, sometimes reaching a maximum at an intermediate velocity. After this maximum is reached, throughput will decrease rapidly with increasing velocity.

Reproducibility and smoothness of squeegee motion are essential for good printing.

Equipment Design. Many of the variables already discussed are related to the basic design of the screen printer. Included are precision and reproducibility of the screen-substrate, spacing and control of squeegee velocity, angle of attack, and pressure. Other variables related to design will not be covered.

New Techniques. The trend in thick film hybrids is to smaller circuits with greater line densities. The factors of line width and spacing become more important in the higher density circuits.

Conventional mesh screens can be used to print 10-mil lines on 20-mil centers, but this requires considerable care and special inks.

Much of the difficulty in fine-line printing is associated with the mesh screens. Etched screens in which the pattern is defined by etching have many small openings (Figure 5-13). Open masks have shown great promise for accurate printing, and improved emulsion systems on fine-mesh screens are also proving remarkably good at fine-line printing.

Modified printing cycles have also been developed that require much less screen substrate spacing. The "contact" printing technique is less affected by spacing variations.

As mentioned earlier, special inks are required for fine-line printing. Modifications of the organic additions are necessary to give desirable rheological properties for fine line work. That means in general a highly thixotropic system. The functional materials must also be modified to produce the best possible conductivities so that resistance of the thin, narrow lines will not be a problem.

Using all of the improvements mentioned it is now possible to print 3 to 5-mil lines on 8 to 10-mil centers.

Chapter 6

FIRING THICK FILMS

The desirable physical and electrical properties of thick films are developed by chemical reactions that occur during an appropriate thermal processing—usually referred to as *firing*. An understanding of these reactions is basic to good control of the process.

In this chapter we discuss many of the chemical reactions that can occur during firing and important aspects of the equipment used in the process.

The most general form of equation that we can write is:

$$\text{reactants} \rightarrow \text{intermediates} \rightarrow \text{products} \qquad (6\text{-}1)$$

The rate at which the reactants are converted to products is influenced by many variables. Concentration of the reactants, intermediates and products, physical form of the reactants, environment in which the reaction is being carried out, time, and temperature are all important.

For a specific ink system, many of these variables are fixed, and we must concern ourselves primarily with time and temperature to control the rate of the reactions. Temperature is the really significant variable. For instance, it is observed experimentally that a 10° rise in temperature can double or triple the reaction rate. This can be formally expressed by the equation:

$$\text{reaction rate} = Ae^{-\frac{B}{T}} \qquad (6\text{-}2)$$

where A, B = constants

T = absolute temperature

The reactions taking place during firing can be classified as reactions between

1. Ink components
2. Ink components and the substrate
3. Ink components and the furnace atmosphere
4. Components of different inks in contact with each other during firing.

The easiest way to cover this subject is to list the specific major reactions that occur in each of the three ink types.

CONDUCTOR INK REACTIONS

Reactions between Ink Components. *1. Reactions between Functional Metals.* The reactions of the metals is limited to sintering and alloying. The electrical properties of the composite will vary widely depending on the type of contacts between metal particles. At low firing temperatures, there may be no chemical reaction taking place and only point contacts will exist. At intermediate firing temperatures, sintering and solid state alloying will occur. Both of these processes will modify the metal contacts. At higher processing temperatures, melting can occur with formation of nearly homogeneous junctions.

In general the resistivity of the conductor composite will decrease with increasing firing temperature as the quality of the sintered contacts improve. At higher firing temperature after melting has occurred, there may be an increase in resistivity due to agglomeration of the individual particles. This agglomeration can lead to poor soldering characteristics for the composite because of surface depletion of the metal layer. Any alloy formation is likely to cause some increase in resistivity.

2. Reactions between Functional Metals and Permanent Binders. Conductor inks use primarily noble metals as functional materials. These metals are not particularly reactive with the other ink constituents. If the metal phase does form an oxide by reaction with either the furnace atmosphere or a glass component, then there is a possibility that this oxide will be soluble in the glass. Since this reaction is confined to the surface of the metal particles, it can affect the nature of the particle contacts. An increase in resistivity would be expected because of increased contact resistance.

3. Reactions between Functional Metals and Temporary Binders. Incomplete removal of the organic system will lead to formation of carbon at firing temperatures. This carbon can form surface carbides with the metal particles leading to increased contact resistance.

4. Reactions between Permanent Binder Components. The permanent binder glass are normally *fritted* before incorporation in the ink. The fritting process is one of melting followed by rapid water quenching of the glass. Any chemical reactions between glass components will usually be completed during fritting. It is possible that unreacted oxides may be included in the ink formulation. Glass forming reactions between these oxides can be expected at firing temperatures.

5. Reactions between Permanent and Temporary Binders. Incomplete removal and subsequent carbonization of the temporary binder can lead to glass phase reactions. As an example, the reaction of carbon with lead oxide is

$$PbO + C \rightarrow Pb + \overline{CO} \uparrow^{\text{gas}} \qquad (6\text{-}3)$$

The CO gas produced in this reaction can cause pinholes and other discontinuities in the composite.

Reactions between Ink Components and the Substrate. *1. Functional Metals.* There is no appreciable reaction between the metal and alumina grains of the substrate. There is some possibility of reactions between an oxidized metal and the glassy phase of the substrate. (This type of reaction accounts for the adhesion of molymanganese metallization systems.)

2. Permanent Binders. There is a very limited solubility of the alumina of the substrate in the permanent binder glasses and extensive mutual solubility of the glassy phase of the substrate and the permanent binder. These interactions determine the bond strength of the conductor to the substrate and are thus of considerable import.

3. Temporary Binders. There is little possibility of reactions between the organic systems and the substrate.

Reactions between Ink Components and the Furnace Atmosphere. *1. Functional Metals.* The furnace atmosphere can vary from strongly oxidizing to strongly reducing. In an oxidizing atmosphere there is the possibility of the reaction

$$\text{metal} + O_2 \rightarrow \text{metal oxide} \qquad (6\text{-}4)$$

The formation of this oxide will be confined to the outer layer of the metal particles and can lead to increased contact resistance of the metal particles and poor solderability. The air (atmosphere) normally used for firing could also cause formation of nitrides, which would have the same effect as oxides in increasing resistivity. A strongly reducing atmosphere will have little effect on the functional metals.

2. Permanent Binders. An oxidizing atmosphere will not react with the glass. A reducing atmosphere can cause the reduction reactions already discussed (formula 6-3). Incomplete binder burn out or solvent fumes from nearby operations can lead to a reducing condition.

3. Temporary Binders. The organic additives are volatile and are normally removed during drying and firing as vapors. There exists always the possibility of carbonization or decomposition of the temporary binders at firing temperatures, leading to a reducive condition.

Reaction between Components of Different Ink Systems. The manufacture of a thick film hybrid circuit will require several firing steps with intermediate screenings. The possibility always exists of interactions between overlapping films during these firings. A typical example is the diffusion of the metal phase of a conductor into a resistor. The results of this diffusion will be altered electrical properties for both composites. Pd-Ag-PdO resistor systems and Ag conductor compositions are not compatible because of diffusion of the silver from conductor to resistor. In principle all of the other reaction described can also occur when two or more ink systems are in contact during firing.

To complete the discussion of conductor reactions, we can make the following observations:

1. At normal firing temperatures and with proper atmosphere control, the only important reactions in the conductor inks are sintering and alloying of the metal particles and reactions of the permanent binders with the glassy substrate phase.

2. Higher firing temperatures can lead to decreased solderability and increased resistance due oxidation and melting and resulting agglomeration of the metal particles.

RESISTOR INKS

There are a larger number of components in a typical resistor ink and the possibilities for more complex and more numerous reactions are increased when compared with conductor systems.

The effect of the resistor composition reactions on the electrical properties is much more pronounced. This implies that close control of the firing process will be necessary for reproducible results. Reaction possibilities in the resistor inks are:

Reactions between Ink Components. *1. Between Functional Materials.* The functional materials of the resistor interact in much the same way as those of the conductor. The larger number of components and the reduction in the ratio of functional materials to permanent binders combine to make the reaction picture much more complicated.

For instance, in conductor inks only metals are used as functional materials, while in resistors, oxides are also included in the functional group. A conductor may contain 85 wt % metal, while a resistor may contain as little as 20 wt % of functional materials.

In a conductor system we could visualize a model in which the metal particles were in intimate contact throughout the composite. The distribution of the metal phase in a resistor cannot be viewed so simply. One extreme for the distribution would be a layer of metal particles formed at the composite-substrate interface. This distribution would occur because of gravity separation of the denser metal particles. It is also possible to prepare resistor inks in which the metal phase is dispersed throughout the composite.

In the first example we would expect conductivity paths similar to those in the conductor. Increased resistance of the composite would occur simply because the thickness of the conductive layer would be much less. The inclusion of oxide particles as functional materials in this layer would also tend to increase its resistance.

In the case where the resistor ink functional materials are uniformly distributed, no clear picture of conduction mechanism has been deduced. It is presumed that the metal particles are surrounded by thin layers of glass which become semiconducting due to the high voltage drop across the glass phase.

Another reaction possible in resistor systems is decomposition of a functional component. The reaction $PdO \rightarrow Pd + 1\frac{1}{2} O_2$ (formula 6-4) occurs at temperatures above 875°C in air.

2. *Reactions between Functional Components and Permanent Binders.* The electrical properties of the thallium oxide resistor systems are controlled by reactions of the thallium oxide particles with the glass binders. The reactions consist of the formation of a reaction layer of intermediate properties on the thallium oxide particles. The semiconducting properties of this layer determine the electrical properties.

Other resistor systems contain oxide functional materials and there is always the possibility of reaction between the oxide and the permanent binders. Systems with Pd metal present a special problem because it is easily oxidized. Reactions of the type

$$PbO \text{ (glass)} + Pd \rightarrow Pb + PdO \qquad (6\text{-}5)$$

are possible in these systems. Reducible glass systems are usually not used in resistor formulations for this reason.

3. Functional Components and Temporary Binders. The entrapment of organics leading to carbonization at firing temperatures presents the same problems for resistors as described for conductors. The inclusion of the easily reduced PbO is an additional concern in resistor formulations. The reaction would be

$$PdO + C \rightarrow Pd + \overline{CO} \qquad (6\text{-}6)$$

4. Permanent Binders and Temporary Binders. The use of reduction resistant glasses in resistor formulations minimizes the possibility of interactions between the binder systems.

Reaction between Ink Components and the Substrate. The only reaction that is of any consequence is between the permanent binder and the glassy phase of the substrate. The larger amounts and different composition of the glass in the resistor as compared to the conductor will affect the reactions to some extent. It is doubtful that lack of adhesion is a problem as far as resistor composites are concerned.

Reactions between Resistor Ink Components and the Furnace Atmosphere.

1. Functional Materials. Oxidation and decomposition of the various functional materials of the resistor during firing plays an important role in determining the resistivity of the composite. These reactions are especially important in systems containing unstable materials such as Pd and PdO.

2. Permanent Binders. The glass used as permanent binders in the resistors are usually more resistant to reduction by the furnace atmosphere than those used in conductor inks.

3. Temporary Binders. The temporary binder systems are similar to those used in conductor formulation and no new reactions occur.

Reactions between Components of Different Inks. The possibilities of interaction of different inks have already been covered in the section on conductors. These reactions are of major importance in very short resistors where a reaction zone of different resistivity accounts for a significant portion of the total length of the resistor.

Summary of Resistor Reactions. The following points should be remembered:

1. There are *many* reaction possibilities with the resistor ink systems. Each of these reactions can have a great influence on a particular electrical property. Especially complicated are the systems that contain unstable functional materials such as Pd and PdO.

2. Processing of resistors (in particular, firing) is critical. The reactions rates are greatly affected by temperature and reproducible results demand close tolerance firing.

3. Reactions between the functional materials play a more important role in resistors than in conductors.

4. Control of furnace atmosphere is important in resistor firing, especially in the Pd-PdO containing inks.

DIELECTRIC INK REACTIONS

There is little point in making a formal list of reactions in dielectric inks, since the possibilities have been described in preceding sections. Some special points about these inks are worth mentioning:

1. In high permittivity systems based on $BaTiO_3$ there is considerable reaction between $BaTiO_3$ and the permanent binders. Because of this the dielectric properties are sensitive to firing cycle.

2. In both types of dielectric systems pinholes and other structural imperfections in the film can lead to short circuits which will render the crossover or capacitor useless.

Any reaction between the functional materials and glass, the glass and temporary binder, or glass and furnace atmosphere that evolves a gas, must be avoided.

The entrapment of carbon in the film can also lead to premature failure of the dielectric.

SOLDER REACTIONS

While not properly a subject for discussion in this section on firing reactions, some mention should be made of the reaction that can occur during and after soldering. The two possible types of reactions are solution of the functional phase of conductors and resistors in the solder and formation of intermetallic compounds between solder and the functional materials.

In both silver-containing conductors and Pd-PdO-Ag, resistor systems' loss of silver during soldering is common. High temperatures or long-time exposures to solder will lead to a large loss of silver from the composite. This so-called solder leaching can drastically affect the conductivity and solderability of the conductor and will lead to large changes in the electrical properties of the resistor systems. A great deal of effort has been spent in developing composite systems with high resistance to leaching. Solder composition changes are also a possible solution to this problem. The simple trick of adding silver to the solder to slow down leaching has been partially successful.

The formation of intermetallic compounds in the body of the conductor is likely to be the cause of loss of adhesion in certain palladium-based conductor systems. The formation of the intermetallic leads to a large change in volume and the bonds between the substrate and the conductor are severely weakened. (This reaction can occur over a period of time *after* initial soldering.)

From this brief coverage, it should be apparent that strict attention must be paid to the soldering process (Figure 6-1).

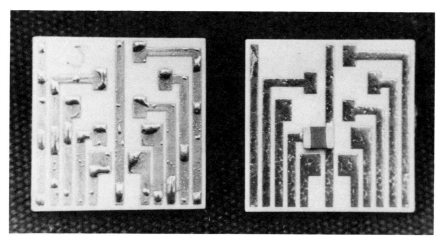

Figure 6-1 "Solder leaching." The silver conductor on the left is totally dewetted, while the palladium silver pattern on the right is still in good shape (same soldering time for both). (Photograph by State of the Art, Inc.)

THE FIRING PROCESS

We have described many of the possible reactions that take place during drying and firing of the thick film composites. The great number of reactions and their sensitivity to variations in firing temperature, time in the furnace, and furnace atmosphere point up the need for close control of the firing step. The control can be obtained only with equipment designed and operated properly.

In our discussion of the firing we break the process into three operations—drying, organic binder removal, and high temperature firing.

Drying. The thick film ink contains large amounts of organic additives which were added to promote easily controllable screening. They must be removed before the final high temperature firing. The drying process is carried out at low temperatures (usually 125°C maximum). During the production process, the thick film circuit will at times normally undergo several separate drying steps before firing. After each drying the part can be handled gingerly and additional elements of the circuit screened.

The drying process requires relatively simple equipment. Close control of the drying step is necessary to produce a good product. Imperfections introduced by improper drying—blisters, cracks, and crazing—will not completely disappear during firing and can lead to device failure. Drying too fast or too high a temperature will promote slumping or spreading of some compositions.

It is possible to dry the print at room temperature, but this would be very time consuming since the compositions are purposely formulated for slow drying to keep the screen from blinding. Small ovens or infrared lamps may be used for batch drying, but the results are usually variable. A good low temperature tunnel kiln with resistance or radiant heating and belt feed will give the best results. Adequate ventilation during drying is a must. (Figure 6-2).

Organic Binder Removal. The drying process removes only the most volatile organics. There is still a large amount of organic material left in the composite after drying. This must be removed at relatively low temperatures to prevent carbonization. In general, this removal is carried out as part of the final firing process.

Firing can be done in batch ovens, but it is almost impossible to get reproducible results. Most firing is carried out in a multizone tunnel kiln (belt furnace). The temperature profile must provide for an adequate period at low temperatures so that all organic binder is removed. Countercurrent flow of air (or an atmosphere) is also necessary to prevent organic fumes from entering the high temperature zone.

High Temperature Firing. As we have already explained, the important properties of the composite are determined by the reactions that take place in high temperature zone of the kiln. The kiln profile must be accurately controlled if good results are to be obtained. A typical temperature profile is shown in Figure 6-3.

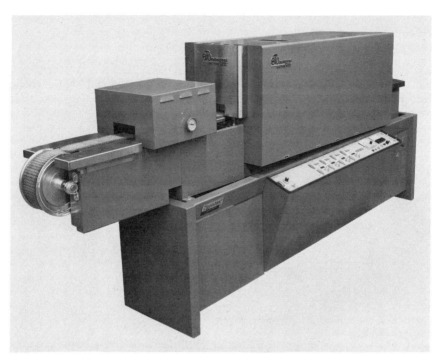

Figure 6-2 Dryer unit mounted on a thick film furnace. (Photograph courtesy BTU Corporation.)

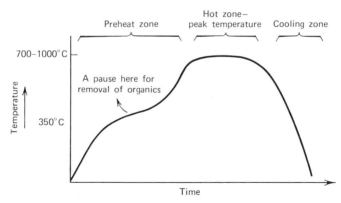

Figure 6-3 Time-temperature profile of a thick film furnace.

THICK FILM FURNACE

The thick film furnace consists of the following functional units: shell, belt assembly, heating elements, and temperature controls (Figures 6-4, 6-5, and 6-6).

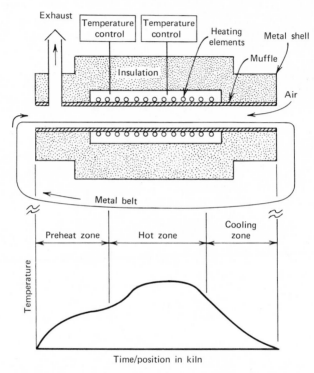

Figure 6-4 Cross section of a simplified thick film furnace (kiln).

Furnace Shell. The kilns vary from small laboratory models 3 to 4 ft in length to high capacity furnaces up to 20 ft long. The shell consists of a framework or supporting structure, a sheet metal enclosure around the furnace insulation, insulating material, and a muffle that defines the active furnace volume. The insulation can be standard refractory brick, loose packing, or castable material. The muffle is usually a ceramic (mullite) or fused quartz tube of rectangular or circular cross section. The muffle is used to protect parts from contamination from the furnace refractories

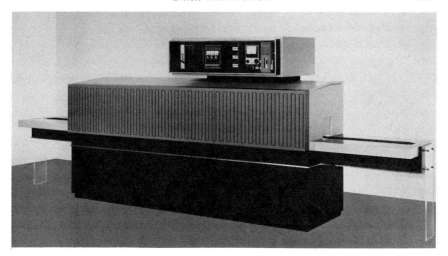

Figure 6-5 Laboratory-size thick film furnace. (Courtesy Thermco Products Company.)

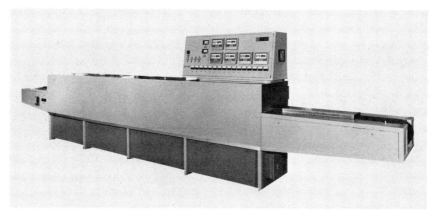

Figure 6-6 Production-size thick film furnace. (Courtesy Watkins-Johnson.)

and windings and more importantly to provide a uniform temperature distribution, as well as to contain and control the flow of the atmosphere (Figure 6-7).

The furnace frame will normally be provided with adjustments so that the inlet end of the furnace can be raised. This creates a "chimney" effect and promotes a countercurrent flow of air through the furnace. If the air stream velocity is high enough, no back diffusion of organic volatiles into the hot zone will occur. It is possible to adapt many thick film kilns to nitrogen or other inert atmospheres for firing packages. Forced air circu-

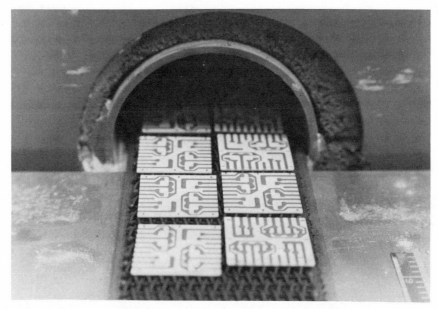

Figure 6-7 Entrance of a small thick film furnace. Note circular muffle. (Baffle gate has been removed to show muffle.) (Photograph by State of the Art, Inc.)

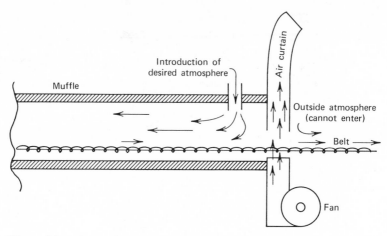

Figure 6-8 Air curtain at exit of kiln serves to seal off outside atmosphere.

lation is also possible and is often used to maintain very exact flow and compositions. This is accomplished by use of air curtains behind which dry air or other atmospheres are introduced. Air curtains can be also used to seal off this firing zone from the preheat zone to keep products of combustion out of the hot zone (Figure 6-8).

Belt Assembly. The continuous chain mesh belts used for thick film work are usually oxidation-resistant stainless steels. Above 1000°C their oxidation rate is too high for continuous operation. If temperatures from 1000 to 1200°C are desired, a nichrome belt can be used. There is no inexpensive belt material available for higher temperature operation. The belts are normally driven by a stepless motor control that provides belt speeds from 0.5 to 6 in./min. Accurate control of belt speed is critical for good firing.

Heating Elements. Proprietory alloys of nickel chromium and other refractory metals are used as resistance elements in most kilns. The elements can be wound on refractory spacers fitted around the muffle or they may be the heavier linked hairpin type buried in a castable refractory.

To establish a proper temperature profile, the kiln should have multiple zones. Each zone usually has its own set of heating elements.

Temperature Controls. Each set of windings has a separate power supply and temperature controller. The four-zone configuration with stepless SCR power supplies and digital set point controllers is popular. A close to ideal temperature profile with ±2°C control can be obtained with this setup.

The controllers normally use platinum-platinum, 10% rhodium thermocouple buried near the windings to sense the temperature. One or more additional thermocouples will be connected to an overtemperature protection device that shuts the furnace down in case of a malfunction. It is important to note that the control thermocouples are not located near the belt on which the parts rest. This means the thermocouples do not indicate the actual firing temperature. The only way to establish the temperature profile accurately is to use a traveling thermocouple. This is usually inserted with a dummy load in the furnace. This traveling thermocouple and a strip chart recorder will give an accurate temperature profile of the kiln (Figure 6-9).

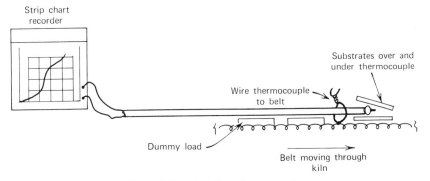

Figure 6-9 Traveling thermocouple.

Furnace Operation. The thick film furnaces available today are rugged and almost foolproof. Their operation is simple—turn on the furnace, set the controllers, and wait for temperature equilibrium. The profile can then be checked with the traveling thermocouple and necessary control adjustments made. This is a trial and error process that requires patience to achieve the proper profile. Changing the profile can take several hours. It is usually faster to go from a profile with a lower hot zone temperature to one with a higher hot zone temperature.

In changing profiles it must be noted that the reproducibility for a given set of controller settings is not perfect and it is always best to check with a traveling thermocouple. There will also be variations when operating at one profile setting for long periods of time and it is advisable to periodically check the furnace with the traveling thermocouple.

Arriving at the *original* proper profile is done by making electrical evaluations of the thick film elements, backed up by a traveling thermocouple measurement so that the proper profile can be recognized. A "proper profile" is one that produces the desired properties. It will probably be slightly different in different kilns.

SUMMARY

Keep in mind that most of the thick film reactions going on are *incomplete* reactions. The reactions will continue with time and proceed at rates that are a *power* function of temperature. Time and temperature are thus extremely important controls in taking the desired reaction just so far—and no further.

Chapter 7

PROPERTIES OF THICK FILM COMPONENTS

The *processes* and *raw materials* used to produce thick film circuits have been discussed. It is time to look at some of the important electrical and physical properties of the components.

In the coverage here the terminology is usually that found in product literature. Descriptions of the measuring technique for obtaining data are given as space permits. No attempt is made to discuss the selection of inks for specific applications.

CONDUCTOR PROPERTIES

Sheet Resistivity. Sheet resistivities for most conductor systems range from 0.002 to 0.15 $\Omega/\square$/mil. The inks high in silver generally have the lowest resistivities and platinum-gold alloys the highest. Only rarely (given good design) will sheet resistivity be a factor in conductor ink selection.

Solderability, Bondability, and Adhesion. The use of conductors for bonding pads and terminations make these factors extremely important in the choice of inks.

There are two areas that must be considered—the adhesion of the conductor to the substrate and the adhesion of the lead or discrete device to the conductor.

The strength of the bond between the device or lead and the conductor is a function of the particular method of attachment. It is difficult to obtain any quantative data describing the bonding processes. Often when consulting the literature only such terms as "good," "bad," or "fair" will be used in describing the behavior of a specific ink system with regard to a particular bonding technique.

When solderability is considered, an important criterion is the conductor's resistance to solder leaching. In general pure silver or gold systems are very prone to leaching. Alloy systems have significantly better resistance to damage. Many suppliers will give the minimum time in which the conductor will dewet when held in the solder bath. These times vary from a few seconds to several minutes. (See Tables 7-1 and 7-2 and Figure 7-1.)

Table 7-1 Conductor Leaching

Type of Conductor	Time in Solder to Dewetting (sec)
DuPont #7553 Pt/Au	300
DuPont #8227 Pd/Au	80
DuPont #8267 Pd/Au	180
DuPont #8151 Pd/Ag	80
Silver conductors	<10

Source. DuPont sales literature.

The adhesion of the conductor to the substrate is not well understood. The relation of the many materials and processing parameters to the strength of the bond can only be guessed at in most cases. Two techniques are used to measure adhesion—the nail head pull and the ribbon peel test. (See Figure 7-2).

In the nail head test a small wire with a flattened head is soldered to the conductor. The free end of the wire is attached to a device that measures the force necessary to break the bond. The peel test uses a ribbon or a lead soldered to the conductor. The ribbon is "peeled" from the conductor by applying a force at right angles to the conductor. The values of these tests are subject to considerable variation. Care must be taken to determine the failure mode—that is, whether the ribbon or nail head pulls off from the ceramic, the conductor itself fails, the ceramic-conductor

Table 7-2 Solderability (5-mil Lines, Pd/Sn Eutectic
Solder, Kester 1544 Flux)

	EMCA	EMCA
	Pd/Ag #422	Pd/Ag #424
Time to wet at 200°C (sec)	5	3
Time to wet at 200°C after 15-min refire at 550°C (sec)	15	6

Source. EMCA sales literature.

Note. Pd/Ag alloys tend to oxidize and have poor solder acceptance upon low temperature refiring. This table shows how this
characteristic can be improved—at some sacrifice in leaching
resistance. (See Figure 7-1.)

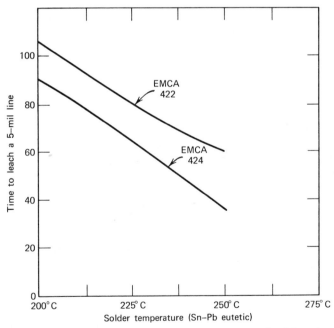

Figure 7-1 The effect of solder temperature on leaching time.
(*Source.* EMCA product literature.)

Table 7-3   **Various Ways of Reporting Adhesion Properties of Thick Film Conductors**

Paste	Strength	Method
DuPont 8267 Pd/Au	20–30 lb/in.	90° peel
DP 8650 Pd/Au	5 lb	90° peel on an 80-mil² pad
EMCA #421 Pd/Ag	>4000 psi	Tensile—0.1 in.² pad
	>2500 psi	Peel—0.1 in.² pad
ESL #9600 Pd/Ag	"Very good"	—
Owens-Illinois #6120-S Pd/Ag	>2000 psi	Pull-on 100-mil-diameter pad

Source. Supplier sales literature.

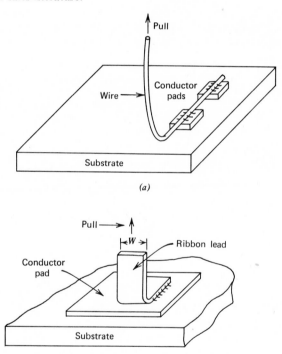

(a)

(b)

Figure 7-2   Various adhesion tests. (*a*) DuPont peel test (pulling wire on several 80-mil pads). Results: pounds per pull. (*b*) Ribbon peel test. Results: pounds per inch of ribbon width. (*c*) Tensile strength test. Pull on 100-mil² square or circular pad. Use nail head configuration. Same size as conductor pad. Results: pounds per square inch. (*d*) "Scotch tape" test. Pull fast. Results: "pass" or "fail."

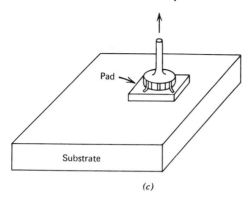

(c)

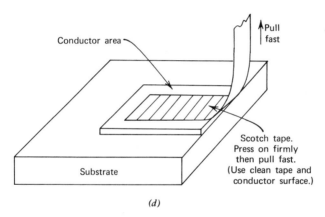

(d)

Figure 7-2 (Continued).

bond fails, or the ceramic fails. All of these types of failures will occur and each has a characteristic value. Values of force required in the peel test vary with the width of ribbon. They usually range from 1 to 30 lb for a 1-in.-wide ribbon. Considerably different readings are obtained if a nail head pull test is made. (See Table 7-3 for details on the variation in adhesion rata.) Another important characteristic of conductor compositions is adhesion of soldered joints *after* high temperature storage. Little is available in supplier's literature on this characteristic. (Table 7-4.)

Compatibility. Conductor compatibility with other inks used in the process must be considered. Quantative data are not available, and this property is described in qualitative terms in the literature. One should be especially

**Table 7-4   Loss of Adhesion during High-Temperature Storage of
Soldered Conductors**

	100-hr Storage at 125°C			148-hr Storage at 150°C	
Paste No.	Before (lbs)	After (lbs)	Paste No.	Before (lbs)	After (lbs)
DP8420 (Pd/Ag)	4–6	1–3	DP8650 (Pt/Au)	~5	~4.5
DP8430 (Pd/Ag)	4–6	1–3	DP8651 (Pt/Au)	4–5	4–5
DP8440 Pd/Ag	4–6	2–3	DP8685 (Pt/Au)	~4.5	3.5–4.5
DP8451 Pd/An	~4	~4			

Source. DuPont sales literature.

careful about compatibility when compositions from different ink manufacturers are used.

Line Definition. The fired line width is a function of the ink composition *and* the screening and firing process. Product literature will usually contain estimates of the best results attainable with a particular system. At present 5-mil lines with 5-mil spacings are considered the practical lower limit as far as the literature is concerned, but careful screening makes 3 × 3 possible (See Figure 7-3.)

Stability. An important consideration for any thick film component is its stability in storage and service. Many tests involving variations in service and storage cycles have been devised, among them thermal and load cycling in different environments, including high humidity. The conductivities of most cermet conductors vary little in these tests. The substrate bond strength and conductor device or lead bond strengths do show severe degradation with certain conductor compositions. The reaction between the conductor and resistor, dielectric, or other circuit elements can be, and often is, accelerated by such tests. A typical example would be silver migration under high voltage and high humidity. If silver compositions are used as resistor terminations, large changes in resistance can occur because of this phenomenon. The loss of substrate adhesion of soldered conductor systems under high-temperature storage conditions has already been cited. These effects are attributable to the same type of chemical reactions that take

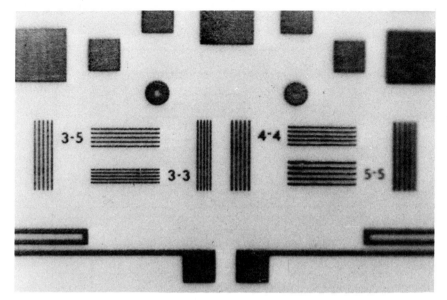

Figure 7-3 Fine-line printing. The numbers represent line width/line spacing. This is about the best that can be done with screens (325-mesh screen here) with thick film. (Printing by Electroscience Laboratories; photograph by State of the Art, Inc.)

place during processing. They take place much more slowly due to the lower temperatures of operation and storage.

RESISTOR PROPERTIES

Resistive elements require a much more detailed electrical characterization than the conductors. The important properties are described below.

Sheet Resistivity. Inks are available with sheet resistivities of 1 $\Omega/\square/$mil to 10 M$\Omega/\square/$mil. (See Figure 1-4.) Each of the many ink systems contains a series of inks with the same base composition but different ratios of functional materials to permanent binders. It is possible to blend inks to produce intermediate values (Figure 7-5), but the user should be careful to get a good mixture and not to mix so hard that the characteristics are changed (see Figure 7-6). The values the manufacturer lists for sheet resistivity are only nominal values and you can expect to get results that vary as much as $\pm 50\%$ from the listed sheet resistivity.

Temperature Coefficient of Resistance. The TCR of a thick film resistor can be negative, positive, or zero over a particular temperature range.

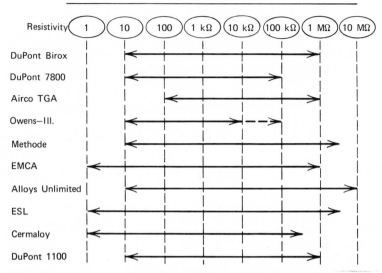

Figure 7-4 The range of sheet resistivities available from various United States paste manufacturers.

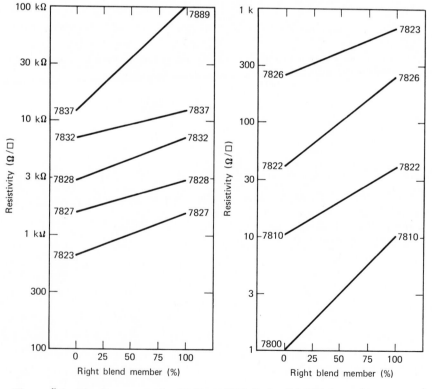

Figure 7-5 Blending curves for DuPont 7800 Series Pd-PdO-Ag resistor compositions. (*Source.* DuPont product literature.)

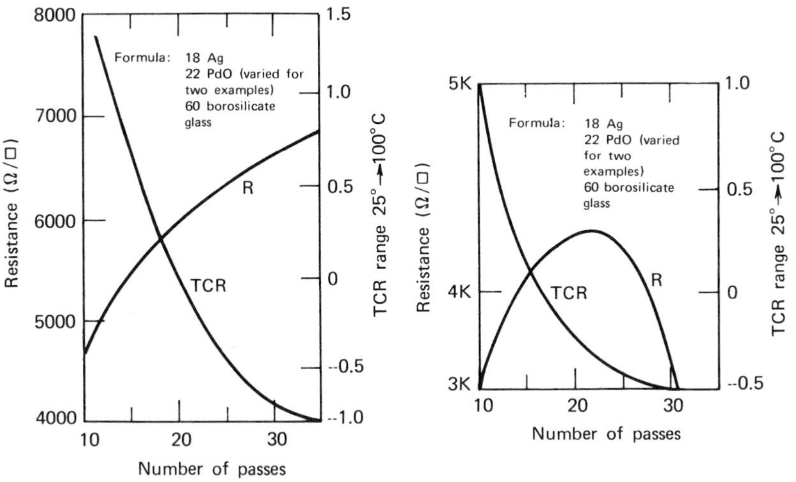

Figure 7-6 Effect of milling on two medium-resistance Ag-PdO-glass compositions. [*Source.* L. F. Miller (IBM), "Glaze Resistor Paste Preparation," *Proceedings of 1970 Electronic Components Conference,* 1970.]

We have already discussed the materials properties that contribute to the TCR.

The value is usually determined by measuring resistance at two temperatures. The TCR in parts per million (ppm/°C) is given by the relation

$$\text{TCR} = \frac{R_2 - R_1}{T_2 - T_1} \times 10^6 \tag{1}$$

The TCR is dependent on processing, the sheet resistance of .. ink, and the measurement temperature range. In general the inks with lower sheet resistances will have large positive TCR, inks of intermediate sheet resistance smaller negative or positive values, and high sheet resistivity inks large negative values. (See Figures 7-7 and 7-8.) This is because low-resistivity inks are high in metal content (positive TCR) and high-resistivity inks tend to be high in oxide content (negative TCR).

For most applications, it is desirable to have a small TCR. Commercial inks range in TCR from +500 to −500 ppm/°C. With good processing techniques and the proper ink, it is possible to maintain a TCR of less than ±50 ppm/°C over the temperature range of −55° to 125°C.

From the TCR curves shown here it should be evident that extrapolation of the TCR outside the temperature range used in its determination involves considerable risk because the curves can completely turn around over a small temperature range.

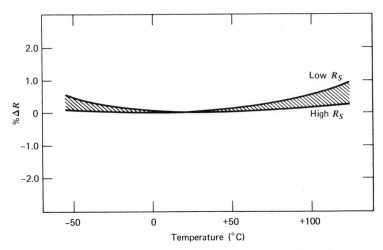

Figure 7-7 Effect of temperature on resistance—a stable resistor composition. (DuPont Birox®. *Source.* DuPont product literature.)

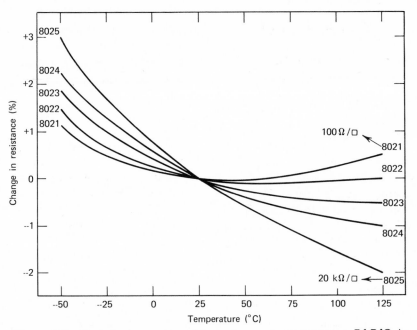

Figure 7-8 Typical change in resistance versus temperature; a Pd-PdO-Ag resistor series. (DuPont 8000 series. *Source.* DuPont product literature.)

TCR tracking is sometimes specified in the literature. This usually refers to the values of TCR obtained for similar resistors on the same substrate. It is possible to obtain tracking of better than 5 ppm.

Voltage Coefficient. A thick film resistor will have a different resistance value for different DC levels. The voltage coefficient, VCR, is calculated from the formula

$$\text{VCR (in ppm/V)} = \frac{R_2 - R_1}{V_2 - V_1} \times 10^6 \tag{2}$$

The values of VCR for common thick film resistors are 20 to 50 ppm/V. Extrapolation of the VCR slightly outside the measured range is permissible.

Noise. Small fluctuations in voltage, current or resistance when an AC voltage is applied to the resistor are referred to as noise. The noise is more properly called current noise and is related to complicated interactions between the atoms and conduction electrons in the resistor. Since the noise is influenced by imperfections, hot spots, and point contact effects, it should not be surprising that screen-on resistors have inherently higher noise outputs than some other types of resistors. The amount of noise is inversely proportional to the area of the resistor and inversely proportional to its resistance.

Measurement of noise output is quite complicated. The accepted technique uses a particular instrument as a standard—the Quanteck Noise Meter, Model 315. In the measurement, the noise output of the resistor is compared to an internal standard. The comparative value is reported as

$$10 \log \frac{\text{noise (sample)}}{\text{noise (standard)}}$$

This unit is called a decibel. The noise is related to frequency range and will have units of decibels per decade of frequency. As an example, a resistor with a noise output of -20 dB/decade has a noise level 100 times lower than the "standard" noise over a particular decade of frequency. (The standard is a noise figure of 1 μV/V.) As already mentioned, the measurement is "complicated" and it is dangerous to put too much emphasis on comparative noise measurements that are only slightly different. (See Table 7-5 and Figure 7-9.) Typical values range from -30 to $+30$ dB. Larger valued resistors are usually noisier.

Solder Resistance. The short time exposure of resistors to solder during a dipping process will often cause irreversible changes in certain electrical

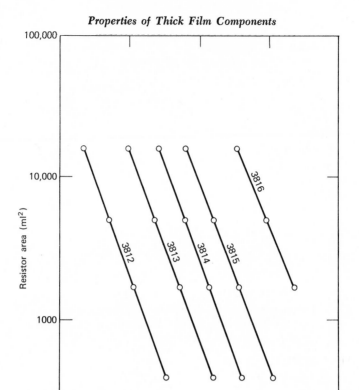

Figure 7-9 Noise index as a function of resistor area. [ESL 3800 Series (higher numbers are those with higher sheet resistance). *Source.* S. J. Stein and J. B. Garvin (ESL), "The Influence of Geometry and Conductive Termination on Thick Film Resistors," *Proceedings of 1970 Electronic Components Conference,* 1970.]

properties. The changes are related to both thermal shock and compositional changes caused by solder leaching—that is, the dissolution of some of the cermet elements in the solder.

Quantative evaluation of solder resistance is not always feasible. Qualitative descriptions will be often found in the literature. Table 7-6 shows effects on resistivity of a very stable system. Silver-containing systems will have some solder leaching problems. Very low resistivity compositions have enough metal at the surface to pick up some solder and drop resistance

Table 7-5 Reported Noise in Various Commercial
Resistor Compositions

Manufacturer	Sheet Resistance	
	100 Ω/□	100 KΩ/□
DuPont (Birox)	−30 dB	0 dB
DuPont (7800)	−18	+22
Airco (TGA)	−30	−2
Bourns	−33	0
Methode	−27	+15
EMCA	−30	+12
Alloys	−35	+15

Source. Supplier product literature.

Table 7-6 Typical Resistance Changes on
Solder Dipping* (DuPont Birox)

Resistivity	Percent Resistance	
	3-sec Immersion	10-sec Immersion
30 Ω/□	−0.14	−0.17
300 Ω/□	−0.14	−0.02
1 kΩ/□	−0.00	−0.05
10 kΩ/□	−0.07	−0.09
100 kΩ/□	−0.07	0.00

Source. DuPont product literature.
* Complete immersion in 62 Sn/36 Pb/2 Ag solder at
215°C for times indicated. All resistors untrimmed.

considerably. Flux remnants can act on resistor compositions under certain
conditions—usually acting as a reducing agent, lowering resistance.

Compatibility and Susceptibility to Processing. The problems of compatibility already mentioned for conductor systems are magnified considerably
in resistors. The multiple firings, encapsulation, and trimming all can
produce considerable temporary and permanent changes in the important
electrical properties.

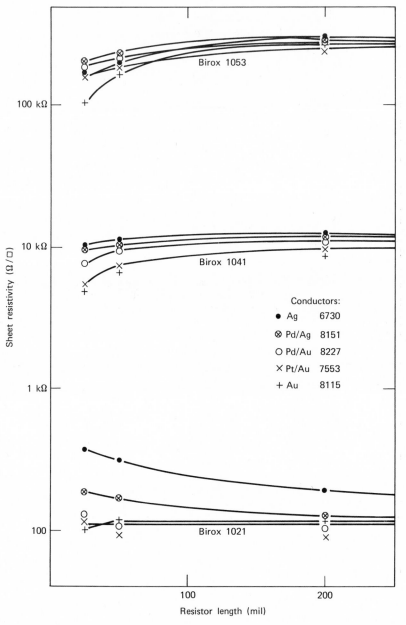

Figure 7-10 Sheet resistivity versus resistor length—the conductor/resistor interface effect. (DuPont Birox®. *Source.* DuPont product literature.)

It is impossible for product literature to pay more than lip service to these problems because they are very specific to a particular process.

In regard to compatibility evaluations, supplier data sheets will list ratings for particular inks, including information about which specific conductor and dielectric systems are compatible with the ink. Typical changes due to encapsulation will also be quoted.

One of the most important compatibility situations to consider is the reaction at resistor and conductor interface. This has a strong influence if the resistors are very short. Figure 7-10 shows interface reaction effects. Note that different results are obtained with different conductor compositions. These results are for "compatibile" conductor/resistor systems. Consider the effect of using a "noncompatible" conductor! Use of conductors from a source other than the resistor ink source can have catastrophic results (some intersupplier combinations, it should be noted, *are* compatible).

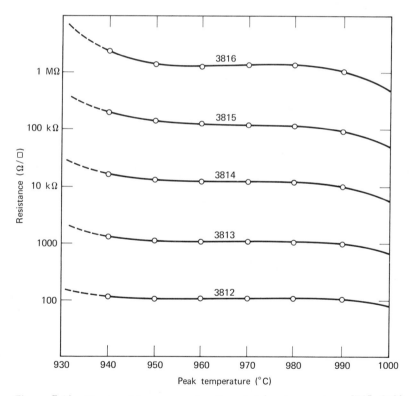

Figure 7-11 Sheet resistance as a function of firing temperature. [ESL 3800 Series. *Source.* S. J. Stein and J. B. Garvin (ESL), "The Influence of Geometry and Conductive Termination on Thick Film Resistors," *Proceedings of 1970 Electronic Components Conference,* 1970.]

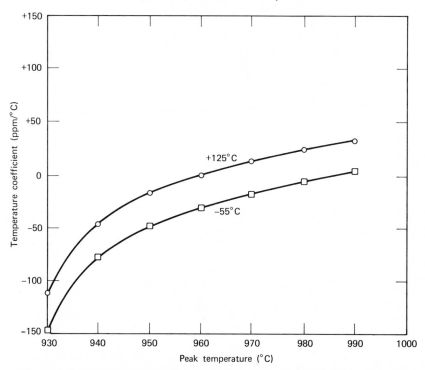

Figure 7-12   Temperature coefficient (TCR) as a function of firing temperature. [ESL 3800 Series. *Source.* S. J. Stein and J. B. Garvin (ESL), "The Influence of Geometry and Conductive Termination on Thick Film Resistors," *Proceedings of 1970 Electronic Components Conference,* 1970.]

Figures 7-11 through 7-17 show some of the effects of processing resistors. They are very much self explanatory and should serve to remind (or convince) the reader that his results depend on processing very heavily.

Stability. The change of resistance properties with time would normally be undesirable. (Examples of desirable changes are the lowering of TCR and noise levels.) There are many types of tests specified by both industrial and military users of thick film circuits. Their purpose is to evaluate component behavior with time under different environmental conditions. It is assumed that these tests will have predictive value relative to the life and performance of the circuit under actual storage and operation conditions. The tests fall into two broad categories—one in which no electrical load is impressed on the unit and the other in which the part is loaded. The more important no-load tests include the following:

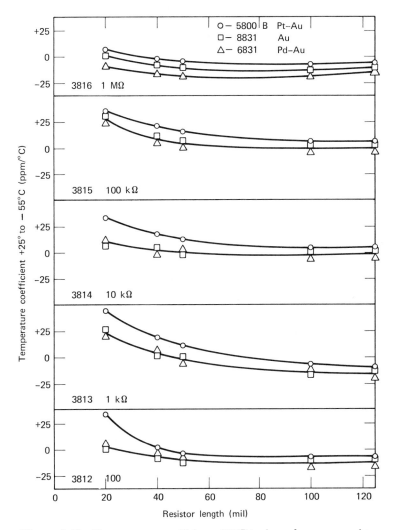

Figure 7-13 Temperature coefficient (TCR) dependence on resistor length and termination material. [ESL 3800 Series. *Source.* S. J. Stein and J. B. Garvin (ESL), "The Influence of Geometry and Conductive Termination on Thick Film Resistors," *Proceedings of 1970 Electronic Components Conference,* 1970.]

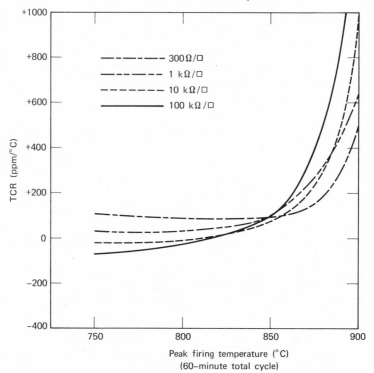

Figure 7-14 Temperature coefficient dependence on peak firing temperature. (DuPont Birox®. *Source.* DuPont product literature.)

Drift. Determination of resistance change after storage of elevated temperatures (up to 200°C) for long periods of time (a few hours to > 1000 hr).

Low-Temperature Exposure. Changes in electrical characteristics may be induced by exposing units to cryogentic temperatures (down to -170°C).

Thermal Cycling. Rapid changes in temperature may cause electrical changes. Typical test specifications call for five cycles of a -55° to 105°C change.

Humidity Exposure. The exposure to high-humidity ambients can cause electrical changes. Typical tests call for exposure times of 250 to 1000 hr at relative humidities up to 95%. The temperatures may range up to 100°C.

The test in which load is impressed can involve variations of the same procedures used in the no-load test. They include the following:

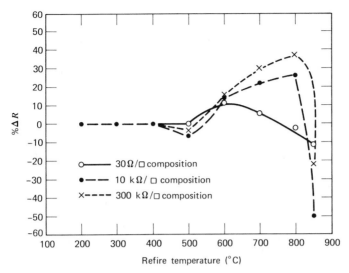

Figure 7-15 Effects of refiring on sheet resistivity. (DuPont Birox®. *Source.* DuPont product literature.)

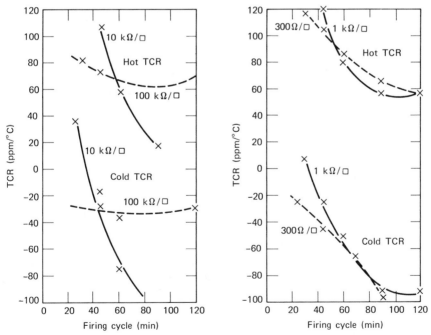

Figure 7-16 Effects of length of firing cycle on temperature coefficient. (DuPont Birox®. *Source.* DuPont product literature.)

149

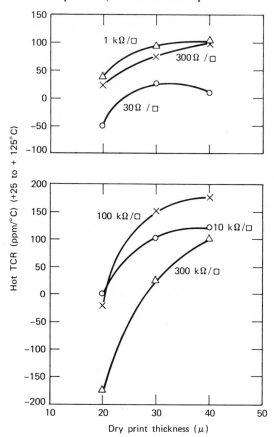

Figure 7-17 Effect of print thickness on temperature coefficient. (DuPont Birox®. *Source*. DuPont product literature.)

Load Life. Long-time exposure to high temperature at some fixed load. A common specification is 1000 hr at 125°C with a loading of 25 W/in.^{2} of resistor area. A high humidity ambient (at a lower temperature) may also be specified in a variation of this test. (Figures 7-18 to 7-21.)

DIELECTRICS

The measurement of the dielectric properties of the thick film crossover and capacitor materials is not a simple matter. Great care should be used in interpretation of the data presented in the product literature.

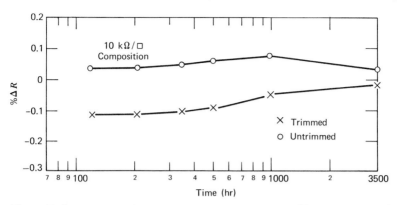

Figure 7-18 Resistance drift under load, trimmed and untrimmed (30 W/in.², 125°C ambient). (DuPont Birox®. *Source.* DuPont product literature.)

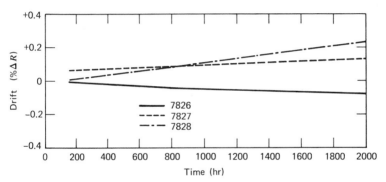

Figure 7-19 Resistance drift, unencapsulated and untrimmed. (DuPont 7800 Series. *Source:* DuPont product literature.)

Dielectric Constant. The dielectric constant of thick films will range from 6 to about 1200. The application will dictate the K value used. Crossovers use low-K materials while capacitors need materials with higher K's.

It is really misleading to refer to the "dielectric constant" of the material because K will not always be constant. For the lower-K inks the values are nearly constant and vary only slightly with temperature, measuring voltage and frequency. The higher-K materials derived from $BaTiO_3$ ceramics have K's that are more dependent on temperature and the method of measurement. (Figure 7-22.)

Temperature Coefficient. The temperature coefficient of capacitance (TCC) can vary from a few ppm/°C to 20 to 30% over a temperature range

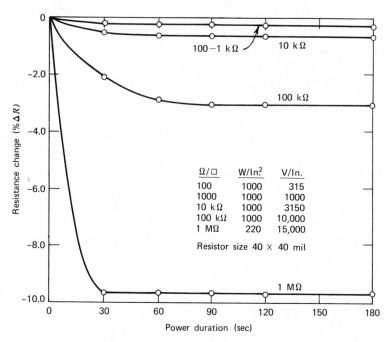

Figure 7-20 Effects of voltage and power overloads. [ESL 3800 Series. *Source.* S. J. Stein and J. B. Garvin (ESL), "The Influence of Geometry and Conductive Termination on Thick Film Resistors," *Proceedings of 1970 Electronic Components Conference,* 1970.]

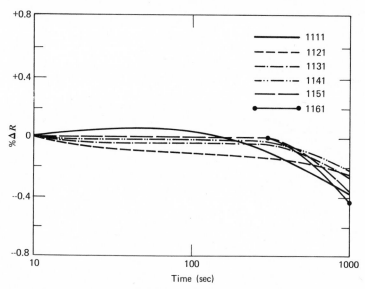

Figure 7-21 Resistance change in hot nitrogen (390°C). (DuPont 1100 Series. *Source.* DuPont product literature.)

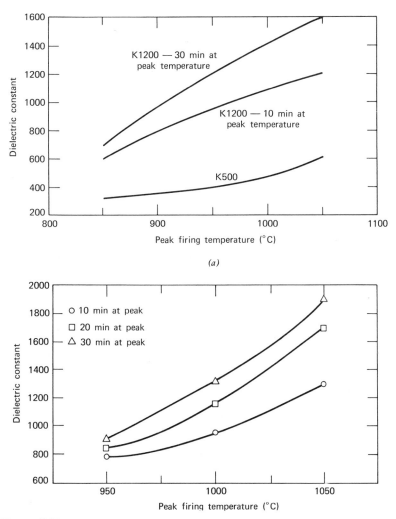

Figure 7-22 Effect of peak firing temperature and time on dielectric constant. (*a*) DuPont K1200 and K500 compositions. (*Source.* DuPont product literature.) (*b*) ESL 4510 compositions. (*Source.* ESL product literature.)

—55° to 125°C. The higher dielectric constant inks will have higher coefficients. (Figure 7-23.)

Voltage Coefficients. The high-*K* inks are sensitive to AC and DC bias levels. The effect of AC voltages is to increase the *K* while DC biases can result in a decrease of up to 20 to 30% in *K* at a level of 50 V/mil (for higher-*K* systems). (Figure 7-24.)

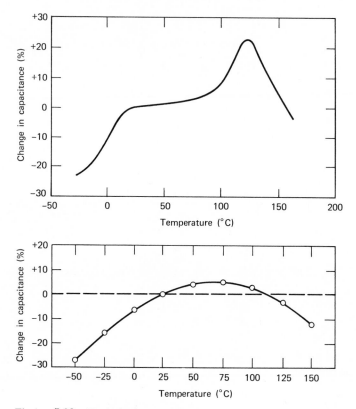

Figure 7-23 Typical change in capacitance with temperature.
(*a*) DuPont K1200. (*b*) ESL 4510 (*K* = 1000). (*Source.* Supplier product literature.)

Measuring Frequency. The high-*K* inks will have different *K*'s depending on the frequency of measurement. At 50 MHz the *K* may be decreased by as much as 10 to 20% from the value measured at 1 kHz. (Figure 7-25.)

Dissipation Factor. The dissipation factor, usually given in %, is an indication of the losses taking place in the dielectric. These losses are always associated with generation of heat. The low-*K* crossover materials will have very low dissipation factors; less than 0.1% is typical. The high-*K* materials will have dissipation factors that can exceed 2 to 3%. The dissipation factor depends, as does *K*, on frequency, bias voltage, and temperature.

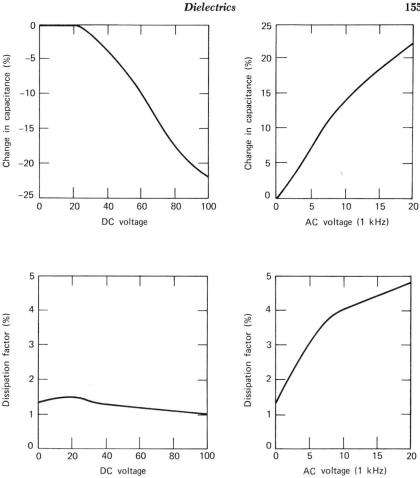

Figure 7-24 Effect of DC and AC voltage on capacitance and dissipation factor. DuPont K500. Approximately 2-mil-thick dielectric. (*Source.* DuPont product literature.)

It is very sensitive to processing, and care must be exercised to prevent contamination of the dielectric film during screening and firing. (Figure 7-26.)

Insulation Resistance. This is a value obtained by calculating the resistance of the dielectric with a specific DC voltage applied. Most dielectric films will have an insulation resistance greater than 10^{10} Ω when measured with 10 V DC.

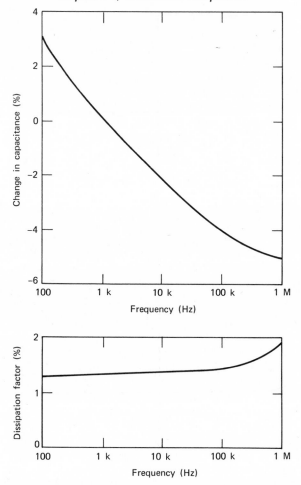

Figure 7-25 Effects of frequency on K and on dissipation factor. (DuPont K500 composition. *Source.* DuPont product literature.)

Breakdown Strength. The DC fields necessary to cause breakdown in a sample are usually quoted in the literature. Values above 250 V/mil are common.

Compatibility. Since the dielectrics are in intimate contact with conductor and resistor composites, extreme care must be exercised in selection and processing of these inks. Figure 7-27 illustrates this very well.

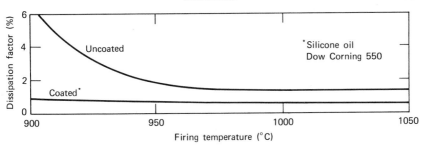

Figure 7-26 Effect of firing temperature on dissipation factor. (DuPont K50 dielectric. *Source.* DuPont product literature.)

Stability. In general the same problems of resistor stability exist with the thick film capacitors. Long-time test cycles must be devised that give information on specific changes in the important properties of the dielectric films. Especially critical are the large changes in K and dissipation factor that can occur in the higher-K materials. There is a considerable body of test methods related to discrete ceramic capacitors which are applicable to thick film dielectrics.

(*Note.* The reader will note a concentration of performance data from DuPont and ESL. We are not trying to give these firms special attention;

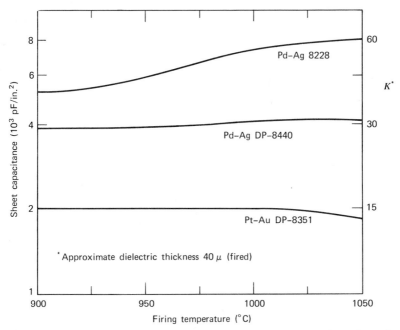

Figure 7-27 Sheet capacitance versus firing temperature for various electrode compositions. (DuPont K50 dielectric. *Source.* DuPont product literature.)

it is just that published performance data on thick film products are so rare. With few exceptions, the suppliers of thick film compositions deserve no compliments when it comes to letting the consumer know how their materials behave. If better performance data from the published literature of other suppliers had been available, they would have been welcomed, and used.)

Chapter 8

TRIMMING THICK FILM ELEMENTS

In this chapter we mention briefly the control of final value by processing, but the main thrust concerns postprocessing adjustments—trimming.

Control of the final element value starts with the original design. The choice of the ohms per square rating of the resistor composition, the aspect ratio chosen, and the area of the capacitor are some of the more obvious ways of controlling value. We point out that decisions at this early point can affect the final values of resistors or capacitors in several important ways.

Process control also plays a major role. We have already seen that the printing process and the firing process have considerable effect on the final values of a run of thick film elements.

Because of the nature of thick film materials and processes makes consistent manufacture of close tolerance resistors and capacitors difficult, if not impossible, and because close tolerance element capability is essential for wide application of thick film technology, trimming techniques for thick film elements are extremely important. Much of the "strength" of thick film technology lies in the fact that accurate and inexpensive trimming methods have been available for some time for resistors. Methods for trimming capacitors are now becoming known—adding even more "strength" to thick film technology.

159

CHARACTERIZATION OF A BATCH
OF THICK FILM ELEMENTS

When a thick film producer manufactures resistors or capacitors, he is producing not just one, but a whole batch. He is interested not so much in the specific value of any one of the resistors or capacitors, but in the *batch* characteristics of his lot.

A batch of elements has two important characteristics: (1) the "nominal" value of the lot and (2) the "spread" of values of individual elements around the nominal. Identification of the former involves use of a numerical average, a modal value or a mean value. The latter usually involves standard deviation calculations, or at least a simple indication of the range between the highest and the lowest value.

If the values of resistance (to use the example of a resistor instead of a capacitor) of a batch of circuits were to be recorded on a *distribution diagram* as shown in Figure 8-1, the resulting "silhouette" of the distribution

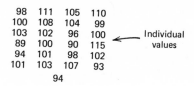

```
98   111  105  110
100  108  104   99
103  102   96  100  ←  Individual
 89  100   90  115       values
 94  101   98  102
101  103  107   93
          94
```

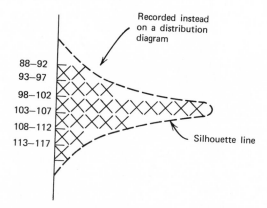

Figure 8-1 The distribution diagram. The recording of values on a distribution diagram (a histogram) makes it easier to understand batch characteristics.

diagram can be used to judge spread and nominal quite easily. Use of such diagrams in thick film production operations is recommended as an easy and quick way to visualize the batch characteristics of a lot of thick film resistors or capacitors. The individual "cells" cover ranges of 5% or less. Lots with large spread, or skewed distributions, can easily be spotted (be careful of applying standard deviation calculations to skewed distributions). Figure 8-2 shows that different spreads and differently shaped distributions can be easily seen.

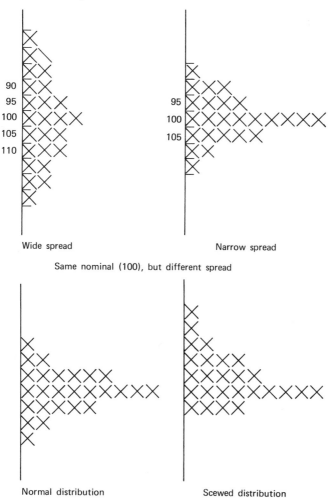

Figure 8-2 Distribution diagrams of batches of varying characteristics. Visual differences between spread and nonnormal distributions are indicated.

CONTROL OF WHERE THE NOMINAL VALUE WILL BE

Some firms might choose to call the modal value (most common) as their nominal, others the arithmetic average. Regardless of which approach is used, it is obvious that having the untrimmed nominal value as close to the final value as possible would be advantageous (faster trimming, less upset, etc.). At times the producer might choose to *not trim* resistors, depending instead on good firing control to reach the proper value. Controlling placement of nominal is of great importance here.

Among the many things that can happen to make a batch of thick film elements have a nominal turn out to be something other than what was planned are the following:

1. Kiln temperature is "off."
2. Thickness of element is off.
3. Wrong number of squares or wrong area is used.
4. Screen setup is not correct.
5. Composition has a different value than is indicated by the level on the container.

Discussion of these various situations follows. It is our aim here to convince the reader that accurate control of the nominal value of a batch is quite complex—a fact that seems to escape many beginners.

Kiln Temperature is "Off." Some of the best resistor compositions are very sensitive to firing temperature, as are the higher dielectric constant capacitor dielectric formulations. (For details, see chapters on materials and firing.) For example, the higher-resistivity inks from DuPont's excellently performing Birox® resistor compositions give a variation in resistance of up to $3\frac{1}{2}\%/°C$. Missing the temperature when firing these materials by only $5°$ can result in a nominal value being off target by over 15%. (Other compositions are not so sensitive, but they may not have some of Birox's excellent performance characteristics either.)

Modern thick film firing furnaces can hold temperature variations to a minimum, and can come back to a temperature used at an earlier setting very closely, but if a long period of time elapses between firing different batches, the temperature may be somewhat different—as it can be also if identical temperature settings are used in different kilns. Thermocouples age, profiles change slightly from one kiln to the next, and a specific setting for one kiln may not result in the same temperature as the same setting in another kiln because of slightly different thermocouple placement or draft settings. Any one of these can lead to missing a nominal value by a considerable margin if a thick film composition is temperature-sensitive—and many of the best systems are *very* sensitive.

Other thick film compositions are sensitive to variations in time at temperature, and thus are quite sensitive to changes in profile and belt speed. Some are sensitive to very slight atmospheric changes. Changes in an element's output, burned out element sections, changes in draft settings, and changes in ambient atmosphere (impurities or humidity) all can produce significant changes in the nominal value that will be realized in a batch of thick film resistors or capacitors. These parameters *must* be understood and controlled if nominal values of batches of thick film elements are to be closed to targeted values.

Thickness of Element is Off. A composition with a changed viscosity or with a changed screen-printing setup (such as snap-off distance) will cause a change in the amount of material left on the substrate. This will effect nominal values of either resistors or capacitors in proportion to the difference in thickness printed.

Print thickness is also a function of element geometry. As a resistor gets very short, for instance, there is a tendency for the thickness to increase because the screen is held slightly off the substrate by the underlying conductor pads (Figure 8-3a). As a pattern gets narrower (say less than 40 mils), there is a tendency for the thickness to first increase, and then as the width is decreased below 20 mils or so, print thickness decreases. This line width dependency has to do with the relative amount of material left on the screen emulsion compared to the substrate. It depends on whether the pattern width is wide enough for the print thickness to be dependent on screen mesh alone or screen mesh plus emulsion. This width/thickness relationship is illustrated in Figure 8-3b. Unless pattern size is taken into consideration when laying out the resistor or capacitor pattern, the thickness can be something other than originally planned, and the nominal value of the element will be different.

Wrong Area is Used. A capacitor will have the wrong area, or a resistor the wrong number of squares unless the amount by which the printed pattern differs from the screen pattern is known and planned for. If the termination pads of a resistor spread (or slump) 5 mils, the length of the resistor could be 10 mils less than originally planned. Added to this, the printed resistor may be 10 mils wider for the same reason, and the final printed resistor will have a nominal considerably different than originally planned. This is illustrated in Figure 8-4. Unless the producer knows the amount his compositions will spread or slump and maintains processing

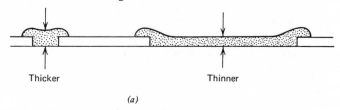

Thicker   Thinner

(a)

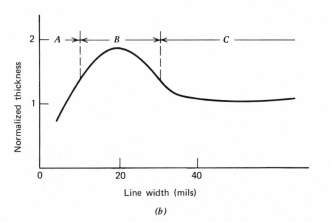

(b)

Figure 8-3 Line width and line length effect on print thickness. (a) Variations in thickness with length of pattern. (b) Effects of line width on thickness. A, Thickness reduced because of material staying with the screen. B, Print thickness a function of emulsion thickness. C, Print thickness a function of screen wire thickness rather than emulsion. (*Source.* L. F. Miller, "Paste Transfer in the Screening Process," *Solid State Technology,* June 1969.)

conditions to avoid variation in spread, his nominals will vary from time to time and will certainly be different than the targeted value.

Screen Setup is Not Correct. Different snap-off settings can produce different shear rates, leading to viscosity changes that result in printing different thicknesses. Ottaviano of GE, in a paper given at the 1969 ISHM Conference ("Repeatability in Screen Printing Hybrid Microcircuits," p. 253), reported a nominal value shift of up to 8% higher as the snap-off distance was decreased from a "regular" 34 mils to 24 mils. This is because the slower snap-off speed allows more ink to stay with the screen rather than on the substrate. With snap-off distance increased from 34 to 54 mils, the viscosity at snap-off was lowered enough so that extra ink stayed on the substrate and lowered resistance by 24%.

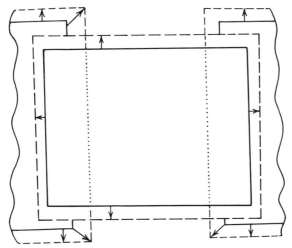

Figure 8-4 Illustration of how slumping can change the actual printed area from the planned area. Solid line: artwork; where one 50×50 mil resistor was planned. Dashed line: actual pattern; a 5-mil slump on a 50×50 mil resistor results in a 40×60 mil resistor and a 33% reduction in resistance.

Poor registration can result in altered effective electrode areas for thick film capacitors. A sloppy screen printer setup can also affect the amount of slump, which results in changed areas. Any one of these can change the amount of area of the composition being printed, so that the nominal value of the production batch of elements will be "off."

The Composition Produces a Different Value Than the Label on the Bottle Indicates. Probably, this is the thing that "bugs" inexperienced thick film producers more than anything else. The immediate reaction to getting 8000 $\Omega/\square$ out of a bottle of resistor paste that states that the supplier got exactly 14,370 $\Omega/\square$ is to put the blame on the ink producer. But this is seldom where the blame belongs. Perhaps coming this close (8000 instead of 14,370) the most that can be expected. In fact, when one reviews all the points mentioned here, and covered in more detail in the preceding chapters, coming so close sounds quite good. The goal is not so much to get the same value that the producer reports, but to miss by the same amount every time.

The user must learn to accept the fact that thick film compositions in his operation will *always* be different from what the ink maker reports. There are so many ways and so many places in which the producer's process can be different from the test procedures of the paste maker that similar values should not be *expected*. The thick film circuit producer should know exactly how his results will differ. Once he knows how his processes affect each of the many different compositions he will be using and once he can produce the same value repeatedly regardless of differences from the manufacturer's value, he is ready to do a good job of controlling the nominal value of his resistor and capacitor production.

To hit a nominal value target reasonably closely, a thick film producer must go through an extensive evaluation of his materials. In the case of resistors, he will run a series of tests with each resistor composition for

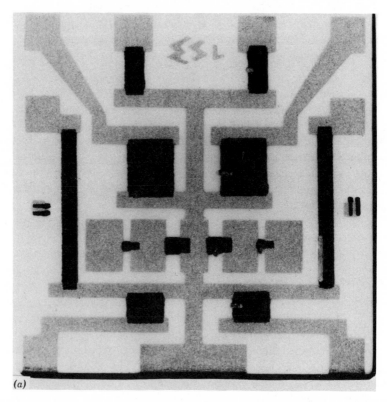

(a)

Figure 8-5 Resistor test and evaluation patterns. (a) Electro Science Laboratories (photograph courtesy of ESL). (b) Sperry Gyroscope Division, Sperry Rand (courtesy of Sperry Gyroscope). (c) Technetics, Inc. (photograph by State of the Art, Inc.). (d) DuPont Company (photograph by State of the Art, Inc.).

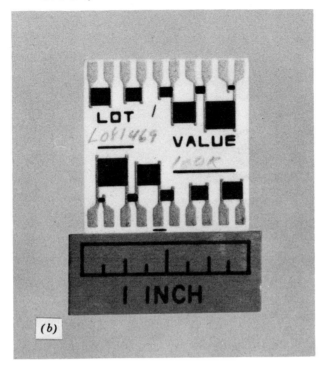

Figure 8-5 (Continued).

each of the various termination materials. These tests will include large and small resistors, long resistors, short resistors, narrow resistors, and wide resistors. The literature is full of test patterns designed for making these evaluations. Several are shown in Figure 8-5.

It should be obvious that a thorough evaluation of all of the many compositions used under all the normal variations that could be expected in a plant is a very extensive and expensive undertaking. Many thick film producers have never attempted to become thoroughly acquainted with their compositions and processes and thus are forced to accept conditions under which the nominal value realized in production is widely different from the expected value. Unfortunately for him, the uninformed producer must compete with informed producers who hit targets the first time and avoid time-consuming and expensive reruns and retooling. Flying by the seat of the pants can be exciting, but the days when this could be done are passing in the thick film industry.

Other Problem Areas. Different brands of substrates can produce different resistivities. Storage of unfired resistors for varying lengths of time in varying

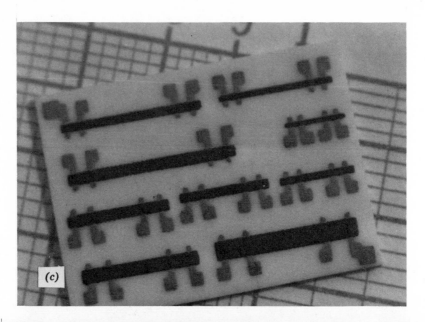

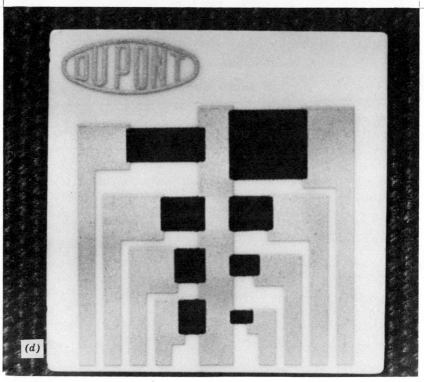

Figure 8-5 *(Continued).*

humidities and atmospheres can have an effect on the nominal value realized. Storage of the paste on a roller mill (used to avoid settling) can change resistance over a long period of time. Varying paint mill treatments (if a mill is used in blending) can change resistivity. There is a trend toward small size components and as resistors get smaller and smaller, the resistor/conductor interface reactions have assumed increased importance. Knowing these effects is essential. The list of factors that influence the realized nominal value is endless. Time and the scope of this text allow no more than scratching the surface.

CONTROLLING THE SPREAD OF THICK FILM COMPONENTS

Controlling the resistor-to-resistor (or capacitor-to-capacitor) variation within a lot (spread) is often different from controlling the nominal value. Efforts to keep the spread "tight" are usually worthwhile. It becomes extremely important if attempts are to be made to produce elements without trimming. Even if trimming is planned, a tight or narrow spread will produce a uniform trim time that results in maximization of trimming rates and more uniform secondary characteristics such as TCR tracking and noise.

Thick film element spread can become large in the following ways:

1. Component is small.
2. Substrate-to-screen separation varies.
3. Temperature control in kiln is poor.

Component is Too Small. We have just discussed the role that small size (very short or very narrow resistors, e.g.) can play in throwing the nominal value off the computed target value. In addition, small size tends to increase the spread of a batch of components. The reason for this is that small variations in print width have a much greater effect on area with small parts than with large parts. For example, a 2-mil variation in a 10-mil² pattern changes area by about 40%, whereas the same variation on a 100-mil pattern changes total area by only 4%. Actual experience is tabulated in Table 8-1. The table also shows that printing methods that define the pattern better, as in the case of the metal mask screen, will reduce spread considerably. Figure 8-6 shows results of test series where a similar increase in spread was demonstrated. Note that printing the resistor first (8-6*b*) tightened the distribution. The reason is that it is more difficult

Table 8-1   Influence of Size and Screen Type
on Spread

Resistor Size	Spread (Wire Mesh)	Spread (Metal Mask)
10 × 10 mils	±64%	±32%
20 × 20 mils	±26%	±13%
30 × 30 mils	±16%	± 9%

to do a precision print over the slightly uneven surface that exists when the conductor terminations are printed first.

Substrate-to-Screen Separation Varies. The Ottaviano study, referenced above, showed that a variation in snap-off distance could change the resistance of a thick film resistor by as much as 1%/mil of snap-off variation. Normal variations in substrate thickness and in camber has the effect of changing the snap-off distance. Figure 8-7. illustrates an extreme situation, where a thin, but flat, substrate gives a snap-off distance of 6 mils more than a thick, but cambered, substrate from the same lot. Such differences are within commonly accepted commercial substrate specifications. A spread of ±3% could be expected from this variation alone. Some users resort to extra sorting of as-received substrates to cut down on the variation in resistor or capacitor values caused by nonuniform substrates.

Temperature Control in Kiln is Poor. In a furnace with improperly located thermocouple, or one that is not functioning properly, the work temperature can swing a few degrees back and forth from a nominal control value. If this swing is slow, resistors or capacitors going through the hot zone at different times will get different temperature treatment. In the example used earlier in this chapter (when discussing how temperature being "off" can shift the nominal value) changes in resistance values of up to $3\frac{1}{2}\%/°C$ were cited. A swing in temperature of only 3° during the firing of a batch of resistors will thus cause identical components to have values vary by up to 10%. This amounts to a spread of +5% or −5%.

Other Factors. The examples given are only three of the many factors that influence the spread in values of thick film resistors and capacitors. A screen that is ghosting, variations in squeegee pressure, variations in the surface of a substrate, and many other factors have a bearing on spread.

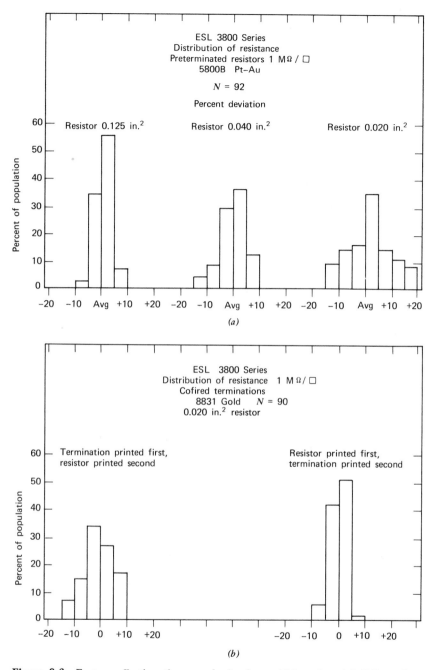

Figure 8-6 Factors affecting the spread of values within a lot. (*a*) Effect of resistor size on spread. (*b*) Effect on spread of preprinted resistors (resistors printed *before* the conductors are printed) versus that of postprinted ones. (*Source.* S. J. Stein and J. V. Garvin, "The Influence of Geometry and Conductive Terminations on Thick Film Resistors," 1970 ISHM Proceedings, p. 198.)

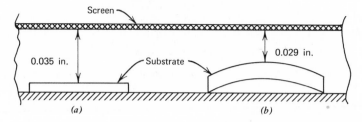

Figure 8-7 The influence of variations in substrate thickness and camber on snap-off distance. (*a*) A 23-mil flat substrate gives 0.35-in. snap-off distance. (*b*) A 26-mil substrate with a 0.003-in. chamber gives a 0.029-in. snap-off distance.

SUMMARY—CONTROLLING SPREAD AND NOMINAL OF THICK FILM ELEMENTS

It should be quite obvious by now that the factors at work in causing variations in the nominal value from lot to lot are different from those causing variations within the lot. Controlling spread and controlling the nominal value are two distinct things. Controlling either one is a complex matter.

The task of producing ±10% element now should seem much more difficult than it might have before we catalogued the many ways of producing variations in spread and nominal. It must be kept in mind that to produce a 10% tolerance part, *both* spread and nominal must be well within the 10% limit. The amount of spread *plus* the amount the nominal is off target must total less than 10%—otherwise out-of-tolerance parts will be produced. For example, if the spread is +6% to −6% (very tight), the nominal must be within 4% of the target value (this takes excellent marksmanship).

Producing ±10% resistors or capacitors "as fired" is obviously quite difficult. Conditions must be ideal, and the design of the element must be optimized (for resistors, aspect ratios close to 1, fairly large size, etc.). Printing to ±20% is not always easy. The average thick film producer probably produces elements that fall in the range of plus or minus 30% to 40%. Some producers claim ability to produce 10% and even 5% tolerance units without trimming, but cost and yields of such production are not given. Costs are probably not low, and yields are probably poor. It may be that such efforts amount to technological showmanship and/or economic foolishness.

Thick film paste makers often describe the quality of their compositions in terms of the tight tolerance resistors or capacitors that can be produced with their materials. These claims must be taken with a grain of salt. The tolerance capabilities mentioned usually include *only* the spread; nothing is said about how far the target is or might be missed. The results of their tests also need considerable amplification, including data about the size of the pattern used and other processing parameters. Tight spreads are usually attributable as much to good element design and processing capabilities as to the raw material.

TRIMMING THICK FILM ELEMENTS

Trimming is Essential. It is assumed that by now the reader is convinced that trimming is necessary to economically produce most thick film resistors or capacitors. Without trimming only the loosest of tolerances can be economically realized.

Fortunately, trimming technology for resistors has been available for many years, and is now becoming known for capacitors. The available techniques and equipment make possible precision trimming at extremely low costs (see a discussion of cost analysis in Chapter 13). The existence of techniques for low-cost precision trimming of resistors has been responsible for much of the vitality of thick film industry. The trimming capabilities now becoming available for thick film capacitors are another positive factor promising continuing vitality of thick film technology.

Trimming Techniques. Trimming resistors differs from trimming capacitors. In the case of resistors, adjustments can be made by cutting slots or grooves that change the aspect ratio. Resistors are trimmed "up"—starting with a low value and removing portions of the resistor until the value of resistance increases to the final desired level. Capacitors are trimmed "down"—starting with extra capacitance. Capacitance trimming involving large percentage changes is not quite as easy as it is with resistors because all of the excess electrode area must be removed from a capacitor, whereas only a small area need be removed in a resistor. Without special geometry, a capacitor's capacitance can be changed 50% only by removing 50% of the electrode, whereas a resistor can be changed by a similar amount by cutting a very narrow slot—perhaps a few percent of the total area. Resistors can therefore be trimmed faster. (Figure 8-8). The most common techniques for resistor trimming are *air-abrasive* trimming and *laser* trimming. Capacitor trimming is done almost exclusively with air-abrasive at present. Other trimming methods that are or have been used range from simple "erasing" by abrasive rubbing (hand) through use of motor-driven abrasive wheels (automated erasing), diamond needle scratching,

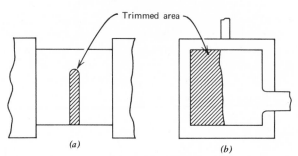

Figure 8-8 Trimming of capacitors versus trimming of resistors, illustrating the amount of trimming required to change value by 50%. (*a*) Resistor trimmed from 100 to 200 Ω. (*b*) Capacitor trimmed from 200 to 100 pF.

ultrasonic machining, arc discharge, anodic reactions, pulsed voltage, and RF trimming. None of these other methods are presently used to any extent for thick film trimming although some are used for thin film trimming.

The Two Basic Approaches to Trimming. Trimming involves changing resistance or capacitance from what one *has* to what one *wants*. This can be done by (1) changing the material properties (resistivity or dielectric constant) or (2) changing the geometry. All of the trimming methods mentioned use one of the two approaches. Changing *geometry* by material removal has proved to be the only practical approach to date for thick film.

Trimming by Changing Material Properties. This can be accomplished by changing the chemical or structural makeup of the element. Arc discharge trimming of resistors is an example of this approach; so is voltage pulse trimming. Little *individual* element trimming is currently done in thick film using this approach, but an important tool often utilized is "batch trimming" of thick film resistors or capacitors. The *entire batch* is altered slightly by a refiring treatment. For instance, if resistor values are all a bit high, a second firing can reduce the nominal resistance, thereby eliminating nontrimmable highs. High dielectric constant ceramic materials can be trimmed upward by refiring at higher temperatures. Figure 8-9 shows the effects of refiring (note that TCR also changes).

Trimming by Changing Geometry. This is by far the most common approach to thick film resistor and. capacitor trimming. With thick film resistors the geometry can be changed by changing the thickness of the

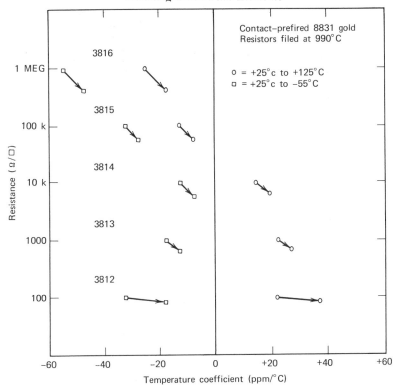

Figure 8-9 The effect of batch trimming (refiring) on temperature coefficient and resistance. (*Source:* S. J. Stein and J. V. Garvin, "The Influence of Geometry and Conductive Terminations on Thick Film Resistors," 1970 ISHM Proceedings, p. 198.)

resistor (as with an abrasive "rubbing") or by changing the width of the resistor (or, to be more exact, changing the aspect ratio).

Capacitors are trimmed by removing portions of one electrode and thus changing the active or effective area (remember, $C = KA/t$?).

Figure 8-10 shows an early thick film trimmer.

A Trimming Complication. Something that should be kept in mind is that when resistance or capacitance is changed, other characteristics of the element will almost surely also change. The temperature coefficient, the humidity resistance, noise output, and power handling capabilities are likely to be altered.

In the case of resistors, the temperature coefficient can be changed because the edge portion of the resistor (which has a higher glass content

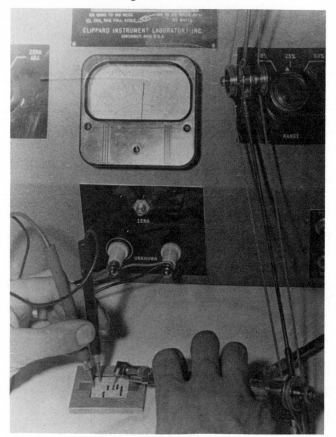

Figure 8-10 Early thick film resistor trimming. Dental equipment was used for grinding and probing done by hand. (Photograph courtesy of H. Simon, Airco Speer Electronics.)

and a more positive TCR) will be removed (leaving the more negative center of the resistor). Noise levels will change because of exposed rough edges. Thick film resistors have a dense surface that offers considerable humidity protection. Air-abrasive trimming opens up this "seal," so that moisture or atmosphere can more easily affect the trimmed resistor. Laser trimming has a resealing action because of the extremely high temperatures created locally, and thus avoids some of the humidity problems.

It is beyond the scope of this book to discuss in detail the "side effects" of trimming, but the reader should be aware of the fact that they do exist. The best attitude to have about the effect of trimming on secondary element parameters is to recognize that trimming will have a definite effect on *all* parameters of interest and that the effect will be "bad." If one takes this attitude, there will be no unpleasant surprises. Finding out what the effects are is largely up to the producer, because his process is a prime determinant of these effects. The materials suppliers can help to some extent; but in the end, the producer must inform himself of the side effects of trimming through extensive evaluation tests of the materials he is using and of his processes. This testing tends to be time consuming and expensive, and many producers have not done it. Embarrassment is in store for those who avoid becoming familiar with their processes and materials.

Setting Target Values. When resistor patterns are initially laid out, a target value is set that is sufficiently below the final trimmed value desired; this ensures that under all but the worst conditions all of the resistors of the batch will be below the final value. The reverse is true for capacitors—the target is set higher.

As resistors get smaller, as more compositions (different ones) are fired at the same time, and as the number of resistors per circuit increases, the target value usually must be set lower and lower. For simple circuits where only one composition is being used and all of the resistors are fairly large, the target might be as high as 80% of the final value. For complex circuits with very small resistors, the target may be only 50%. It is important for the producer to know his process capabilities so that the targets are set no lower than need be, but low enough to avoid no highs. Setting targets too high will result in untrimmable high values and expensive scrap or rework. Setting the targets too low will result in excessive trimming time and degraded resistor performance. With heavily trimmed resistors the TCR will be more erratic, resistance to atmosphere and humidity will be poorer, and hot spots will be more likely.

The same applies to capacitor trimming—targets are set higher for more erratic formulations, smaller areas, and so on.

Air-Abrasive Trimming. An air-abrasive trimmer is a specialized sandblasting device. (Figures 8-11 and 8-12.) Probes sense the resistance or capacitance during trimming. Trimming proceeds by material removal (the body of the resistor or the top electrode of the capacitor) which changes the element's value. Trimmers have arrangements for automatically moving the trimming head over a predetermined path at a controlled speed. When the trimmed value reaches the desired stop point, the air supply of the sandblaster is cut off and trimming stops. The distance of the nozzle from the element being trimmed determines to some extent the width of the cut, although this is decided primarily by the shape and size of the nozzle. The amount of sand being fed into the system and the amount and pressure of the

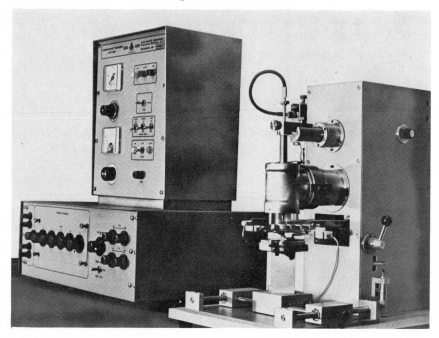

Figure 8-11 Laboratory model of an air-abrasive trimmer. (Courtesy of S. S. White Division, Penwalt Corporation.)

air are adjustable, so that the rate of trimming, width of cut, and speed must all be adjustable as well. (Figures 8-13; 8-14 and 8-15.)

Overshoot. When the resistance-sensing system signals that target resistance has been reached, it activates a signal that closes off the air supply, and the sandblasting stops. Air-abrasive trimmers have a "problem" in that when the signal to cut off the air supply is given, the compressed air and abrasive grit remaining in the conduit between the cutoff valve and the nozzle tip must run out before trimming action stops entirely. This lag between signal and the actual end of trimming can be up to 50 msec. It is called *overshoot*. Since in a givèn setup the amount of overshoot tends to be the same from one trim to the next, it can, to a great extent, be compensated for; simply find out what the overshoot is and stop the trimming by that amount prior to the final desired value. For instance, with 30-Ω overshoot, to make a 1000-Ω resistor, stop at 970 Ω, and the overshoot will cause the trimmer to "coast into" the 1000-Ω value.

Resistor Trimming—Width of Cut. Figure 8-16 shows three possible widths of cut that could be made to trim a resistor. Very narrow cuts do not

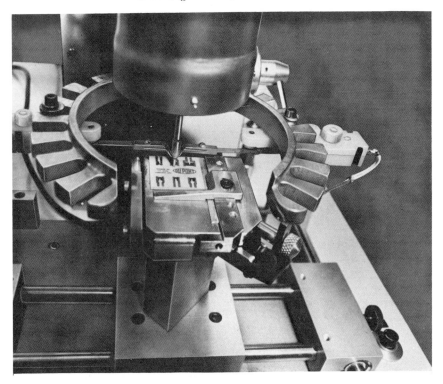

Figure 8-12   Close-up of a laboratory model of air-abrasive trimmer, showing probe head and nozzle. (Courtesy of S. S. White Division, Penwalt Corporation.)

cause resistance change early in the cut nearly as much as late in the cut. Overshoot in the case of a narrow cut that is proceeding fairly rapidly—as when the producer is trying to trim at a high rate—can be excessive. Even with compensation it makes accurate trimming difficult. It is possible, in fact, if the speed of the cut is too high and the cut is narrow, to cut completely through a resistor. For narrow cuts, the cutting speed must be slowed down to control overshoot. Wider cuts lessen the effect of overshoot considerably, but are slow and use abrasive excessively. This is one of the reasons that high-aspect ratios are not desirable. Low-aspect ratios are easier to trim.

Precision Trimming. During air-abrasive trimming the resistor is "upset" to some extent by the localized heating caused by abrasive action and by the repeated pummeling of the high-speed abrasive particles. Therefore, the value of the resistor at the actual time of trimming is somewhat different

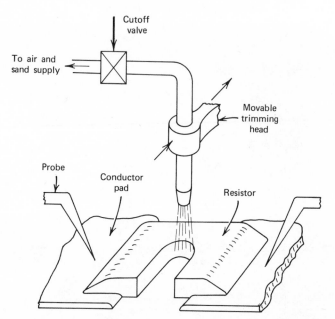

Figure 8-13 Schematic of an air-abrasive trimming system.

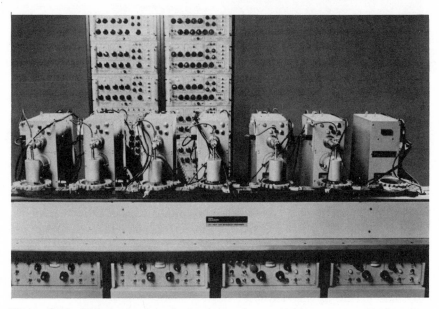

Figure 8-14 High-production air-abrasive resistor trimming system—12,000 trims per hour. (Courtesy of S. S. White Division, Penwalt Corporation.)

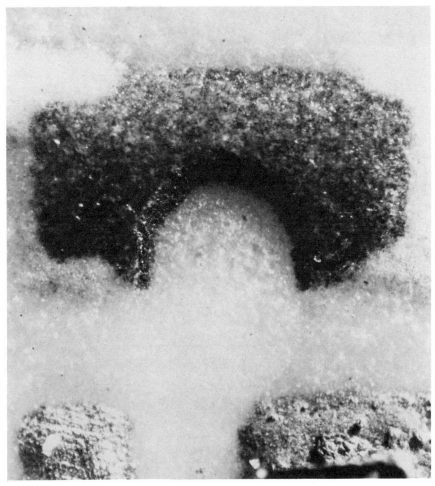

Figure 8-15 Close-up of an air-abrasive-trimmed resistor (177×). (Courtesy of S. S. White Division, Penwalt Corporation.)

from the value immediately after trimming stops, and after trimming stops there is a slow change in resistance over a period of hours. This places a limitation on accuracy. The biased reading during trimming is somewhat like overshoot in that the error tends to be the same and setting a slightly different target to compensate for this corrects a large portion of the error. The aging effect is tougher to compensate for, although compensation for this can be cranked into the original cutoff if the aging correction is known. Another approach is illustrated in Figure 8-17. A rough cut is made first—say to within ½% of the final value. After aging overnight, a second

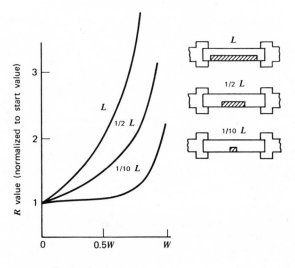

Depth of cut—normalized
to resistor width

Showing generation of data for
curve above

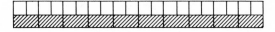

Full length cut
Start: 10 squares. Half way: 20 squares

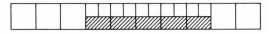

Half length cut
Start: 10 squares. Half way: 15 squares

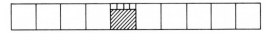

1/10—Length cut
Start: 10 squares. Three quarters: 13 squares

Figure 8-16 Trimmed resistance value versus depth of cut for various-width nozzles. (*Source.* Sanders, "Process Information for the Design of Automatic Resistor Trimming Equipment," *1969 ISHM Proceedings,* p. 197.)

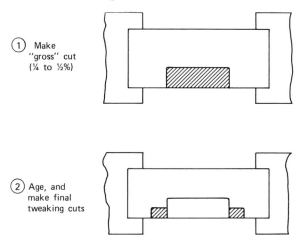

① Make "gross" cut (¼ to ½%)

② Age, and make final tweaking cuts

Figure 8-17 An approach to precision trimming. Final trims are made after aging.

"tweaking" cut is made to bring the resistance up to its final value. For trimming to $\frac{1}{10}\%$ tolerance, such a procedure is probably necessary, but for looser tolerances ($\frac{1}{4}\%$ and over) the more expensive double trimming can be avoided with most thick film resistor compositions. A similar approach can be used for precision capacitor trimming. Different resistor compositions of course behave differently during trimming, and the amount of resistor upset during trimming can vary considerably.

For many circuits, trimming to a specific value is not as important as is exactly matching ratios. A resistor or capacitor trimmer can always match ratios closer than it can trim to absolute values. Typically, if a trimming system can trim to $\frac{1}{4}\%$ absolute, it will have little trouble matching ratios to about $\frac{1}{10}\%$.

Another important factor is maintaining tracking capabilities. If all of the resistors on a substrate are of the same composition, the untrimmed resistors will track very closely with either temperature or time. Improper design (layout) and trimming can damage this built-in tracking capability, however.

If high precision trimming (close matching, close tracking, and close absolute values) is attempted, as in the case of ladder networks, special care must be taken, starting with the way the resistor circuit is laid out. For close tracking, it is important that all of the resistors maintain uniform temperature—therefore the power rating (watts per square inch) must be kept at an absolutely uniform level. Otherwise, one resistor will operate at a different temperature than its mates, and the resistance ratio will change somewhat. (To the extent that a zero TC composition is available, the need for uniform resistor temperatures is lessened.) The resistors should be laid out so that the amount of trim to be made is uniform from one resistor to the next and the least possible trimming is done. This means that target values will be set much closer to the final value for circuits such as this, and more care will have to be taken to keep tight spreads and to hold nominals close to the target.

Trimming Power Resistors. Figure 8-18 shows how, in a typical trimming situation, a resistor that starts with three squares finishes up as four unequal

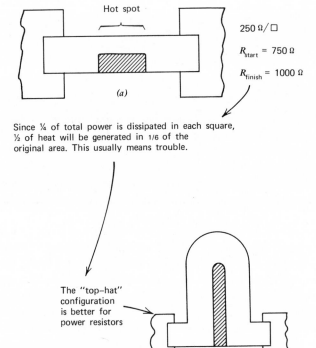

Figure 8-18 Trimming power resistors. (*a*) Heat generation density depends on trimming geometry. (*b*) The "Top-hat" form is desired because it avoids hot spots.

squares where one-half of the heat dissipated will be dumped into only one-sixth of the resistor area. If the original power dissipation calculations anticipated this situation, no harm is done, but a hot spot might develop otherwise. The hot spot would degrade resistor performance and perhaps damage other parts in the circuit.

Higher-aspect ratios such as illustrated in Figure 8-16 are in general undesirable for power resistors because of the likelihood of hot spots. The "top-hat" configuration is much more attractive because it trims out to squares of uniform size with uniform heat dissipation throughout the resistor.

Capacitor Trimming. Air-abrasive trimming of capacitors is more complicated than trimming resistors. The complication is illustrated in Figure 8-19. If a capacitor trim proceeds in a manner similar to resistor trimming,

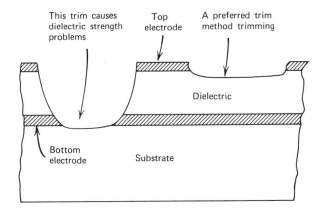

Figure 8-19 Capacitor trimming; cutting all the way through causes problems that can be avoided by removing only the top electrode.

where the entire structure down to the substrate is removed, the trimmed capacitor is left with the two electrodes separated only by the thin dielectric layer. Furthermore, it is possible that some of the top electrode material has been imbedded in the walls of the dielectric so that shorts or dielectric weaknesses are made even more likely. A capacitor trimmed in this manner has reduced dielectric strength, and its reliability has been severely decreased. A protective coating (glass or plastic) can be placed over the "wound," but this is not totally satisfactory. It will not bring the capacitor back to its original dielectric strength levels, and it will also change the capacitance slightly, which makes precision trimming difficult.

A preferred method of capacitor trimming is to remove only the top electrode, leaving the dielectric (at least most of it) in place. This is a much more delicate trimming task. A manually controlled visual trim can be quick enough to move the trimming head on to new territory as the metal is removed, before the dielectric is gone; with an automatic trim, this is more difficult.

Automatic trims for capacitors, short of programming extremely complicated trimming head movements, depend on the use of special abrasives that are to some extent selective. They will remove the metal, but will not remove the dielectric at nearly the same rate. This allows an automatic trim cycle to proceed with a good chance of avoiding abrading all the way through to the bottom electrode. Wide trimming nozzles are used to permit cutting a wide swath. (See Figure 8-20.)

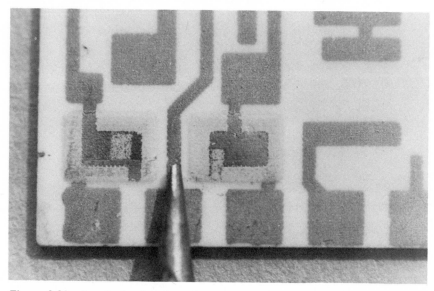

Figure 8-20 An air-abrasive-trimmed thick film capacitor. Note that only the top electrode has been removed. (Photograph by State of the Art, Inc.)

The processor can help a capacitor trimming operation by using a top electrode composition that abrades easier, by putting it on thinner, and perhaps even by making the dielectric a bit thicker where he wants to trim. Above all, he must be careful to produce uniform top electrodes so that they will abrade in a uniform manner.

High dielectric materials are harder to trim to precision values in that they are upset more during the trimming. Precise values are largely meaningless with high K compositions because they are so voltage and temperature sensitive, and so time sensitive, that a precision value at one particular point does not mean much. A 10% tolerance is about as close as one would want to trim the higher dielectric constant compositions—perhaps 5% in rare cases. The lower dielectric constant compositions are much stabler, and precision trims can be made with greater ease. One percent tolerance is not difficult except for very low-capacitance values where accurate capacitance measurement becomes difficult.

The industry still has a lot to learn about capacitor trimming. Until 1971, commercial trimming systems were not available, and only those who cared to go through internal development programs could trim capacitors. Trimming systems are now coming on the market and capacitor trimming will no doubt become much more widespread. Adding this capability to thick film's "bag of tricks" should result in many very advantageous situations for thick film.

LASER TRIMMING

The laser has, in the past couple of years, gone from a trimming approach that "offered a lot of promise" to a solid reality. It has certain advantages that ensure its place as a popular trimming method. Many firms now offer a variety of laser trimmers. (Figures 8-21, 8-22 and 8-23.)

The laser trimmer channels its energy into a small beam that focuses

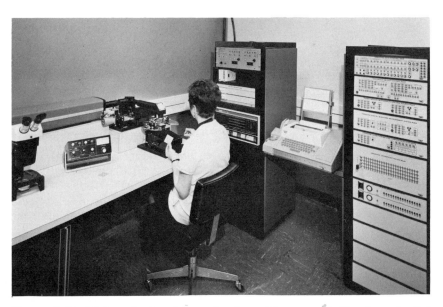

Figure 8-21 High-production laser trimming. (Courtesy of Teradyne Applied Systems.)

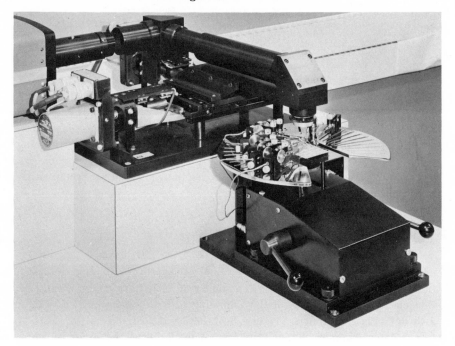

Figure 8-22 Trimming lead for laser trimming. (Courtesy of Teradyne Applied Systems.)

in the plane of the resistor. The concentrated energy vaporizes the resistor material in a small area. The beam can be rapidly moved in an X or Y direction by manipulating mirrors, by table movement, or by laser lead movement. The ease of movement of the beam has led to one of the advantages of a laser trimming system: the ability to trim several different resistors with one setup. A laser beam can move on to trim a second, a third, and a dozen or more different resistors on a single substrate by means of a numerically programmed beam movement arrangement. All of the resistors on an entire circuit can be trimmed in this way in a few seconds. (Air-abrasive systems can trim more than one resistor also, but the system is more awkward—single-station trimmers in tandem with mechanical transfers between stations.)

Either the YAG or the CO_2 laser can be used with thick film, and it is not entirely clear which is better. The YAG has the advantage of working on both thin and thick film, but the CO_2 has advantages of its own and is often preferred for thick film. One advantage is that focal length limitations are smaller and a CO_2 laser can trim warped substrates.

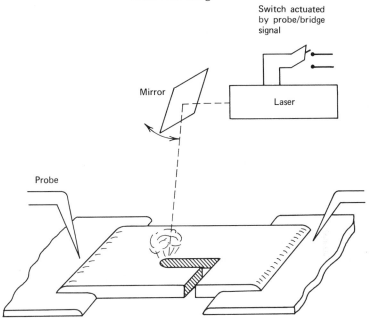

Figure 8-23 Schematic of a laser trimming system.

Trimming with a laser proceeds via a series of short pulses (100 μsec or so). During the pulse, a plasma is formed whose conductivity lowers the resistance sensed. In order for the sensing system to know what has happened, the laser must stop long enough for a reading to be made. This may sound complicated, but it is easily accomplished electronically.

A laser, in spite of its stop-and-go style, can trim at the rate of several inches per second, whereas an air-abrasive can trim only at the rate of a very few inches per minute. For this reason, laser trimmers hold an inherent speed advantage.

The laser trimmer has another *very* important advantage over air-abrasive trimmers. Air-abrasive particles bounce at high speed off the resistor being trimmed and often turn into destructive missiles. An abrasive particle traveling at high speed, as in a trimming bounce, can severely damage an active device if it is hit in a vulnerable spot. This means that dynamic trimming wits air-abrasive is almost impossible unless the devices are protected (not always easy to do at this stage). A further problem with using an abrasive in dynamic trimming has to do with overshoot. Dynamic trimming is thus being left almost entirely to laser trimming systems. Since dynamic trimming is so important to thick film, the laser's place is assured—even though the laser systems are much more expensive than air-abrasive trimmers.

Figure 8-16 showed that narrow cuts in high-aspect ratio resistors are difficult to trim because the rate of resistance change with respect to cutting speed was very high. The laser beam makes a cut that is even narrower than the smallest air-abrasive nozzle. Thus a verticle cut would limit the laser's trimming accuracy (at least for rapid cutting) in spite of the fact that the laser's overshoot is practically nil. To get around this problem, most laser trimmers can make an L-cut, where the cut is perpendicular to the resistor length until it is about halfway through, then parallel until the stop value is reached. Some laser makers say that a perpendicular cut is for "rough trimming" and the parallel cut is for "fine trimming." This is not quite correct; the turn is often made before the value changes very much at all, and most of the resistance change occurs during the parallel cut. Without L-cut capabilities, the laser would be impractical for high aspect ratios. If a laser trimmer cannot make L-cuts, resistors have to be designed with aspect ratios of less than one (such as top-hats) in order to achieve accurate trimming. (Figures 8-24 and 8-21.)

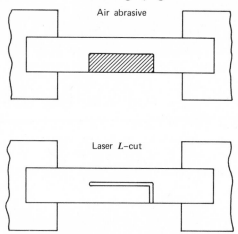

Figure 8-24 Comparison of the geometry of air-abrasive resistor trimming with that of laser trimming. The trimming is from four squares to six squares.

Laser-trimmed thick film resistors are likely to be less affected by atmosphere and humidity problems in later life because there is a fusion seal of sorts made by the very high localized temperatures. To some extent the trim cut is resealed. Lasers reportedly upset the resistance less during trimming so that (when properly set up) they have better precision trimming capabilities.

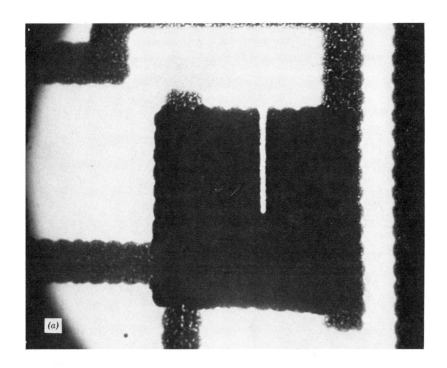

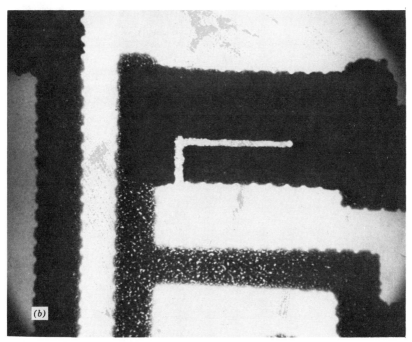

Figure 8-25 Laser-trimmed resistors (transmitted light micrographs approximately 60×). (*a*) A straight cut for a low-aspect ratio resistor. (*b*) An L-cut for a high-aspect resistor. (*c*) Mulitple plunge cuts for improved accuracy without retention to L-cuts. (Courtesy of Teradyne Applied Systems.)

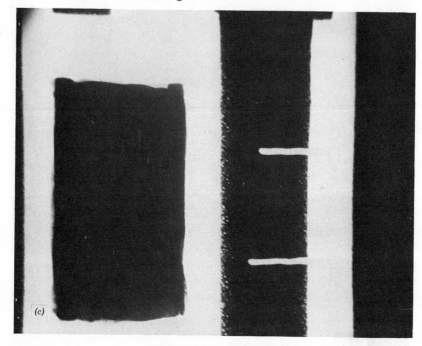

Figure 8-25 (Continued).

Laser trimmers are not without some problems. If the beam is improperly focused, or if the power output is too high, the substrate underneath can be damaged (e.g., cracked) and large changes in resistance will occur after trimming. The need for L-cut capabilities, operator protection from the beam, and safeguards against other similar problems keeps the cost of laser trimmers high compared to air-abrasive trimmers.

Laser trimmers have not been used for trimming capacitors to date.

Chapter 9

BONDING AND SOLDERING

Chip and Wire Bonding of Active Devices

The various procedures in use for attaching semiconductor chips to substrates are discussed in the first part of this chapter 9. Soldering will be taken up in the second part of the chapter. There are three areas to be covered in our discussion of bonding:

1. *Die or chip bonding*—methods for attaching silicon IC chips to the substrate.
2. *Wire bonding*—methods for stringing wires from the surface of the silicon chip to the pads on the substrate.
3. *Face bonding and other approaches,* designed to get around some of the limitations of chip and wire bonding.

Figure 9-1 illutrates these various types of bonding.

DIE BONDING (CHIP BONDING)

Of the various types of bonding to be covered in this chapter, chip bonding is perhaps the "easiest" and certainly the least controversial. Another way of putting this is to say that wire bonding causes more problems and more

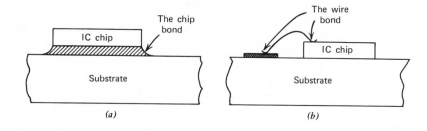

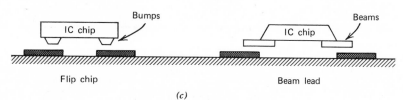

Figure 9-1 Types of IC bonding. (*a*) Chip bonding. (*b*) Wire bonding. (*c*) Face bonding.

is being done to eliminate these problems—hence more controversy also exists. Chip bonding of course has its problems and complexities, but at least the available technologies are meeting IC needs without being pushed so hard. Several highly satisfactory methods are available.

DIE BONDING REQUIREMENTS

The most obvious requirement for a die or chip bond is that of mechanical attachment of the silicon device to the substrate. The bond must be strong enough to hold the chip in place during subsequent assembly operations and in final use.

At times there must also be an electrical path through the bond from the chip to the substrate. This a relatively common feature of single transistor or diode mounting, but not for IC chips.

The bond must be able to carry off heat generated on the chip. Thermal conductivity or thermal resistance of the bond is therefore of interest when there is heat being generated on the chip.

Chip bonds can be judged by how well they satisfy these three requirements. Since different applications have different requirements, the criteria vary from application to application. The basic bonding approach must be matched to the particular application.

The four die bonding methods in use today are (1) eutectic bonding, (2) solder bonding, (3) glass bonding, and (4) plastic bonding.

EUTECTIC BONDING

Eutectic bonding today is the most widely used method of attaching semiconductor chips to the package or to the substrate. It makes use of the fact that silicon (from the IC chip) and gold (from the mounting pad) form a eutectic at 370°C (if brought into close contact with each other). This is a very "good" temperature—hot enough to allow several other heatings at successively lower temperatures to attach other kinds of devices (including wire bonding), but still not hot enough to damage most silicon devices through exposure to heat (unless the substrate and device are held at this temperature for a long time). Figure 9-2 is a phase diagram of the gold-silicon system, showing the eutectic at 370°C.

An advantage of the gold-silicon eutectic bond is the simple metallurgy involved. Silicon is available from the back of the chip and gold is available in a great variety of packages and substrates ranging from gold plated on metal packages to gold deposited on insulating substrates by thick or thin film techniques or by plating.

A potential problem arises with this simple system, however: once the melting starts, it continues until the supply of material to be melted is exhausted (gold normally) or until the temperature is reduced below the eutectic temperature. This places limitations on the length of time the chip can be held above the eutectic temperature and sets of minimum for the amount of gold. These conditions are easily met when single chips are being bonded, but can cause difficulty when many chips are bonded on the same substrate or when extensive rework is necessary.

Some producers feel that the best bonds are made by using tiny alloy "preforms" (punched from thin sheets) of the eutectic alloy. The preforms are placed on the heated (to about 400°C) substrate pad where they melt at once. The silicon chip is then placed on the molten eutectic mix. A bond is made in much the same way as solder makes a bond.

Preforms are often used when a bond of other than gold/silicon is desired. Gold-tin preforms give a lower bonding temperature for heat-sensitive chips. Gallium, antimony, and indium preforms can be used where making (or *not* making) a junction in the base of the chip is desirable. Gallium and indium alloys make *n*-type materials and would thus create a junction for a *p*-type chip or would *not* make a junction in an *n*-type chip. Antimony

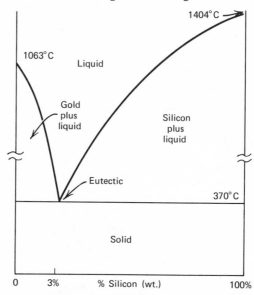

Figure 9-2   The gold-silicon phase diagram.

is a *p*-type dopant and would make a junction in an *n*-type chip. Other than the gold-tin alloy, these special preform materials are not used to any extent in IC fabrication.

Most bonding today is done *without* the preform, using instead the silicon in the chip and gold from the substrate pad to form a eutectic bond. It is necessary to make intimate contact before melting will start. This is usually accomplished by having the bonding machine "scrub" the chip into the gold by moving it back and forth under pressure. The scrubbing abrades away oxides and dirt, producing an intimate contact between the gold and the silicon. The scrubbing movement can be either mechanical, which is the most popular, or ultrasonic. The pressure required is high, so that there is a chance of breakage for very large chips; alloy preforms are therefore preferred for large chips (or for high-reliability bonds). When no preforms are used, there must be an adequate coating of gold on the pad—otherwise the supply will run out before the bond is completed and adhesion will be low (or nonexistent). Many silicon chips are furnished with a gold coating on their backs to aid in forming the eutectic.

EUTECTIC BONDING EQUIPMENT

Machines have been designed by many firms to aid in the chip bonding process. IC chips are small, and extremely accurate and precise equipment is needed. The cost of a chip bonder runs from as low as $800 for one that can be operated by a dextrous girl with tweezers to pick up and place the chips to about $4000 for a simple production model bonder. Automated versions cost much more. All chip bonding machines have certain basic features. (Figures 9-3 and 9-4.)

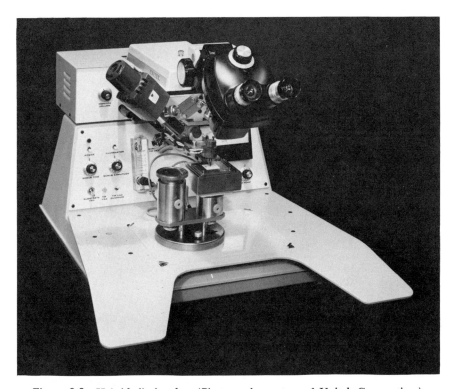

Figure 9-3 Hybrid die bonder. (Photograph courtesy of Unitek Corporation.)

1. A Chip Storage Tray. Chips to be bonded are placed on a movable tray. The surface of the tray is often a mirror so that the bottom of the pickup tool can be seen (by reflection) through a viewing microscope. The alignment of the chip and the pickup tool is accomplished by hand manipulation of the storage tray—sliding it over a smooth surface allows rapid and accurate alignment.

2. A Viewing Microscope. Monolithic IC chips are small and they must be positioned very accurately prior to pickup. A microscope is usually required. Some die bonders have microscopes with cross hairs which are used for aligning the chips. Other designs achieve alignment by looking

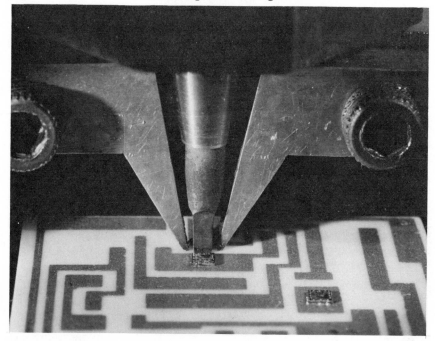

Figure 9-4 Close-up of a hybrid die bonder. The fingers on each side of the chip holder are for heating the area beneath the chip. The rest of the substrate is kept at temperatures well below the gold-silicon eutectic. (Courtesy of Unitek Corporation.)

at the bottom on the pickup tool via a reflection from the chip storage tray.

3. A Vacuum Pickup Tool. All but the least expensive die bonders have pickup tools. They pick up the aligned chip, holding it by vacuum while it is transported to the mounting area on the substrate or the package. Pickup tools are constructed so that only the edge of the chip is touched. Damage to the face of the chip by touching with the tool is thus avoided.

4. A Transport Mechanism. The two basic transport arrangements used in die bonders are (1) a stationary pickup with movable die storage tray and substrate heater stage or (2) a stationary chip tray and heater stage, but a movable pickup tool. In either case, the pickup tool and the stage must somehow be maneuvered into accurate alignment so that the chip will be in its proper position when lowered.

5. A "Scrubber." A mechanical vibrator or an ultrasonic vibrator is connected to the pickup tool. When the chip is lowered into place and pressure is applied, the scrubber vibration starts. It produces good metallurgical contact so that eutectics can form rapidly and uniformly.

6. A Heated Stage. This is a temperature-controlled device that holds the package or substrate in position during bonding. Many bonders have stages that hold more than one package; one package can then be brought up to heat while bonding is taking place on another. They often have provisions for furnishing a "gas blanket" of forming gas (10% H_2-90% N_2) to keep the metallization on the heated IC chip from oxidizing.

Some bonders designed for multichip bonding hold the stage just below the eutectic rather than just above. They rely on final heating by means of a hot air jet directed at the area where bonding is taking place. The rest of the substrate or package is thus kept below the liquidus and the problems of holding for excessive time at excessive temperatures are avoided.

Bonders designed for multichip packages have stages that can be shifted accurately between one bond and the next to enable the pickup tool to descend to a new location. These bonders have chip storage tray arrangements that can accommodate several different chips.

Typical Chip Bonding Sequence. Figure 9-5 shows a typical bonding sequence. The stage holds the package (substrate) so that when it is swung under the chip pickup tool, the chip can be lowered exactly into position. Other versions have movable pickup arms and stationary stages.

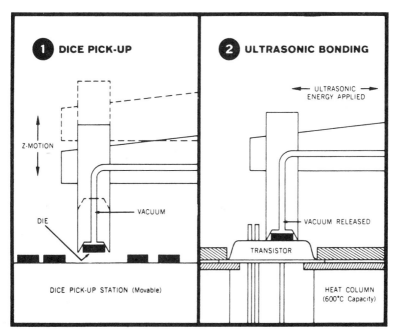

Figure 9-5 Chip bonding sequence. (Courtesy of Axion Corporation.)

A typical sequence of bonding is as follows:

1. The operator orients the chip under the bonding tip, utilizing the mirror surface of the chip storage tray.

2. The "Z motion" of the pickup tool is actuated with a hand or a foot switch. The tool lowers itself, and vacuum picks up the chip (by its edges). The pickup tool moves back up to position.

3. The operator slides the work column (heated stage) into position under the pickup tool.

4. The pickup tool is lowered into place by means of a switch. Upon contacting the substrate, a timed mechanical or ultrasonic scrub starts (usually in less than a second). The pickup tool continues holding the chip to the pad under pressure for a timed bonding period (usually several seconds).

5. When the bond cycle is finished, the pickup tool retracts, the operator slides or swings the heated stage away, moves the chip storage tray back under the pickup tool, removes the substrate with its bonded chip, loads the new substrate or package on the heated stage, and a new cycle starts.

The time required for making a bond varies considerably, depending on the degree of automation of the various movements and the skill of the operator. Most bonders can complete several bonds per minute under good conditions.

Solder Bonding. This is a technique sometimes used in hybrid IC operations. The basic approach is very similar to the gold-silicon eutectic bonding operation where preforms of gold-silicon eutectic were used. Other metal systems with lower melting temperatures can be utilized. Perhaps the most common is 80% gold/20% tin with a eutectic melting point of 280°C. Other solders could be used with melting points all the way down to the 183°C of 63% tin/37% lead eutectic.

Besides using preforms of the solder, other solder application methods are available. Reflow of pretinned pads and screen-printed solder application are both popular techniques in the thick film hybrid industry. Gold-silicon eutectic compositions can be screen-printed also—an approach that is often faster than placing individual preforms. (See the second part of this chapter for more information on soldering.)

What is an advantage of soft solders over the gold silicon eutectic—the lower melting temperature—can also be a disadvantage. Each packaging process has its temperature hierarchy, starting with the first operation at the highest temperature and finishing with the last and lowest temperature operation. To avoid upsetting the work of the previous operation, each successive temperature has to be lower (usually). A good general rule of thumb is that at least 50°C must separate each operation. Finally, the last operation should be at least 50°C (using the same rule of thumb) from the highest service temperature the finished device will see. Since many devices run 50°C or so above ambient (because they produce heat) and ambients can be as high as 125°C, choosing a low-temperature chip bonding solder makes it difficult or impossible to have many subsequent operations.

Chips that are bonded with solder (along with eutectic bonding, which is no more than a special kind of soldering) have the advantage of being easily removed. This is accomplished by simply bringing the package to the melting temperature of the solder. The chips then can be picked off the pad.

Glass Bonding. Glass is another material that can be used to bond semiconductor chips. It has three limitations, however. First, it is an electrical insulator, hence cannot serve where there must be an electrical contact between the substrate and the chip back. Second, it is not so good a thermal conductor, hence cannot be used if large amounts of power are to be dissipated. Third, the temperatures required for the bond are higher than in other bonding methods—approximately 500°C. Some semiconductor devices would experience degradation of their electrical performance at these temperatures. In spite of these limitations, occasionally glass can be used at no disadvantage. It is most often employed in high production situations where only one chip is to be bonded.

The substrate is furnished with the areas where the chip is to be attached coated with a screen-printed layer of glass. The substrate is heated in the work stage of a bonding machine, as described above, until the glass softens. The chip is then picked up and deposited on the soft glass.

Glass bonding also makes possible a good thermal expansion match, and some packaging schemes allow simultaneous bonding of the chip and attachment of the lead frame. (This was a popular approach with some of the high-volume, plastic-encapsulated, dual-in-line packages, although it is now more common to simultaneously use glass to attach the leads and gold eutectic bonding to attach the chip.)

Plastic Bonding. The fourth method of bonding silicon chips utilizes organic materials. Organic "glues" have not turned out to be unreliable, as might have been expected, and organic bonding (primarily epoxy materials) is relatively and increasingly popular. For many hybrid producers, this is the preferred technique.

The advantages of organic bonding are that (1) the process is relatively simple and straightforward, (2) the bonds are strong and reliable, and

(3) low curing temperatures can be used, thus avoiding the possibility of degradation of the active device's characteristics. The disadvantages are that organic materials have poor heat dumping capabilities and, when repair is needed, the chips are hard to remove.

Thermocompression bonding temperatures can damage plastic bonds; ultrasonic wire bonding is therefore more commonly used. Outgassing of some types gives trouble in hermetically sealed packages.

As already mentioned, epoxy is the most commonly used bonding material. It is very strong and will take high operating temperatures. It is applied by screen printing, by hand or automatic dispensing of small drops, or by the use of preforms. Metal fillers are often utilized to increase the thermal or to impart electrical conductivity.

Summary—Chip Bonding. Bonding of chips is comparatively straightforward (compared with some of the other packaging operations). Several good bonding methods exist, the gold-silicon eutectic and the epoxy bonding methods being the most popular.

WIRE BONDING

Making electrical contact from the metallized pads on the integrated circuit to the metallized pads on the substrate is a very important part of building a hybrid IC. About the only way to accomplish this (at present) is a rather laborious, one-at-a-time, stringing of fine aluminum or gold wires from the surface of the silicon chip to the substrate metallization. Because of the small size of the silicon chip, the wires used must be very fine (only about 1 mil in diameter). Thus the wiring is a very delicate job. One-at-a-time wiring (delicate or not) is just what ICs are supposed to get away from. It suffers from the main problems of one-at-a-time hand wiring: high expense (complicated by its delicate nature) and poor reliability. Wire bonding is the weakest step in the entire process of IC making. Fully half of all field failures come from wire bonding faults. There is much pressure to replace the present technique with something less expensive and more reliable. Approaches designed to eliminate fly wire bonding difficulties are discussed in the final section of this chapter.

CLASSIFICATION OF WIRE BONDING METHODS

Figure 9-6 shows the different kinds of wire bonding and the various configurations used. The terminology is often somewhat confusing. It is hoped

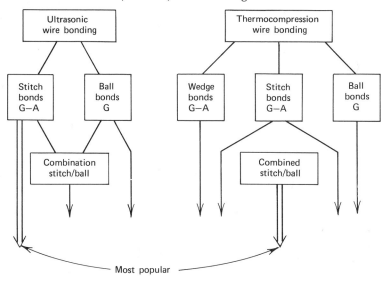

Figure 9-6 Wire bonding classification.

that the chart will help to remove some of the confusion. (The letters G or A that appear on the chart refer to the kinds of wire that can be used with the various bonding approaches—gold wire or aluminum wire.)

Wire Used. Gold or aluminum wire is used for bonding because both metals are soft and malleable. This property leads to high adhesion coefficients. Gold and aluminum are relatively compatible with package or substrate metallization (gold, palladium, platinum, etc.) and with chip metallization (aluminum) although we shall see that "relatively compatible" two-metal systems can also cause problems.

Thermocompression Bonding. This is the oldest technique and is probably the most popular today. The very name "thermocompression bonding" tells something about how the bond is made. When the gold or aluminum wire is placed on a metallized area of a heated substrate chip, the heat will soften the metal. Pressure, applied with a hard metal tool, causes the wire to deform and spread. With this deformation and spreading, plus the intimate pressure contact, surface oxides are broken, and the two separate metal systems are welded together. The temperature during bonding is about 300° to 90°C below the gold-silicon eutectic temperature, so that the eutectic bond is in no danger of melting. A thermocompression wire bonder is shown in Figures 9-7 and 9-8. Figure 9-9 illustrates TC bonding action.

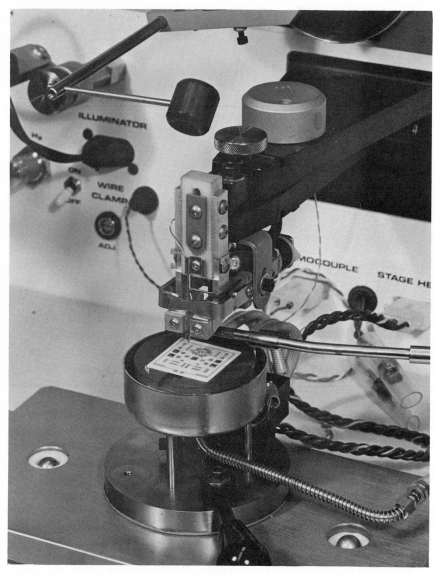

Figure 9-7 Thermocompression wire bonder—details of the work area. (Courtesy of Unitek Corporation.)

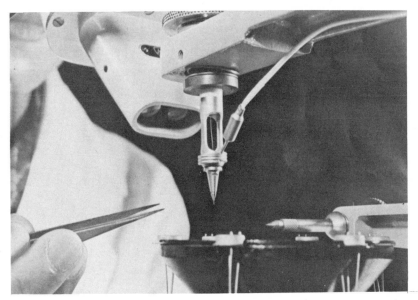

Figure 9-8 Another view of thermocompression wire bonder work area. Note capillary holding wire. Hydrogen cutting torch is on the right. (Photograph courtesy of Tempress Division, Sola Basic.)

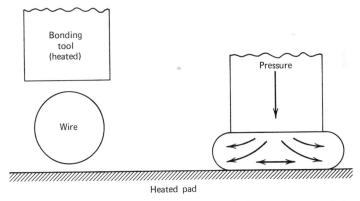

Figure 9-9 The thermocompression wire bond, showing how metal deformation takes place during the bond.

Ultrasonic Bonding. With ultrasonic bonding, the energy needed to make a bond is furnished by rapidly (ultrasonically) rubbing the wire against the bonding pad. Friction causes very high localized temperatures—enough to lead to melting and the formation of intermetallics. The major advantages of ultrasonic bonding are that (1) the chip does not have to be heated, so that there is no possibility of degradation, and (2) chips bonded by lower temperature solders will not be heated past the melting point of their bond. (Figures 9-10 and 9-11.)

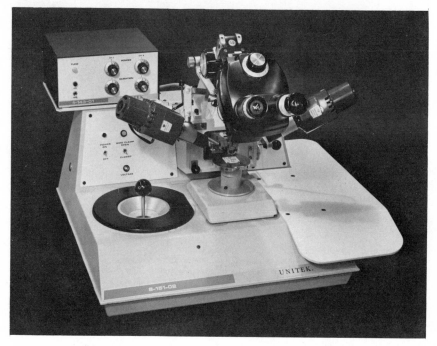

Figure 9-10   Ultrasonic wire bonder. (Courtesy of Unitek Corporation.)

Ultrasonic bonding is newer than thermocompression bonding, its development being prompted by some of the problems encountered with thermocompression bonding, such as the various "plagues" and device degradation caused by heating.

Aluminum wire is preferred to gold wire for ultrasonic bonding because it softens at lower temperatures. The thin oxide coating present on any aluminum surface is considered advantageous because it acts as a cutting medium to help remove contamination on the pad surface and increases friction coefficients (thus producing more localized heating).

Tool pressure is critical in ultrasonic bonding. It influences the resonance of the system. The ultrasonic transducer driving the tool must resonate in order to efficiently produce bonding energy. It is sometimes difficult to set and maintain proper resonant frequency. Some bonding equipment gets around this difficulty by sweeping through a frequency range, thus ensuring some time at resonance.

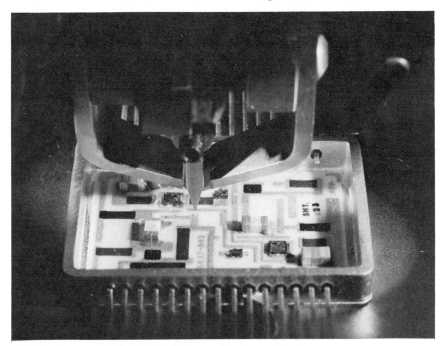

Figure 9-11 Close-up of an ultrasonic bonder at work on a hybrid circuit. Note that bonding is done after discretes have been soldered into place. (Courtesy of Unitek Corporation.)

Ultrasonic bonders offer clear advantages in some aspects but tend to be somewhat more difficult to set up and keep operating.

Wedge Bonding. The first bonders used separate devices to feed and hold the wire. The pressure needed to make the bond was furnished by a hard metal wedge that was brought down on the wire. This method has largely been replaced by ball and stitch bonding in which the tool for applying pressure is combined with the "capillary" wire feed tool. Wedge bonding is still used for very fine wires ($\frac{1}{2}$ mil). (Figure 9-12.)

Ball Bonding. Ball bonding takes advantage of an easy way to cut the wire after a bond has been made. The wire is passed through a hydrogen flame. The heat melts the wire. The molten metal forms a ball. This can be done with gold wire only (aluminum will oxidize, and ball formation is poor). (Figure 9-13.)

Figure 9-14 shows how a ball bond is attached to the pad on the silicon chip. As pressure is applied through the thermocompression bonding tool,

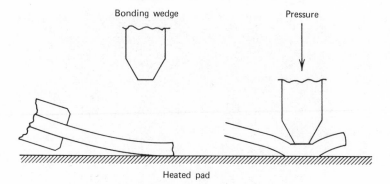

Bonding wedge

Pressure

Heated pad

Figure 9-12 Wedge bonding.

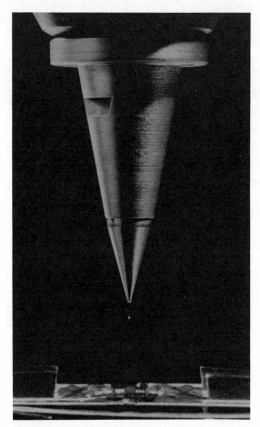

Figure 9-13 Close-up of a ball bonder's capillary with ball formed on the wire, ready to make the bond. (Photograph courtesy of Unitek Corporation.)

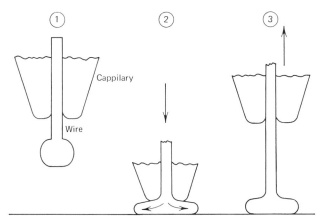

Figure 9-14 The ball bond.

the ball spreads out to about twice its diameter, and a very reliable bond is produced. Note that in the case of ball bonding, the tool (capillary) that applies the bonding pressure also feeds the wire.

Stitch Bonding. Stitch bonding is done with either gold or aluminum wire and with either thermocompression or ultrasonic bonding. The bonding tool/wire feeder (capillary) applies pressure to wire that protrudes from the end of the capillary. As the bond is completed, the wire deforms and widens along a length of approximately two to three wire diameters. When done properly, this type of bond is as strong and as reliable as the ball bond. A somewhat differently shaped bonding pad is needed, however, to accommodate the length of wire to be bonded (and for the small bit of wire that sticks out beyond the bond). An advantage of stitch bonding is that successive bonds can be made (as in making stitches with a needle). (Figures 9-15 and 9-16.)

Breaking Bonds. The normal way of breaking off the wire with a stitch bonder is to pull it apart. The wire breaks at the edge of the bond where there is a discontinuity in the wire diameter. This pulling force can sometimes disrupt a poor bond. It is possible to make two stitch bonds in a row so that only the second bond experiences the tensile pull.

Ball bonders use a stitch bond to make the second bond (on the substrate pad). After the stitch bond is made, the capillary feeder pulls back and a flame cut is made. This leaves a pigtail "flying in the breeze." (Figure 9-17.) These pigtails can be pulled off with tweezers. An alternate approach with the second bond of a ball bonder is to pull the lead off and *then* pass the

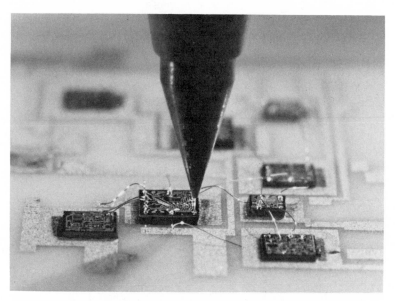

Figure 9-15 A thermocompression ball bonder making practice bonds. Note stitch bonds in center foreground. This bonder is equipped with an automatic "tail puller." (Photograph courtesy of Unitek Corporation.)

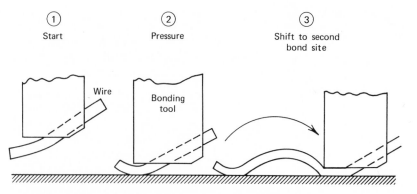

Figure 9-16 The stitch bond. The tool is shown in ultrasonic configuration.

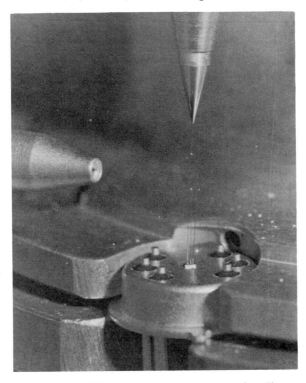

Figure 9-17 "Pigtails"—ready to be pulled. (Photograph courtesy of Tempress Division, Sola Basic.)

broken stub protruding from the capillary through a flame making a new ball for the next bond to the silicon chip. Ball bonders are always "hybrid" in that they use a combination of stitch and ball bonding. (Figure 9-18.)

Wire Bonding Equipment. All wire bonding equipment shares similar features.

1. Work Holders. A stage to hold the work. The stage is heated in thermocompression bonders and unheated in ultrasonic bonders. The work holder is connected to a micromanipulator so that the chip or substrate pad where the bond is to be made can be brought under the bonding tool.

2. Viewing Microscope. Binocular microscopes are essential because of the need for depth perception.

3. Wire Holders. A tool that brings the wire from a storage spool to the bond position. The "capillaries" of the thermocompression bonders have a shaped point so that they will accommodate either the ball or a wire

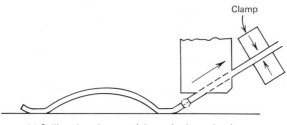

(a) Pulling the wire apart (ultrasonic shown here)

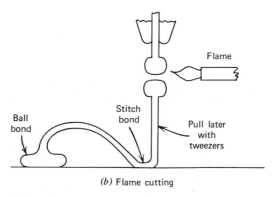

(b) Flame cutting

Figure 9-18   Breaking wire after the bond. (*a*) Stitch bonds (*b*) Ball bonds.

running off to the side for the stitch bond. The ultrasonic bonding tools take the wire through a small hole in the back of the tool. (Figure 9-19.)

4. Motion Capabilities. The vertical motions of a wire bonder are complex and precise. The micromanipulator first brings the chip *approximately* under the tool. For *final position* adjustment, the tool must be brought down to within a few mils above the bonding pad. Too far, and a ball is driven up the mouth of a capillary. If not far enough, close adjustment to proper final position is not possible. Complicating this is the fact that the "search height" varies alternately from the chip to the mounting post or to the substrate pad. Wire bonding machines have cams which automatically lower the bonding capillary to the proper "search" height. Since this search height must alternate from the first bond to the next, different heights are programmed on the cam.

Thermocompression Bonding Sequence. To illustrate the bonding sequence, a series of sketches is shown in Figure 9-20. The sequence illustrated is that of a thermocompression ball bonder with an automatic "tail puller"— probably the most common type of wire bonder used today.

The sequence for gold ball bonding is as follows (Figure 9-20):

1. Using X-Y manipulator, position work. Depress foot switch (a hand switch is located on the micromanipulator on many models) to lower wire ball to "sight" (or search) position.

2. Release foot switch. Heated bonding tip automatically descends, bonds ball to die, rises, and stops. Move work with micropositioner to second bond position.

3. Depress foot switch to lower bonding tip to search position over post of terminal. Release foot switch after final micropositioning adjustments are made—bonding tip descends and stitch-bonds wire to terminal.

4. Bonding tip rises to clutch position.

5. Wire clutch clamps wire. Bonding tip rises, breaking bond at second stitch bond, thereby removing pigtail.

6. Hydrogen torch sweeps flame through wire, forming a gold ball. Steps 3 to 6 are automatic—actuated by releasing switch.

Ultrasonic Bonding Sequence. The sketch series of Figure 9-21 shows the bonding steps made with a typical ultrasonic bonder. This type, together with the gold ball bonder, is the most popular type. Bonders operating with other wire materials or in different modes (as shown in Figure 9-6) are relatively rare.

The sequence of operation in Figure 9-21 is as follows:

1. Using X-Y manipulator knob in the left hand, position work below bonding tip. Actuate switch. Bonding head descends to #1 search position. After final manipulations are made, release switch to bond.

2. Position die under bonding tip with manipulator. Wire feeds through wire brake and bonding tip. Actuate switch to place tip at #2 search height. Release switch to bond when final position adjustments are made.

3. With bonding tip clamping wire on the die: the wire brake pulls the wire back to break it.

4. Bonding head lifts, then wire brake pushes wire through tip into ready-to-bond position.

An advantage of the ball bonder over the ultrasonic is that the bonder can go from the ball bond in any direction to make the second bond. With the ultrasonic bonder, one can leave the first bond site only in a direction in line with the directon of the wire—not off to an angle. This

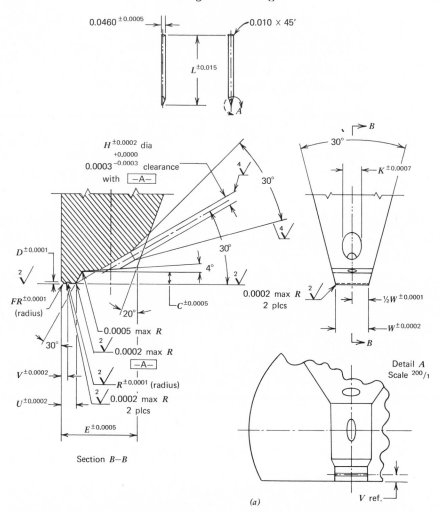

Figure 9-19 Bonding tools (capillaries). (*a*) Ultrasonic (courtesy of Tempress Division, Sola Basic). (*b*) Thermocompression bonding tool (courtesy of Tempress Division, Sola Basic.)

means the work must be positioned so that the second bond site is in line before the first bond is made. The micropositioner usually has a switch to rotate the stage to the proper position. The following scanning electron micrographs (SEM) illustrate dramatically both the ultrasonic wire bonding process and the thermocompression bonding process. We are *particularly* grateful for these fine photos. (They show the potential usefulness of SEMs in reliability studies, inspection techniques, etc.) (Figures 9-22 and 9-23.)

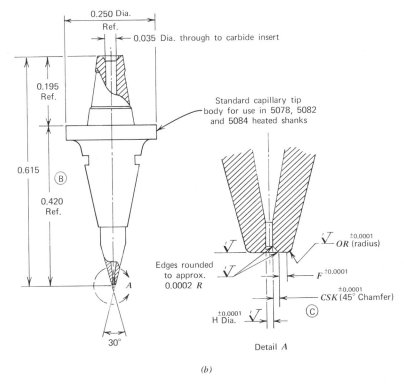

0.250 Dia.
Ref.

0.035 Dia. through to carbide insert

0.195
Ref.

Standard capillary tip
body for use in 5078, 5082
and 5084 heated shanks

0.615

Ⓑ

0.420
Ref.

Edges rounded
to approx.
0.0002 *R*

A

30°

$\overline{\nabla}$ $^{\pm 0.0001}$ *OR* (radius)

F $^{\pm 0.0001}$

$^{\pm 0.0001}$ *CSK* (45° Chamfer)

Ⓒ

$^{\pm 0.0001}$ *H* Dia.

Detail *A*

(b)

Figure 9-19 (Continued).

WIRE BONDING PROBLEMS

It should be no surprise that such a delicate an operation as placing 1-mil wires on pads only a few mils square has its problems. Remarkable progress has been made over the past few years in understanding bonding metallurgy and equipment refinement. Improving accuracy of the pressure applied, the accuracy of positioning the bond, and many other situations rooted in the mechanics of the equipment has greatly reduced problems such as broken leads, bonds that are not strong enough due to lack of pressure, weak leads because of too much pressure, and missed contacts. In spite of the progress, these problems still exist.

Wire bonding is a hand operation. Even in advanced production machines, each bond is placed one at a time by hand. There are semiautomatic aids, but even with these the wire bonding operation is subject to all the problems of human operation. It is quite expensive, both in labor costs,

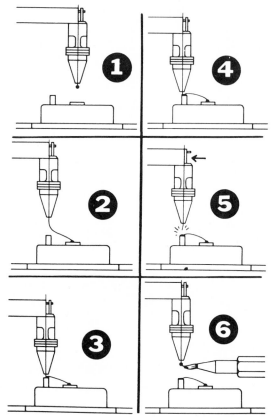

Figure   9-20 The   thermocompression   bonding
sequence. (Courtesy of Axion Corporation.)

and for equipment costs. (Highly automated wire bonders are available
for transistors and other high-volume applications, but are not yet ready
for hybrid operations.)

There are also metallurgical problems that must be faced. With gold
pads or posts on the package and aluminum metallization on the chip,
regardless of whether a gold or an aluminum wire is used, there will always
be one bimetallic joint. Gold-aluminum intermetallics that have undesirable
characteristics can appear. Probably the best known of these intermetallics
is known in the industry as "purple plague" (after the color of the compound AuAl). The color is harmless but replacement of the high ductility
gold or aluminum by a very brittle intermetallic, makes an unreliable bond.
Any flexing or movement of the wire, such as might occur in subsequent
processing, in shock and vibration testing, or in acutal use can result in

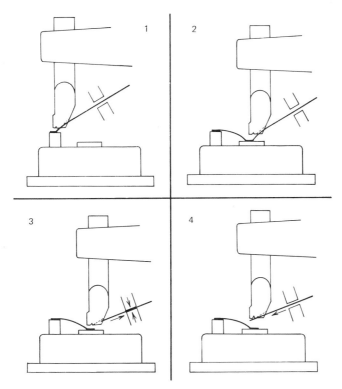

Figure 9-21 The ultrasonic bonding sequence. (Courtesy of Axion Corporation.)

a broken wire lead. There are other intermetallic compounds that can form besides purple plague—all of which result in brittle joints.

OTHER BONDING APPROACHES

We have outlined some of the problems of wire bonding. Tremendous progress has been made in the past few years, and the overall problems of wire bonds have been very much reduced. Even so, IC industry is still burdened with an expensive process which is responsible for about half of all field failures.

Because of this, there have been many attempts to replace chip and wire bonding with a more reliable and/or less expensive technique. At present there are several promising approaches, but none of them have

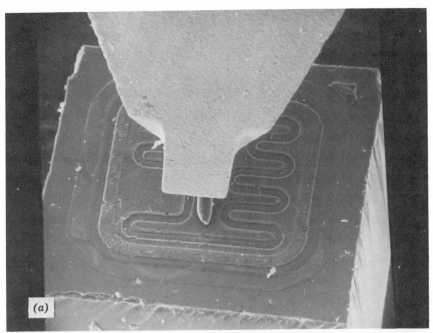

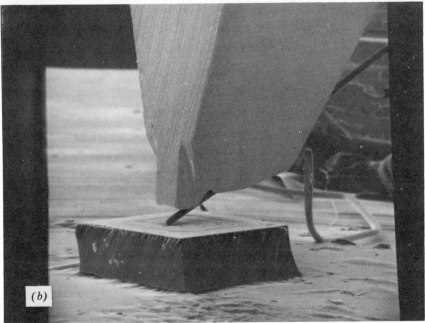

Figure 9-22 SEM photographs of an ultrasonic bond. (*a*) The ultrasonic tool over the silicon chip (150×). (*b*) Side view of ultrasonic tool and chip (70×) (ready to bond). (*c*) Side view of wire under the foot of the tool just prior to bonding (400×). (*d*) The ultrasonic bond (800×). (*e*) Enlarged view of one end of the ultrasonic bond. (Courtesy of Gaiser Tool Company.)

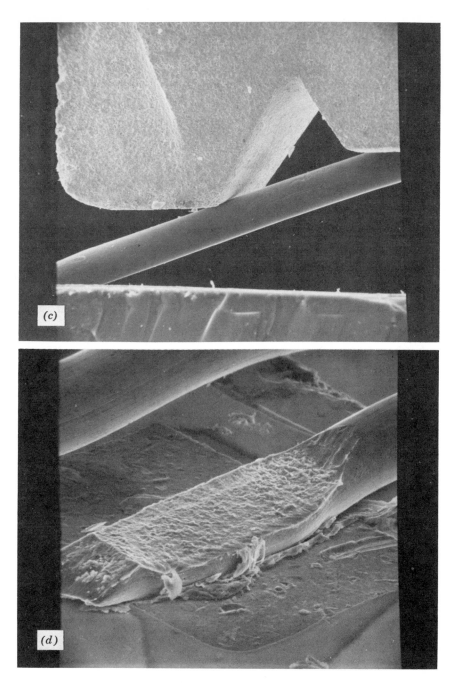

Figure 9-22 (Continued).

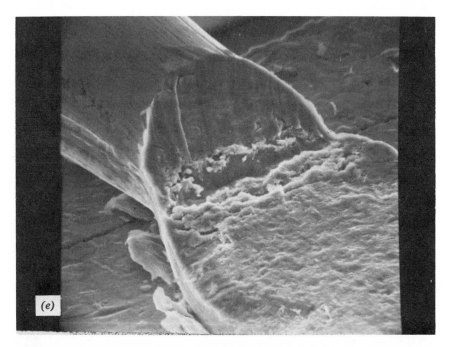

Figure 9-22 (Continued).

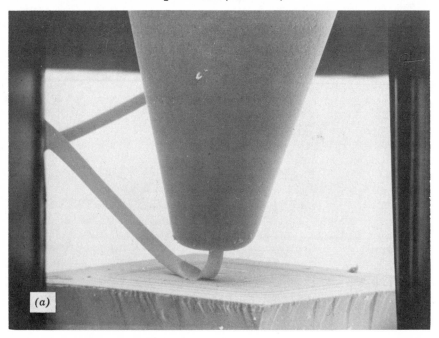

Figure 9-23 Three views of a thermocompression bond. (A bit too much pressure and/or heat here.) (a) 150×. (b) 400×. (c) 1800×.

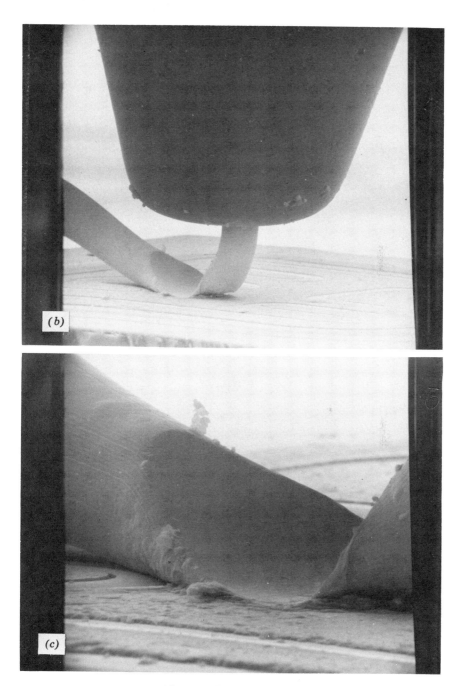

Figure 9-23 (Continued).

221

wide acceptance. They are unable to *equal* the cost of conventional chip and wire bonding in hybrid circuits, let alone result in a cost reduction (a major exception is IBM's in-house flip-chip system which has lower costs). Improvements in reliability *have* been achieved, however.

Most of the new approaches being developed today utilize a *face bonding* approach where the chip is turned upside down so that all the elements and their electrical connections are facing the substrate.

The connections to the mounting pads on the IC chip are all made during the final wafer processing steps. This eliminates half the individual bonds that would have to be made if fly wire bonding was used. All connections to the substrate are made simulatneously during bonding, and the remaining half of the individual one-at-a-time bonds are avoided.

THE FLIP CHIP

One of the earliest approaches to replacing the flying wire bond was the "flip chip." It gets around the one-at-a-time bonding of individual wires by placing metal "mesas" or "bumps" several mils high at the various pad locations on the silicon chip. The chip is flipped over on its face and lowered onto the substrate (over carefully located metallization areas that match the chip pad locations). It is then in a position where pressure or heat can be applied to effect a bond of all interconnects simultaneously. Figure 9-24 shows a transistor flip chip.

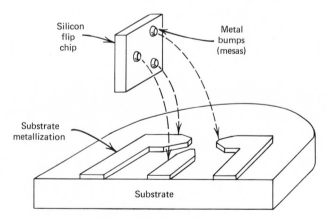

Figure 9-24 The flip chip.

IBM's Solderable Flip Chip. IBM pioneered one version of the flip-chip approach. It has been in very heavy production for some years. It represents just about the only "successful" production adaptation of flip chip as far as realizing production cost reductions. The SLT (solid logic technology) thick film circuits used in IBM's system 360 computers use flip-chip technology for bonding transistors and diodes. A new version (the "controlled collapse" technique) has been developed which will be used to bond complex IC chips.

The IBM flip-chip process starts with a glass-coated (passivated) chip. Holes are etched at the various pad locations to make electrical contact. Figure 9-25 shows the metallurgy of the completed flip chip, which features

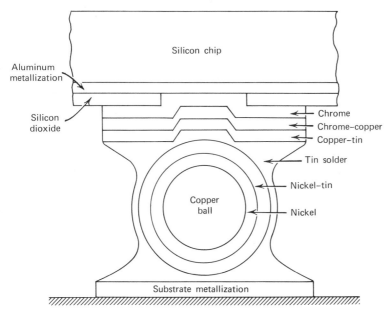

Figure 9-25 The metallization system in an IBM flip chip.

a copper ball resting in the hole. The ball is solder-coated so that when placed on a pretinned substrate pad it will attach itself by reflow. The effort required to develop this process was tremendous. To date its use is confined to IBM's internal needs. (Figure 9-26.)

Non-Solder Bumps. Other techniques for making bumps on a flip chip involve vacuum deposition or plating of mesas of aluminum or gold. Thermocompression or ultrasonic methods are used to bond this type of flip chip. The pressure required to make a good contact causes difficulty in that damage to the chip is possible (especially when there are many contacts

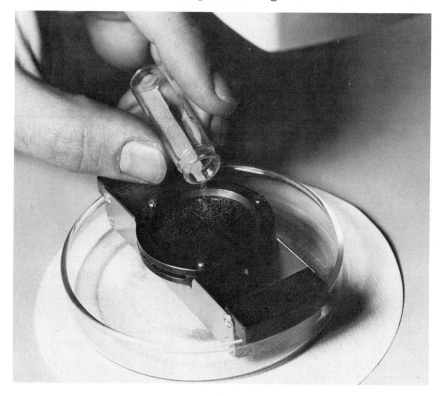

Figure 9-26 Pouring copper balls into locating jig over the silicon wafer. Shaking will cause a ball to drop into each location. (Photograph courtesy of IBM.)

to be made). The requirements for substrate flatness are also quite tight. These and other problems make the future of nonsolder flip chips doubtful.

"Controlled Collapse" Solder Bumps. Perhaps the most promising of the flip-chip approaches involves use of 100% solder bumps. This is the idea behind IBM's "controlled collapse" method. The technique has been recently embraced by others also. Solder is plated up over the contact holes in the chip's glass passivation. Upon heating the wafer, the solder pulls back into a spherical bump (Figure 9-27). When a "solder bump" chip is placed over its position on the substrate and heated, the solder bump melts and combines with a pretinned area on the substrate pad to form a molten column of solder. Surface tension forces of the molten solder pull the unit into exact location (very handy). The nonwettability of the passivated chip surface and of the untinned areas on the substrate keep

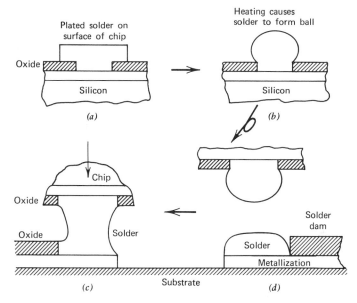

Figure 9-27 The IBM controlled collapse flip chips—100% solder bumps. (*a*, *b*) Forming the solder bumps. (*c*, *d*) Soldering to the substrate.

the chip elevated slightly and keep the solder of one bump from shorting out to the solder in another.

The controlled collapse flip chip technology is becoming increasingly popular. Several firms have developed systems based on this technique for in-house use. Some firms offering to build-up solder bumps "on your own wafer" have been established. (Figures 9-28 and 9-29.)

Advantages and Disadvantages. An advantage of the solder-type flip chips is that they can be easily removed. The ductility of the solder helps in taking up some of the stresses formed via thermal mismatch.

Face-bonded chips such as the flip chip are not efficient in dumping heat. Back-bonded versions transmit heat better because of the increased area connected to the substrate. Face-bonded chips also tend to allow localized hot spots, so that temperature tracking is not so good. (This is a disadvantage with both the flip chip and the beam-lead chip.)

The added processing steps used in making flip chips are expensive. Each step adds to the total processing cost of a wafer and adds to the total losses. To bring a wafer to a ready-to-bond condition (scribed and tested) in flip-chip version adds up to 50% to the cost of the same circuit

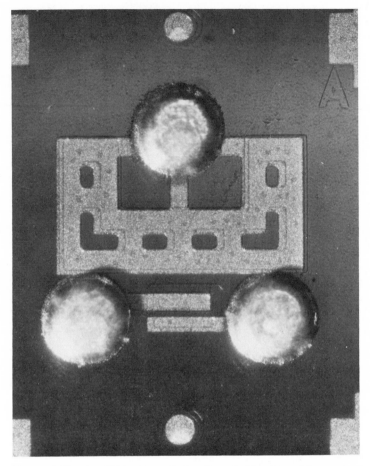

Figure 9-28 An IBM "controlled collapse" flip chip. (Courtesy of IBM.)

made for conventional chip and wire bonding. This is a serious cost disadvantage. Cost savings are possible only in very large operations. It is likely, however, that these costs will decrease and that relatively inexpensive solder bump flip chips will become available to the average user.

BEAM-LEAD CHIPS

The beam-lead chip is the second important approach to eliminating the flying wire lead. Western Electric pioneered the method. Beam-lead devices

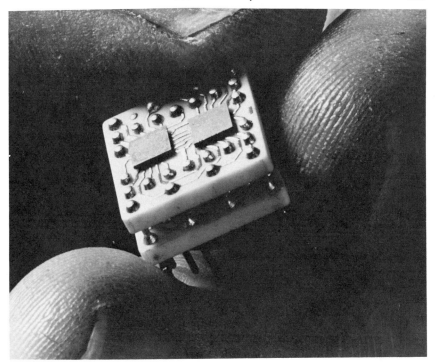

Figure 9-29 Complex IC chips attached via controlled collapse methods on thick film conductor arrays. This is a memory module for the main memory of IBM Sytsem/370 Model 145. This model has 696 memory circuits, replacing the same number of the more conventional ferrite memory cores. (Courtesy of IBM.)

have been chosen for the Safeguard ABM system. Several other IC houses (Texas Instrument, Motorola) that are Safeguard contractors have now developed capabilities in the technology. Raytheon has been offering beam lead devices in increasing variety to the general chip buying market and Texas Instruments announced first versions in 1971. At the time of writing this chapter (early 1971) the beam lead seems to be "winning" over the flip chip as a face-bonding approach available to small producers. Solder bump flip chip developments in the future may change this, however.

Beam-Lead Construction. Figure 9-1 shows the basic construction of a beam-lead chip. The chip is manufactured in such a way that heavy gold beams can be plated while the chip is still in the wafer form. The beams extend out over the edge of the functional area of the chip into nonfunctional areas on the wafer reserved for the leads only. The extra space needed is minimized by means of an interdigitating approach (Figure 9-30). The finished chips are separated from each other by etching the nonfunctional silicon away, leaving the exposed beams. Wafers used for beam leads are much thinner than back-bonded chips because of the back etching require-

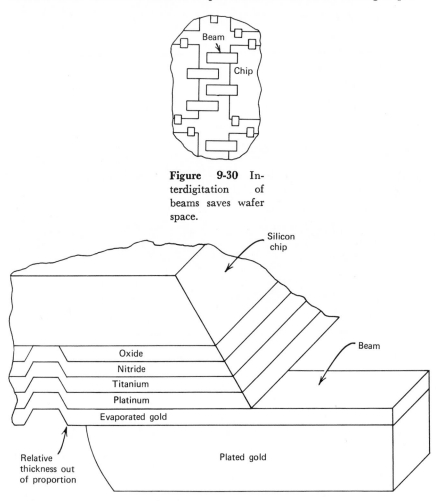

Figure 9-30 Interdigitation of beams saves wafer space.

Figure 9-31 Beam lead metallization details.

ments. The metallization steps of a beam lead device are as complicated as for flip chips. This can be seen in Figure 9-31.

Beam-Lead Attachment. Beam leads can be attached to the substrate by either ultrasonic or thermocompression methods. Thermocompression is the usual approach, however, because it is difficult to get a good ultrasonic bond with gold. Beam attachment is often done one at a time although machines that are able to make simultaneous attachment are now available.

The total pressure required for simultaneous beam attachment can be great, and the flatness requirements for the substrate very stringent without certain features of the bonding equipment that get around this. They make pressure contact to only one or two beams at a time by means of a "wobble" built into the bonding tool. The tool for bonding is cocked to one side so that bonding starts only in one area. As the tool "wobbles" around in a circle, pressure is applied successively to the rest of the beams.

Another beam-lead bonding technique receiving attention is *compliant bonding,* where high pressure is applied to an aluminum sheet that lies over the gold beams. The aluminum deforms, making a seal around the individual gold beams. Very uniform pressure (almost hydraulic in nature) is applied to each gold beam. Although not in wide use at this time, the compliant bonding has considerable promise—primarily because it promotes uniform bonding pressure to all beams, even on somewhat uneven surfaces.

The beams of a beam-lead chip are typically ½ mil thick, 3 mils wide, and 5 mils long. They are spaced on 10-mil centers. This compares to a typical flip chip's bump size of 4 mils—spaced on 8- to 10-mil centers.

Beam-Lead Advantages and Disadvantages. The beam lead can be attached without applying pressure to the chip itself—an advantage over nonsolder flip chips. The beams are visible, so that bonds can be inspected, which is not possible with flip chips.

The beam lead has the extra metallization and processing costs of the flip chip, and also takes up more wafer space; the basic cost of a beam lead chip therefore is probably more than twice that of the same chip made for back bonding. Beam-lead cost is somewhat higher than flip-chip cost.

The beams are quite fragile and are easily bent. Flexing of the beam can cause damage to the insulation between the beam and the silicon, promoting shorts (better handling methods are beginning to overcome this).

The beam lead shares some of the heat-dumping limitations of the flip chip. It is not subject to as many thermal mismatch problems (the beams can flex somewhat).

OTHER APPROACHES

IBM's in-house flip chip and Western Electric's in-house beam lead have been the only successful large scale applications of face bonding to date. Other large semiconductor firms have been at work—evaluating these approaches or developing others of their own. Two techniques that had been disclosed by 1970 are the "spider bonding" approach of Motorola and the "SDT" method of General Electric. Both are strictly in-house methods at this time and are of no more than academic interest to the smaller chip maker or buyer. Motorola has its development in production while GE's is still a laboratory approach. Other major semiconductor houses (GE, Fairchild, Signetics) announced development of their own systems in early 1971. They all use approaches somewhat similar to Motorola's spider bond.

Spider Bonding. Spider bonding is a special version of a beam-lead approach—one that is particularly adaptable to high production volume. Its most attractive feature is that it can use regular chips rather than special chips. According to Motorola (in 1970) the process requires production levels of over a million chips per month with the same pad locations to make it pay off. It is not advantageous unless more than 10 bonds per chip are used. Fewer than 10 bonds are less expensive if made with conventional chip and wire bonding methods.

Spider bonding starts with punching out a "spider"-shaped beam-lead pattern from a strip of thin aluminum sheet (Figure 9-32). The chips are then attached to the strip of aluminum by means of ultrasonic bonding.

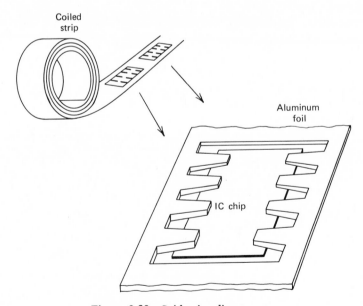

Figure 9-32 Spider bonding.

The chips can be stored at this step until ready to be punched out and bonded to the final package. (GE's "Minimod" system features mounting on 35-mm film; Fairchild's system uses solder bonding.)

The strips are fed into machines that can punch out the chip with its aluminum beams and attach it to the metal lead frame of a DIP. It is intended primarily for high-volume single-chip packages.

General Electric's "STD" Process. In 1970 GE released details of its STD (Semiconductor-Thermoplastic-Dielectric) process. It involves building metal risers over thick or thin film printed substrates, attaching chips via back bonding, laying a sheet of thermoplastic material—fluorinated ethylene propylene (FEP)—over this and applying heat and pressure. Then holes are etched in the FEP so that the risers and the chip faces are exposed (using photolithographic methods). A gold metallization is finally deposited over the top of the plastic and the interconnect pattern is made by conventional etch methods. (Figure 9-33.)

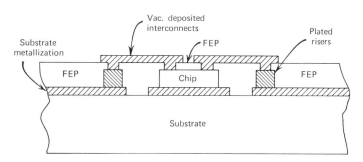

Figure 9-33 GE's STD bonding.

STD has the advantages of not requiring special chips and of using back-bonded methods that give better heat-dumping capabilities and better element tracking. There are probably problems in making good etches through the plastic, in the plastic-metal and plastic-semiconductor interfaces, and in achieving good alignment on enough substrates at one time to make the process economical. If these production problems are overcome, the method holds much promise.

Beam Lead Substrates. Another approach, designed to get around the specially prepared chips required for flip chip and beam lead techniques involves plating beams on the *substrate* rather than on the chip. The chip rests in a hole in the substrate. The chip is first attached to a metal backing (good thermal conductivity) and the substrate with its beams is lowered over the chip. Normal thermocompression bonding is used to make the bond (Figure 9-34).

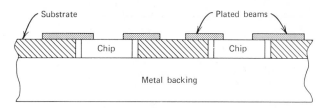

Figure 9-34 MIT's beam-lead substrates.

This process—pioneered at MIT—has the advantage of using the more readily available and less expensive standard chip, but adds a lot of expense to the substrate. It is not clear if the economics of approaches such as this would be attractive.

A similar approach is to bond the chip in a depression in a substrate, fill the surrounding empty volume (the moat) with plastic, and finally plate the entire substrate face to make a metal interconnect pattern.

Summary—Newer Bonding Techniques. None of the new techniques are available to the average chip buyer and to the small semiconductor house. The only methods in production are those developed for private in-house use by large makers of ICs. The most successful has been IBM's flip chip.

In an interesting paper given at the 1970 ISHM Conference in Los Angeles, Kirby of Welwyn Electric relates how a thick film producer set up its own semiconductor production facility and is economically producing solder bump flip chips for internal use. What many feel is possible only in *giant* corporations is apparently becoming practical in much smaller operations. This type of development will probably become more common.

The great majority of today's bonding is done with standard chip and wire techniques. With all its reliability problems—chip and wire are still surprisingly reliable—especially when compared with discrete component methods. In spite of the high costs the IC "revolution" continues. The consensus today is that chip and wire bonding will continue to be the leading bonding approach through much of the next decade.

Table 9-1 is taken from the DuPont *Thick Film Handbook*. It summarizes some of the strong points and weak points of the various bonding approaches.

Table 9-1 Comparison Chart of Face Bonding and Back Bonding

Characteristics	Conventional	Flip Chip	Controlled Collapse	Beam Lead	Spider Bond	STD	Beam-Lead Substrate
Chip cost	Low	High	N.A.	High	Low	Low	Low
Reliability	Good	Excellent	Excellent	Excellent	—	—	—
Chip availability	Excellent	Poor	None	Poor	Excellent	Excellent	Excellent
Bonding cost	High	Low	Lower	Low	Lower	—	—
Bond inspection	Yes	No	No	Yes	Yes	Yes	Yes
Mounting pressure	Some	Heavy	None	None	Some	Some	None
Compactness	Poor	Excellent	Excellent	Good	Fair	Excellent	—
Power handling	Excellent	Poor	Poor	Poor	—	Excellent	Excellent
Tracking	Excellent	Poor	Poor	Poor	—	Excellent	Excellent
Thermal mismatch	Fair	Poor	Fair	Good	—	—	Fair
Special substrates	No	Sometimes	No	No	No	No	Yes
Equipment or processes readily available	Yes	No	No	No	No	No	No
Repairability	Fair	Poor	Good	Good	—	—	Poor
Bond strength	Fair	Strong	Strong	Fair	Fair	—	OK
Chip ruggedness	Excellent	Excellent	Excellent	Fragile	—	Excellent	Excellent

Soldering

Soldering is a method of attaching one metallic materal to another. It has been in use in the electronics industry for some time. Because of its familiarity and because it is a very good way to "stick" things together, soldering has found wide application in thick film hybrid circuits. (Figure 9-35.)

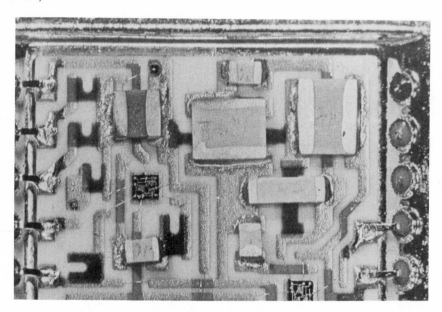

Figure 9-35 Discrete chip capacitors soldered onto a thick film circuit. (Photograph courtesy of CTS Corporation.)

There are two kinds of soldering—" hard soldering" and "soft soldering." Hard solders melt at red heat (also called brazing). Soft solders melt at much lower temperatures. Soft solders are generally soft and ductile, and the hard solders much less so. Our discussion is limited to soft solders.

Soldering starts with heating the parts to be joined past the melting point of the solder. The molten solder then flows, "wetting" the two metal surfaces. Upon cooling back to a solid, the solder holds the two parts together. Since it is a continuous system, electrical resistance is low, so that solder joints are good electrical conductors.

To make a good soldering joint, solder must (1) successfully "wet" the two metals at a temperature low enough so that the materials being joined

are not damaged; (2) it must meet several electrical and physical requirements (such as having strength, low resistance, and enough ductility to
compensate for thermal expansion mismatches); and (3) it must not cause
damage to the joined materials, either during or after soldering. The solder
system must also meet certain economic demands.

WETTING

Soldering consists of joining two metal (or metal-coated) pieces together
by melting a low temperature metallic material between the two pieces
that are to be joined. It is somewhat like gluing two items together, except
that the glue is a metal alloy rather than an organic material.

To get adherence between the solder and the metal, *wetting* must occur;
that is, the molten solder must *wet* the surface of the metal that is to
be soldered. For wetting to occur, there must be a clean surface so that
nothing is between the molten metal and the material that is to be soldered.
Close metal-to-metal contact (obtained with wetting) is necessary to get
strong bonds. The bonding forces come from unsaturated surface bonds
on the surface of the solid metal system. These molecules or atoms must
be able to present themselves *directly* to molten solder.

The degree of solder wetting can be measured by observing the area
over which a drop of solder spreads. Figure 9-36 shows three degrees of

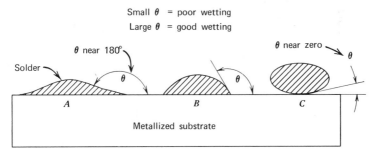

Figure 9-36 Various degrees of wetting. *A*, "good" wetting; *B*, "fair"
wetting; *C*, no wetting.

wetting. In the "good" wetting example, the solder spreads over a large
area. One can think of the unsaturated bonds as *pulling* the molten solder
over ever-increasing areas. In the "in between" example, the "pulling"
done by the available unsaturated bonds is in equilibrium with the opposite
surface tension "pull" of the molten solder. In the "no wetting" example,

surface tension reigns supreme and the "pull" of the unsaturated surface bonds has no effect whatsoever—perhaps because of a film of dirt between the metal and the solder. Wetting will not occur with materials that do not have atoms or molecules at the surface with unsaturated bonds—as for instance oxides.

FLUXES

Fluxes are materials that remove contamination from the surface of the material to be soldered so that wetting can occur. The same unsaturated bonds that will "attract" molten solder molecules will also attract other materials. Most metals under average conditions will collect a thin layer of oxides or tarnishes. These films must be removed so that the process of wetting can proceed. The surface of a metal can also be covered with dirt or grease. Fluxes do not generally remove dirt and oil films, but solvent dips or washing prior to fluxing will remove these materials.

What Fluxes Must Do. Fluxes break up and remove the tarnish layer on the metal surface either by chemical combination or by chemical reduction.

Fluxes also have to protect the surface of the metal *during* the soldering action. At soldering temperatures, oxides will form on unprotected surfaces. The flux must have properties such that it (1) not only removes the oxide that was originally on the surface, but (2) *continues* to keep the surface clean until the solder has melted and flowed over the fluxed surface.

One of the limitations placed on fluxing action is that it cannot be too strong. Fluxes are to remove *only* the oxides and tarnish, not to eat into the metal. They should not be dangerous to personnel. Fluxing action should not continue *after* soldering is completed. No reactions are desired with anything but the tarnish on the metal before, during, or after soldering.

Flux Removal. Although most fluxes are relatively nonreactive after soldering (the heat of soldering serves to deactivate them), it is considered good practice to carefully remove any flux remnants. This is especially true in microcircuit applications.

Types of Fluxes. Three types of fluxes are used in thick film hybrid circuit operations: (1) rosin fluxes, (2) activated rosin fluxes, and (3) gaseous fluxes. (It is also possible to do soldering *without* fluxes if extreme care is taken to clean the components and to keep them clean during soldering. Fluxless soldering is employed to seal flat packs with gold-tin solder so as to avoid the possibility of flux getting inside the sealed package.)

Rosin fluxes are the most common type of flux used in thick film hybrid circuits. "Water white" is the grade usually used. Water-white rosin is made up of a combination of abietic acid and pimaric acid. It is solid at room temperature, melting between 150° and 200°C. Upon melting, the abietic acid will attack metallic oxides, forming a metallic abiet that is soft and "crumbly" and lifts off the surface of the metal very easily. The molten rosin keeps the metal surfaces covered *during soldering,* giving protection from reoxidation. Upon cooling, the rosin hardens again. It is a fair insulator. In noncritical conventional circuits the flux is sometimes left on the soldered joints to act as an insulator, but this should never be considered in thick film circuits. Rosin flux is soluble in many organic solvents and removal is quite easy. Rosin flux is not a strong flux and works only on comparably clean surfaces. Most thick film circuits can be soldered easily with plain water-white rosin fluxes.

For the few instances where plain rosin is not strong enough (as in soldering parts that have been in storage a long time) an *activated* rosin flux can be considered. The activated fluxes contain various chemical addatives (acids and/or halogens) that become highly corrosive at soldering temperatures. An example of an activated flux action would be one that contained an organic halogen. Upon heating, the activator breaks down, one of the products formed being gaseous hydrochloric acid. The strongly corrosive action of the hot acid will attack surface oxides and tarnishes much more violently than will the abietic acid of the plain rosin flux. Since the activator breaks down into gaseous components upon heating, there are (theoretically) no remnants of the activator after soldering. If the soldering cycle is fast, however, all of activator might not have a chance to decompose. Any unreacted flux remnants left on the circuit could in time have a strongly corrosive effect. If an activated flux is needed in a thick film operation, extra care should be taken to make sure there are no remnants left on the circuit.

Gaseous fluxes leave no remnants of any kind and they are extremely strong in their action. Hot hydrogen or forming gas are popular gaseous fluxes. The strong reducing action of the hydrogen reduces a metallic oxide or tarnish back to its original metallic form very rapidly. A problem in using this type of flux with thick film circuits is that many thick film materials, and many discrete devices used on thick film circuits, are very susceptible to reduction. Palladium oxide resistor compositions, for instance, will reduce to palladium metal, making short circuits in the place of resistors. Multilayer ceramic capacitor chips and certain high dielectric constant screen-printed dielectric compositions will partially reduce, giving capacitors that have high dissipation factors and low insulation resistance. Gas fluxes are rarely used in thick film soldering operations, but are often used in die bonding of active devices. If this is the case, the thick film producer must be sure to use nonreducing thick film resistor compositions or protect the resistors by overglazing.

Other fluxes such as inorganic and organic acids, or inorganic salts, are rarely employed in thick film operations.

SOLDER METALLURGY

Kinds of Solder Available. There are many different solder systems used in thick film. Table 9-2 lists several that are in use today. Of all the items listed the various tin-lead system solders are the most widely used. The tin-lead eutectic alloy is the most applied of the tin-lead systems.

Table 9-2   Common Thick Film Solders

Solder System	Plastic Point °C	Flow Point °C	Used For
98% gold–2% silicon	—	370	Chip mounting
88% gold–12% germanium	—	356	Chip mounting
80% gold–20% tin	—	280	Chip mounting and package sealing
97½% lead–2½% silver	—	304	Device mounting
95% lead–5% tin	300	315	Device mounting
96½% tin–3½% silver	—	221	Device mounting
63% tin–37% lead	—	183	Device mounting
62% tin–36% lead–2% silver	—	179	Device mounting

Source. A. R. Kroehs, *Bonding Alloy Placement and Device Attachment by the Use of Metal/Chemical Systems*, Alpha Metals, Inc., 1969 ISHM Proceedings, p. 71.

With a wide choice of alloys available, soldering temperatures can be chosen to give added process flexibility. For instance, a popular solder for attaching ceramic multilayer capacitors is the 95% lead-5% tin. With its 300°C freezing point, it is possible to attach the package lid or to solder leads on with a lower melting point solder without disturbing the capacitor bond.

Tin-Lead Phase Diagram. Figure 9-37 shows the lead-tin phase diagram along with its eutectic (the lowest melting point). Eutectic solders are

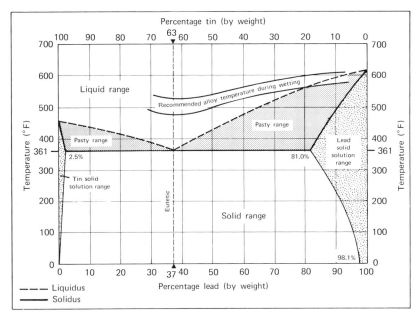

Figure 9-37 Tin-lead phase diagram. (Courtesy Alpha Metals, Inc.)

very desirable over noneutectic solders because the transformation from molten to solid is instantaneous. With noneutectic combinations, there is a "pasty" or a "slushy" range where the solder is part molten and part solid. If the parts being soldered move while in the "slush range," the bond can be damaged (by allowing a void to form in the solder):

SOLDER CONTAMINATION

It is possible to contaminate solder systems with other metals. When this occurs, the properties of both the melt and the final solid system will change. The most common result is to get intermetallic compounds (two-metal compounds) that give the solder a slush range, increase the brittleness of the solid solder, and often raise the melting point. Any of these reactions can degrade the effectiveness of a solder operation.

Silver leaches (dissolves) in tin-lead solders very rapidly. It makes the solder somewhat more brittle, especially when present in levels of several percent. The problem in soldering silver is not so much that the solder joint degrades but that the supply of silver will be exhausted because of the rapidity with which the silver moves into the solder melt. With silver thick film conductors this occurs so rapidly that, in order to avoid excessive leaching, the solder can be molten only a few seconds at temperatures only a few degrees about the liquidus temperature.

Gold intermetallics also form rapidly in tin-lead solder, seriously damaging solder joint quality. Gold-tin intermetallics produce a very brittle solder joint. Gold is not a good material to use for soldering because of this.

Thick film conductor compositions of palladium-silver alloys or platinum-gold alloys greatly slow leaching rates. There is little or no leaching problem with most thick film soldering operations when these alloys are used. (See chapter 7 for conductor performance characteristics during soldering.)

SOLDERING METHODS

Solder Iron. This is sometimes used in thick film hybrid circuits—a carry-over from discrete component assembly practice. Procedure is very much the same except that small irons and fine solder wire are used. It is not a particularly popular method except in repair situations, being slow, unwieldly, and often damaging to the devices being attached.

Solder Reflow. The most popular method today in thick film is solder reflow. Solder is first put on the circuit conductors and on the component to be soldered by dipping the parts in a solder bath. The component is then placed in its proper position on the thick film circuit, held in place by a bit of flux (which is sticky). On heating the solder *remelts* or *reflows* and the part is soldered into place. The flux serves to float off any solder dross that may have formed on the surface of the pretinned parts and substrate. Jigs or weights are sometimes used to hold the parts in place if they have a tendency to shift during soldering. Solder tinning of conductors is often used to ensure high conductivity of long, narrow conductor runs.

Preforms. Small shapes can be stamped out of thin sheets of any solder compositions. These preforms can be placed on the substrate where a device is to be soldered. After the preform is placed, the part to be attached is placed. This can be done on heated substrates, or on cold substrates (heating is done later). Use of preforms is limited primarily to active-device bonding operations and to sealing packages.

Screen-Printed Solder. This is a newer development that has much promise as a thick film soldering method. Finely ground solder and flux are combined with proper vehicles to make a thick film screening ink or paste. This can be screened on the substrate using a pattern that places the solder in only the areas where it is wanted (dipping will coat all conductors unless they are covered up with a solder resist). In order to get enough solder on the substrate, a heavy mesh screen (80-mesh) is used, backed with a metal mask or an extra thick emulsion. The components that are to be attached can be added before the solder paste dries. A short bake hardens the solder paste and the circuit can be handled without dislodging the discrete components. Placing the circuit on a hot plate or running it through a continuous oven will melt the solder. (Figure 9-38.)

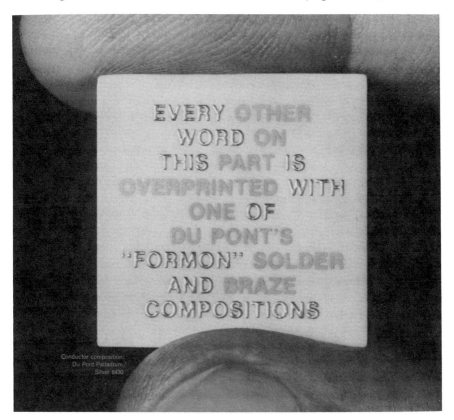

Figure 9-38 The capabilities of screen-printed solder paste. (Photograph courtesy of DuPont.)

The advantage of this type of soldering is that it is compatible with other thick film operations, it is fast and inexpensive as far as labor is concerned, and it lends itself to automatic placement of passive discrete devices. It will undoubtedly play an important role in thick film—especially in high-volume operations.

Chapter 10

DISCRETE DEVICES FOR THICK FILM CIRCUITS

Active Devices

In years past, thick film hybrid circuit manufacturers experienced considerable difficulty in obtaining unencapsulated active chips for their circuits. Miniature plastic packaged transistors and diodes were readily available, but inexpensive compatible packages for silicon ICs were not.

There were many reasons why enencapsulated chips were not available, ranging from a reluctance on the part of the semiconductor manufacturers to sell the chips to firms they viewed as competitors to the fact that encased chips are not easy to test and ship.

The pressure to sell chips in their unencapsulated form was too much for the semiconductor manufacturers to resist, however, and by 1970 unencapsulated active chips had become widely available. The pressures that brought about the improved availability of chips to thick film hybrid makers included suggestions by large customers that continued "foot dragging" in selling chips might result in loss to more cooperative sources of conventionally packaged semiconductor device business, as well as the recognition by progressive semiconductor marketers that here was a potential market that offered possibilities for added profits and growth.

In early 1969 buying active chips was difficult, especially for smaller producers without "clout." By 1970 the "dam had broken," and almost any chip could be obtained from any manufacturer, albeit varying degrees of enthusiasm between different semiconductor suppliers could be noted. By 1971 availability had improved even further. The semiconductor makers were now fully convinced that marketing chips was indeed a highly desirable activity. Marketing channels have improved to the point that various standard active chips are even being stocked by local distributors. Semiconductor producers today are eagerly marketing a wide variety of transistors, diodes, and monolithic ICs in chip form.

Limitations on Active Chip Testing. Static tests on active devices are usually made while the chip is still in the wafer form. These tests are conducted automatically. Bad chips are marked, and after the wafer is broken into individual chips, the rejects are removed.

Dynamic tests on active devices *cannot* be performed in the wafer form. Semiconductor firms are not usually prepared to conduct dynamic tests on separated chips. Dynamic tests done on the chip can be misleading because the performance of a finished device is often affected by the mounting method and the package design. Device performance depends on lead length, lead placement, shielding, and many other things that have nothing to do with chip itself.

Because of testing difficulties the hybrid producer must learn not to specify active chips as though they were the familiar old leaded components. Most chips are bought with *no* dynamic tests performed. (If tested, they will be very expensive. The semiconductor maker will not have good ways of conducting dynamic tests short of mounting the device in a temporary package, running the tests, and then disconnecting the chip.)

Asking for *special* tests is not recommended, but if necessary most suppliers are willing to run special static tests in place of their standard tests, provided they are within the capabilities of their test equipment. Charges for special tests are determined on a "negotiated basis" (which usually means an extra charge).

Getting "Special" Chips. Most semiconductor houses offer their most popular devices in chip form. The majority are willing to negotiate to furnish any of the less popular devices they produce, although these will probably not be as inexpensive—unless a very large purchase is to be made. Most semiconductor firms will also be happy to talk about producing a device in chip form that is *not* part of their regular product line, but such custom specials can be very expensive. Asking for special devices, not normally offered in chip form, should be avoided. To avoid longer delivery and higher prices, make certain that another supplier does not offer in chip form what you are looking for.

Packaging Active Chips for Shipment. Chips are shipped (1) in bulk, (2) in plastic carriers, or (3) in wafer form.

Bulk shipment is not a recommended method of shipping chips unless slight damage would not be objectionable and the user is willing to spend extra time in orienting. The user may also have problems in returning damaged chips if they are shipped in bulk. Bulk shipment of chips is sometimes accomplished by putting the chips inside a closed end straw and inserting the bent straw inside a pill vial. Small amounts thus packaged will shift around less. Up to 1500 small chips can be placed inside such a straw.

Plastic carriers (Figure 10-1) are the recommended method for shipping discrete active chips. Several sizes of carriers are available, with capacities ranging from ten chips to a thousand or more. Each chip is held in the carrier, metallized side up, so they can be visually inspected through the transparent top of the carrier without opening the carrier (provided the manufacturer does not paste a label over the face of the carrier).

Chips shipped in the wafer form offer many advantages to the user. The user can opt for purchasing the unscribed wafer, packed in individual boxes (Figure 10-2). The unscribed wafer can be either unprobed or probed (with the rejects marked). The wafer can also be furnished scribed and broken. The broken chips are packed, held in place in a vacuum-sealed plastic bag. This is more economical than shipping in carriers and is just as safe. However, the user must do visual inspection himself. A price must be negotiated, usually based on a minimum yield, since the producer has removed none of the visual or the electrical rejects.

Figure 10-3 shows the final steps in processing active chips. The ways in which chips can be packaged are also indicated. Seminconductor makers are usually willing to sell chips with any degree of testing and sorting.

The wafer form, for those firms capable of scribing and testing them, is a very economical way of obtaining active devices (it is also a way of hanging on to the last bit of value added). Chips in the wafer form are often more available because most of the testing and shipping problems need not be worked out.

Incoming Inspection of Active Chips. When hybrid circuit producers start to buy silicon chips, a large part of the manufacturing process formerly the responsibility of the semiconductor house is shifted to the hybrid manufacturer. The hybrid maker will want to inspect carefully the incoming chips for visual defects and subject a sample of the lot to electrical tests to make certain that the producer has sorted to specification. If chips are purchased in wafer form, they will have to be inspected by trained inspectors to cull out all the many mechanical and visual defects that can occur.

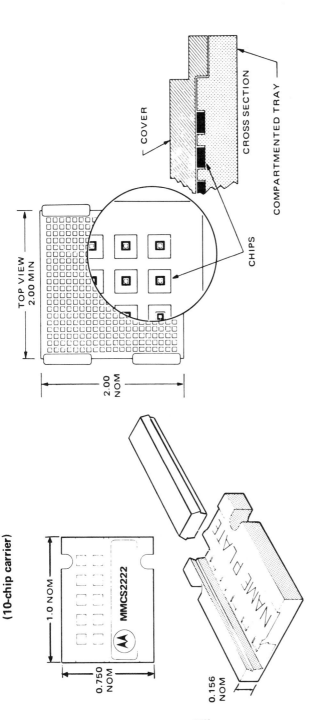

FIGURE 2 – MULTI-PAK

COVER

CROSS SECTION

COMPARTMENTED TRAY

CHIPS

TOP VIEW
2.00 MIN

2.00
NOM

FIGURE 1 – DEKA-PAK

(10-chip carrier)

1.0 NOM

0.750
NOM

MMCS2222

0.156
NOM

NAME PLATE

The Multi-Pak carrier is designed for production use. Two versions are available, one holding 400 small chips, and one holding 100 large chips such as those used for power transistors. All of the carriers are 2 inches square, and are vacuum sealed before shipment.

To accommodate the customer with limited quantity requirements, the Deka-Pak carrier contains individual compartments for 10 chips.

Figure 10-1 Plastic carriers for shipping silicon chips. (Courtesy of Motorola, Inc.)

245

WAFER OPTIONS

Motorola unencapsulated transistors may be obtained in wafer form. The information in Table II gives the various specification verification and packaging options.

TABLE II – Specification Options

WAFERS	Shipping Options
1. Sample probed. Guaranteed minimum yield.	See Figure 6
2. 100% probed. Rejects inked.	See Figure 6
3. 100% probed. Rejects inked, scribed and broken. Wafer is placed between two sheets of mylar or filter paper and vacuum sealed in a plastic bag.	See Figure 5

FIGURE 5 – PLASTIC BAG SHIPMENT SCRIBED

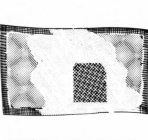

Wafer is 100% probed. Rejects inked, scribed, and broken. Wafer is placed between two sheets of mylar and vacuum sealed in a plastic bag.

FIGURE 6 – WAFER SHIPMENT (UNSCRIBED)

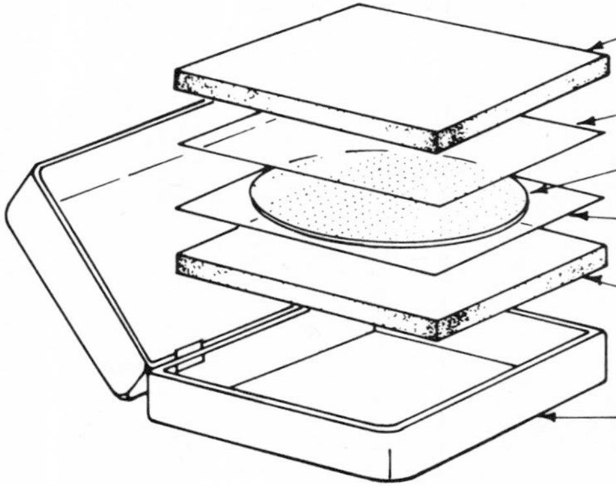

FOAM

MYLAR

WAFER

MYLAR

FOAM

PLASTIC BOX

Wafers are shipped between two layers of mylar, sandwiched between two layers of polyfoam pressed together in a plastic box. This prevents movement or damage to the wafer.

Figure 10-2 Shipping containers for wafers (scribed or unscribed). (Courtesy, Motorola, Inc.)

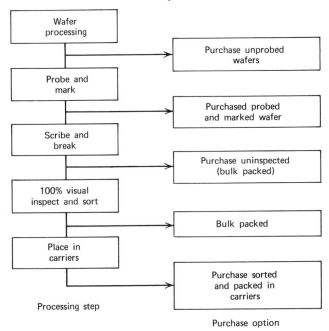

Figure 10-3 The various purchase options available for active devices.

This is a much more involved procedure than is simple incoming inspection for scribed and sorted chips.

It is not the purpose of this book to go into detail on active device inspection criteria; but we are happy to give the reader a hint as to what is involved, quoting from the 1970 Motorola chip catalog which describes the recommended visual inspection procedure. It shows that inspection and testing can be an involved procedure and also suggests the kind of sorting that must be done if one is to become involved in buying wafers instead of chips. The passage below is quoted with permission of Motorola, Inc.

VISUAL INSPECTION

Definition of Terms

Emitter-Base and Collector-Base Junctions. The region where the base and collector, and the emitter and base meet. These junctions will be defined on the surface of the chip as an oxide step.

Diffusion Window. The opening etched through the oxide to permit the diffusion of the emitter and base.

Active Junction. A change in "N" type to "P" type doping or conversely, by a diffusion step. On discrete transistors, there are two active junctions, the collector-base junction and the emitter-base junction.

The Pre-Ohmic Window. The opening etched through the oxide for metalization contact to the emitter and base regions.

Pre-Ohmic Alignment. The positioning of the oxide opening into which the metalization is placed.

Passivated Region. Any region covered by glass (SiO_2), nitride, or other protective dielectric.

Expanded Contact. Any pattern that has metalization crossing a diffused junction.

Attached Foreign Material. A foreign substance that cannot be removed when subjected to a nominal gas flow. Lint, silicon dust, etc., are not considered attached since they can be removed after die mount.

INSPECTION CRITERIA

Visual inspection is performed with a microscope using 40X–80X magnification for Silicon-Power Chips and 100X–125X for other devices.

Scribing Defects

Excess Chip. A chip shall be rejected if a portion of an adjacent chip with metalization is still attached to subject chip.

Scribe Line Limits. A chip shall be rejected if a scribe line touches or crosses an active junction area or a metalized region.

Mechanical Defects

Inspect each chip to insure there are no cracks or breaks that:

Non-Expanded Contacts
    (a) Touch the collector-base junction (NPN).
    (b) Extend through the annular ring (PNP).
Expanded Contacts
    (a) Touch the collector-base junction (NPN).
    (b) Extend through the annular ring (PNP).
    (c) Extend under any metalized bonding pad.

Inspect each chip to insure there are no cracks greater than one mil in length in a passivated region and extending toward an active area. (Does not apply to Silicon Power devices.)

Alignment Defects

Pre-Ohmic Alignment. The chip shall not contain pre-ohmic windows that cross the edge of a diffusion window.

Diffusion Window Alignment. No diffusion window shall touch another diffusion window.

Metalization Alignment. The metalization must be aligned so that at least 50% of the pre-ohmic window is covered with metalization.

Foreign Material Defects

Bridged-Across Metal. A chip shall be rejected when attached foreign material bridges across normally separated metalized areas.

Particle Size Inside Active Area. A chip shall be rejected when attached foreign material greater than 2 mils is found inside collector-base junction or on the emitter-base bonding pads.

Oxide Defects

Exposed Silicon on Junction. A chip shall be rejected if exposed silicon touches or crosses the collector-base junction or the emitter-base junction.

Exposed Silicon Touching Metal. A chip shall be rejected if exposed silicon touches or extends under the bonding pad metalization. (Expanded contacts only.)

Oxide Defect in Active Area. A chip shall be rejected if an oxide defect occurs inside or on the collector-base junction with a major dimension greater than 1 mil. (Does not apply to Silicon Power Devices.)

Oxide Defect Crossing or Touching. A chip shall be rejected if gross oxide defects, evidenced by alternately colored bands (rainbow effect), emit from two separate ohmic contacts and either touch or cross each other; or cross the collector-base junction.

Oxide Defect Under Bonding Pads. A chip shall be rejected if an oxide defect extends under 25% of the bonding pad.

Metalization Defects: Expanded Contacts (Finger Geometries)

Missing Metalization on Bonding Pads. A chip shall be rejected when 25% of the metalization is missing from a bonding pad.

Metalization Width at Oxide Step. Any chip shall be rejected if the metalization width of any finger is reduced greater than 25% at any oxide step. 75% of the metal width must remain.

Metalization Width in First 50 Percent of Finger. A chip shall be rejected if the finger metalization is narrower than 50% of its original design width or if the finger width is reduced greater than 50% due to a severe scratch or void in the first 50% of the finger. A severe scratch is one which exposes the underlying surface.

Fingers Isolated or Missing. A chip, shall be rejected if any finger is not 100% continuous over the first 50% of the finger (from the bonding pad).

Bubbled Metalization. A chip shall be rejected if it exhibits any bubbled metalization on a bonding pad.

Lifted Metalization. A chip shall be rejected if it exhibits any lifted metalization. Slight undercutting causing a lifted appearance is not cause for rejection.

Bridged Metalization. A chip shall be rejected for bridged metal shorting any two normally separated metalized areas.

Metal Corrosion. A chip shall be rejected if it exhibits any corroded metal. Corrosion is a chemical reaction or process causing abnormalities in the metalization. A rough metalization surface is not to be considered corrosion.

Metalization Effects: Nonexpanded Contacts

Missing Metalization. A chip shall be rejected when more than 25% of the metalization is missing from a bonding pad.

Lifted Metalization. A chip shall be rejected if it exhibits any lifted metalization. Slight undercutting causing a lifted appearance is not cause for rejection.

Bubbled Metalization. A chip shall be rejected if it exhibits any bubbled metalization on a bonding pad.

Bridged Metalization. A chip shall be rejected for bridged metal shorting any two normally separated metalized areas.

Narrow Metal Widths in Relation to Design Width. A chip shall be rejected if the metalization is narrower than 50% of its original design width.

Metal Corrosion. A chip shall be rejected if it exhibits any corroded metal. Corrosion is a chemical reaction or process causing abnormalities in the metalization. A rough metalization surface is not to be considered corrosion.

Metalized Annular Ring

Missing Metalization. A chip shall be rejected when a metalized annular ring is not 100% continuous.

Bridged Metalization. A chip shall be rejected for bridged metal shorting the metalized annular ring with any other metalized area.

RECOMMENDED INCOMING INSPECTION PROCEDURES

Motorola assures that the devices will meet the customers' incoming visual inspection when inspected to the visual criteria and LTPD limits specified in the data sheet. Inspection must be performed at the power and magnification indicated. Motorola guarantees dc parameters to LTPD limits specified in the data sheet.

Returned Components

It is suggested that the customer perform incoming inspection in the following sequence:

1. Visual.
2. Test dc electrical parameters.

A. If the lot fails visual inspection, containers must be closed and secured and the entire lot returned to Motorola with a detailed inspection report. In no case will Motorola accept rejected material that the customer has inspected 100%.

B. After the lot has passed incoming visual inspection, samples are selected and subjected to electrical tests of the dc parameters. If samples do not pass the electrical tests, they shall be packaged separately and identified with all the information from the original package of chips. The shipping container must be closed and secured. The entire lot together with the test samples and a detailed inspection report shall be returned to Motorola. In no case will Motorola accept rejected material that the customer has inspected 100%.

Face-Bonded Chips. Face-bonded chips are not so universally available as back-bonded chips. In 1970 and 1971 some standard beam-lead devices became available to the public, first from Raytheon and then from Texas Instruments. Flip chips are largely unavailable in 1971 except as negotiated special purchases, although several firms will furnish these on special orders (primarily solder bump versions). Face-bonded devices, although much used internally by large semiconductor houses (increasingly so) are not generally available to the hybrid circuit maker unless he is involved with heavy usage.

Minicomponents. Another way to use discrete transistors is in the form of minicomponents. The various configurations, several of which are illustrated in Figure 10-4, offer relatively compact packages, thus avoiding the problems (just discussed) of buying and handling uncased chips.

Small IC flat packs can be easily attached to thick film hybrid circuits.

The variety of devices available in minicomponent packaging is somewhat limited, and often the device package (usually plastic) is not always compatible with the package used by the hybrid manufacturer. They are, however, fairly economical, and one can avoid bonding equipment investment. They are also often available at the local distributor—another advantage.

Lids. Another configuration that many users find attractive is the leadless inverted device (LID). The LID is no more than a miniature package

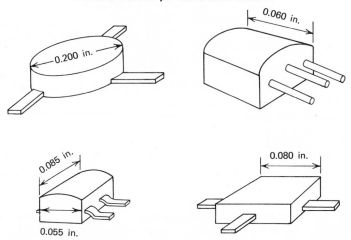

Figure 10-4 Miniature transistor packages suitable for mounting on thick film hybrid circuits as discretes.

especially designed for use in hybrid circuits. Figure 10-5 shows the basic configuration of the LID. LIDs are purchased with the transistor mounted in the LID, covered with epoxy. The hybrid user mounts the LID via reflow solder (in exactly the same way as he would mount ceramic chip capacitors). The major advantages of this configuration are compatibility with other thick film discrete-device mounting methods, ruggedness, and the fact that very small hybrid firms do not have to invest in bonding equipment. They are often used where extensive preassembly testing is needed. The LID is easily replaced. A major disadvantage is that the LID is expensive, compared either to standard minicomponents or to encapsulated chips.

SUMMARY—ACTIVE DEVICES

Almost anything the user needs is available in back-bonded chips—from simple diodes to the most complex IC. Producers of chips are usually willing to perform special DC tests. Dynamic testing of unmounted chips in difficult.

The chip user will find that buying and using unencapsulated chips is quite different from buying conventional active devices. Incoming inspection is considerably different, with different electrical tests and added visual inspection.

An opportunity to push for more value added is available through purchase of devices in the wafer form, but the user has to add scribing and breaking capabilities, and more inspection skills are required.

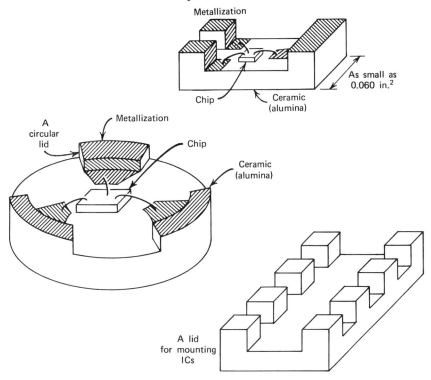

Figure 10-5 Leadless inverted device (LID) configurations (The drawings are not to relative scale.)

Face-bonded devices are becoming available, but are still (early 1971) not *widely* available.

Minicomponents and LIDs often are an attractive source of active devices, especially to the low-volume user or to the firm just getting started.

Passive Devices

Reprinted below is the major part of a paper given by the coauthor Donald W. Hamer at the 1971 IEEE Component Conference at Washington, D.C. It addresses itself to the *reasons* for using passive devices in thick film circuits rather than using thick film technology to make the same components, and thus fits very well into this part of the text. The passages are reprinted by permission of IEEE.

THE USE OF PASSIVE CHIP COMPONENTS IN HYBRID INTEGRATED CIRCUITS

Summary. This paper looks at the reasons a hybrid integrated circuit manufacturer would have for using passive chip components in his designs, rather than using thick or thin integrated circuit technology for fabrication of these elements. Emphasis in this analysis is placed on resistors and capacitors (rather than *all* types of discrete components) and on chips (rather than on minicomponents and other leaded devices).

Introduction. Most supplier literature, published papers, and trade journals articles on passive chips are devoted to describing construction and operating characteristics of various components. This paper covers a somewhat different area: it is an analysis of the *reasons* for using chip components.

Why would a thick or a thin film producer want to turn to discrete chips when he has at hand his own film technology with which to make capacitors and resistor elements? This paper will look at some of the rationale behind making decisions about when to abandon IC film elements for discrete components, or conversely, when to abandon use of chips in favor of making the component via film IC technology.

Chip components are being used sometimes when a careful inspection of the economics involved would argue against use of chips. There are also instances when film elements are made when use of chips would be preferable.

The Reasons for Using Chips. Thick film and thin film technology allows the fabricator IC to make a wide variety of high-performance precision resistors and capacitors—so why use a chip component—especially when it is rather "expensive"?

The situation is different with resistors, as compared to capacitors. This means that a somewhat different process will be followed in deciding when to use resistor chips as compared to that used to decide when to use capacitor chips. The differences arise from the fact that film capabilities versus chip availability for one type of component/element is greatly different from that for the other.

Film Resistors versus Chip Resistors. Thick and thin film IC resistor technology is "strong." Excellent performance capabilities can be realized and trimming capabilities make precision values easily obtainable. On the other hand, the resistor chips commonly available do not offer significantly different characteristics (indeed, thick or thin film technology is usually used to make the chips). In addition, purchase price and mounting labor usually make the chip approach rather "expensive."

Use of discrete resistors in either thick or thin film should be a special situation. The best approach is to assume that the resistors in the circuit will be made by the hybrid film technology—and to look for those special situations where chips are more attractive.

Film Capacitors verus Chip Capacitors. The situation is exactly reversed in the case of capacitors as compared to resistors. Chips of superior operating characteristics are available in a wider range of values, at prices that are usually not so high as are those of chip resistors. At the same time, film technology for capacitors is (at present, at least) not so strong. The characteristics are not so good, close tolerances are not always available because of undeveloped trimming techniques, and high values take up too much space.

Use of discrete capacitor chips in thick or thin film integrated circuits is, therefore, the rule. The fabricator will assume that he will be using chip capacitors and will then look for the special situations where using film technology would be more attractive. This is the opposite situation from that which exists with respect to resistors.

Looking for the Exceptions to the General Rule. There are, of course, times when chip resistors should be used and times when, contrary to the general practice, screen printed or vacuum deposited capacitors are more attractive than chips.

The reasons for using chips instead of film elements can be categorized as follows. Chips are often used (1) because the operating specifications cannot be met otherwise; (2) because they save space; (3) to repair a finished circuit; (4) for convenience, as in breadboarding; (5) to save money.

If a situation fits into one of the foregoing categories, purchase of a chip is preferable to making the circuit with film elements.

To Meet Specifications. There are times when the thick or thin film versions of resistors or capacitors are not able to meet all the performance requirements. The circuit maker then has no choice other than to turn to chips (or to conventional discrete components).

Capacitors. Although film capacitors are fairly good, they often cannot meet the performance requirements such as temperature coefficient, Q, or tolerance.

The multilayer ceramic chip is able to outperform the thick or the thin film elements in many respects—flatter temperature coefficients, higher Q, and so on. Since capacitance trimming is not a widely used or available technique in either thick or thin film hybrid operations, close tolerance requirements often can be met only by use of discrete chips. A large portion of the total usage of ceramic multilayer capacitor chips takes place because the film technologies cannot meet performance requirements.

Resistors. Both thick and thin film IC resistors have excellent performance characteristics. Most discrete chips use either thick or thin film technology in their manufacture, so that there is little to be gained by going to a chip. Thick film circuits can take advantage of some of the lower noise capabilities of thin film chips, and perhaps temperature coefficient also— although the thin film chip makers seldom list standard specifications that indicate their product is significantly different from thick film chip characteristics.

Chip resistors are not commonly used for reasons having to do with inability of the film technologies to meet specifications.

To Save Space. It is probable that more chip capacitors are sold for this reason than for any other. Both the multilayer ceramic capacitor and the tantalum chip are extremely compact.

Chip resistors are also at times used to save space. The situations where this need exists are not frequent, but they do come up often enough to support considerable effort on the part of the chip makers to make very small resistor chips.

Resistors. Thick film chips are often used in thin film hybrid circuits to save space. A thin film resistor of very high value will need considerable length (and will have to do a lot of meandering) in order to reach a high value. Even with thin film's capability of producing narrow lines, too much area is often required for high values. The availability of high sheet resistance materials in thick film allows high values to be produced in only a few squares that will easily fit on a relatively small chip. Megohms and up are readily available in thick film chips only 50 mils square.

Low resistance values can be obtained easily in thin film on a very small chip—20 mils square. Such chips are smaller than can be easily made using thick film techniques, so that there is some opportunity for space saving in thick film hybrid circuits by using a small thin film chip. This situation is not particularly significant, however; most space-saving of resistor chips is concentrated in the use of high resistance value thick film chips in thin film circuits.

Capacitors. The use of capacitor chips to save space is much more widespread than the use of resistor chips for this purpose. The space efficiency of the multilayer ceramic capacitor is made evident in Table 10-1, which compares capacitance values attainable in a given area by several different techniques. For over 2000 pF thin film capacitors use too much space. Thick film makers can use screen-printed high-K compositions up to perhaps 10,000 pF, but then they also have to use chips. For high-performance capacitors, thin film technology is quite effective and is often able to avoid use of discrete chips except for bypass-type applications.

The most important reason for use of chip capacitors is that they save space.

Table 10-1   Comparison of Space Efficiency in Various Capacitor Technologies

Capacitance Available in 5000 mils² (0.050 × 0.100)

Ceramic Multilayer Chip		Thin Film (Silicon Oxide)	Thick Film	
K1200	NPO		K800	Low-K
39,000 pF	1000 pF	1000 pF	5000 pF	150 pF

For Repair Purposes. If a circuit is close to completion, especially when active devices are in place, substitution of a chip resistor or capacitor for a bad film element is usually preferable to throwing the whole circuit out. Overtrimmed resistors and shorted capacitors are the most common reason for using repair chips. A problem that often comes up in these situations is that it is usually difficult to find a place to mount the repair chip. Properly placed mounting pads may not be available.

The number of chips used for this purpose is not large, although the savings they offer to a hybrid manufacturer can be significant.

For Convenience. In this category are several situations where chips are used as a matter of choice. The choice is not always a wise choice.

Breadboarding. It may be convenient to use chip components for breadboarding—even if the final version of the circuit will use screen-printed or vacuum-evaporated elements. Chips made of the same material (i.e., thick film resistor chips) will allow performance of the breadboard circuit to be more true to the final version than would be the case if discrete leaded parts from other functional materials were to be used. The total number of discrete chips sold for this reason is low.

Processing "Convenience." Usage in this category is considerable. Passive chips are often employed to allow the producer to use a preferred process or to avoid a process in which he is not fully capable.

Many chip capacitors are utilized even when screen-printed versions would be more attractive merely because the producer has not mastered the various techniques needed to produce screen-printed thick film capacitors.

IC manufacturers specializing in circuits that are primarily monolithic often have no thick film capability or soldering capability. For these firms silicon substrate chip resistors and capacitors are convenient because they can be bonded eutectically. Standard wire bonding techniques are used to make the electrical connection.

Using chips because they are convenient from a processing standpoint is a practice that should be questioned, except when done as a stopgap measure. The economics of fly wire bonding on purchased discrete chips that could just as well be made using film technologies is not encouraging.

The back-bonded chips, connected by wire bonding techniques, can be quite small. When space must be saved, this design is attractive.

To Save Money. Discrete chips are relatively expensive. The average chip costs approximately 20¢. Chip resistors, although they are inherently very inexpensive to produce, generally cost more than chip capacitors. The reason probably is that the chip resistor is not used to the same extent as the more complex chip capacitor. If really high usage were to develop (not likely), the selling price of the chip resistor (either thick or thin film) could come down to only a few cents.

Elements made by film technology are (or can be) much less expensive than present-day chip prices. Precision thick film resistors can be produced for less than a penny each and thick film capacitors for only a few cents each. Thin film resistor or capacitor elements are more expensive to produce than are the thick film versions, but are still much less expensive than discrete chips. A resistor or capacitor produced by film technology, as part of a hybrid IC, can be produced at costs similar to what mounting alone would cost for a discrete chip.

How, then, can chip resistors and capacitors be used to save money if they cost so much more than the film versions?

There are two general situations where a chip component could be used to replace a film version for economic reasons: (1) in short production runs and (2) when only one or two elements can be made at one time.

Short Runs. It is obvious that if a production run is very short, it would be less expensive to buy a few chips than to pay for the artwork, screen or mask, and the setup labor involved to produce the screen-printed or vacuum-deposited circuit elements. Figure 10-6 shows this situation. The

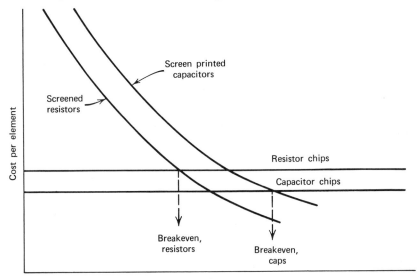

Figure 10-6 Relative costs of discrete chip resistors or capacitors and screen-printed resistors or capacitors as a function of the length of the production run.

cost per component drops very slowly for discrete chips (only volume purchase discounts working). For integrated elements, the costs start at very high levels, but come down rapidly as the tooling cost is spread across a longer production run. The breakeven point is farther out for resistors than for capacitors because of the higher prices for resistor chips and the less costly IC production costs. It the production run is long enough, it is almost always less expensive to produce film versions of resistors. Film capacitors have to "struggle harder" to beat out discrete chips. Some of the high values (where lots of substrate space is used) never become less expensive.

Multiple Elements. Another important factor in the cost of resistor or capacitor film elements is the number of elements that are to be made at the same time. Variable costs are relatively independent, in film ICs, of the number of elements made—no more labor is needed to screen-print ten resistors than to screen-print only one. (There *is* a variable labor cost for trimming resistors and capacitors, however.)

Also, fixed costs can be spread when more than one element is made at the same time. The costs of screens, masks, setup labor, and so on, are mostly independent of the number of resistors or capacitor elements to be processed at any one time.

Figure 10-7 shows this cost structure. Unless the production run is very long, making only one capacitor or one resistor per screening (or evapora-

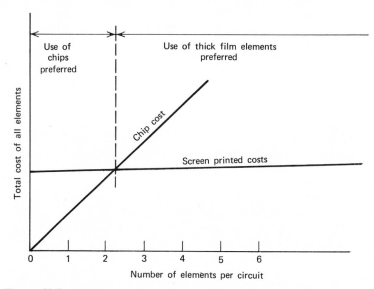

Figure 10-7 Relative costs of discrete chips and screen-printed elements as a function of the number of elements (components) per circuit.

tion) is seldom attractive when compared to the cost for discrete chips. However, if two or three elements can be made at the same time, the advantage shifts toward use of film elements. For several or more, the cost advantage for film elements is very clear.

Other Kinds of Chips, Other Discrete Forms. There are so few other kinds of chips available that an analysis of these has not been included. Because of limited inductance capability in film elements, almost all inductors are *forced* to be in the discrete form.

For discrete forms other than chips, that is, minicomponents, the same rationale would apply as has been given here for chips.

Summary. Table 10–2 shows the situations in which resistor and capacitor chips are employed and the relative amount of the chips used in the industry in the various categories. Most usage occurs because chips are the only way specifications can be met. Many chip capacitors are used to save space, others to save money. Still other reasons exist, but they are of more im-

Table 10-2   Relative Usage of Chip Components in Hybrid ICs

Reason for Using a Chip	Type of Chip*				
	Thin Film Resistors	Thick Film Resistors	Ceramic Caps	Tantalum Chips	Film Capacitor Chips
To meet specifications	M	L	VH	L	VL
To save space	ML	Nil	VH	M	Nil
For repair	L	L	L	L	VL
Breadboarding	L	L	L	L	VL
Back bonding, etc.	M	L	L	Nil	ML
To save money	M	M	MH	Nil	Nil

* M = medium, L = low, H = high, V = very.

portance, in sales volume, to the fabricator of ICs than to the chip producer. More chip capacitors are used than chip resistors.

The discrete chip is filling an important need and will continue to be used in large numbers by the hybrid IC industry.

WHAT IS AVAILABLE IN PASSIVE DEVICES

Figure 10-8 illustrates the most common configurations of discrete passive components: (1) chips used for wire bonding attachment, (2) chips for soldering, (3) "beam lead" type components, and (4) minicomponents.

Passive Devices Compatible with Wire Bonding. Some resistor and capacitor chips are marketed that can be back-mounted (by soldering, epoxy, or eutectic bonding) to the substrate and then connected electrically with the same wire bonding techniques that are used for the active chips. The very small area needed for some values of thin film resistors and capacitors makes fabrication on a silicon substrate (hence eutectic bondable) quite practical. This configuration is attractive for firms that do not have soldering capabilities, or want to avoid soldering, although there is seldom any economic advantage—the chips are expensive and labor costs for bonding are high compared to other chip attachment costs.

Passive Chips for Reflow Soldering. Most passive chips are in this configuration. The multilayer ceramic capacitor can easily be fabricated so that the terminations are on the ends of the chip (Figure 10-10b). Resistor chips also can be made in this manner. The chips can be purchased pre-tinned so that reflow soldering is readily accomplished.

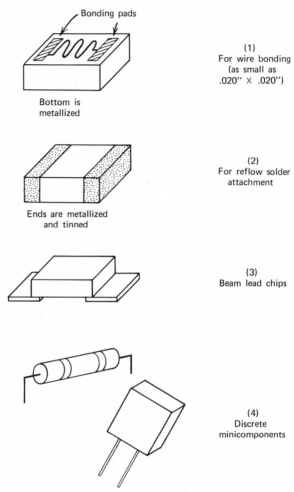

Bonding pads

(1)
For wire bonding
(as small as
.020" × .020")

Bottom is
metallized

(2)
For reflow solder
attachment

Ends are metallized
and tinned

(3)
Beam lead chips

(4)
Discrete
minicomponents

Figure 10-8   Common configurations for discrete passive
components used in thick film hybrid ICs.

Beam-Lead Passive Chips. Some tantalum chips are furnished in this
configuration so that they can be either soldered or welded to the substrate.
The beam-lead configuration is not popular otherwise.

Passive Minicomponents. There are a wide variety of passive devices that
are available only in a minicomponent version. While not totally compatible
with thick film circuits, a minicomponent often represents the only way
a circuit's needs can be met. If this is the case, the user can go ahead—even
if mounting the component requires a substrate with holes for leads. Sub-

strates with holes are available without paying crippling tooling charges, so that the overall cost penalty is not necessarily high.

Some firms use too many minicomponents and thus make their thick film designs (except for a few resistors) something that is little improved from a conventional discrete circuit. Others get overinvolved with seeing how far they can embrace the newer technology, and ignore the "handiness" of the minicomponent. Either of these two extremes is bad.

Types of Capacitors Available. Four types of discrete capacitors are used in thick film: (1) ceramics—the most versatile, the least expensive, and overwhelmingly the most popular; (2) thin film chips—small and rather expensive; and (3) tantalums—only recently available in chip versions designed specifically for hybrid application (very useful for higher capacitances).

Ceramic Chip Capacitors. The miniature ceramic capacitor (the multilayer types, sometimes called "monolithic" ceramic capacitors) have aggressively adapted themselves to use in a hybrid circuit and at present have most of the business. Almost any ceramic capacitor that is available with leads is available in chip form. There are many sizes made especially for use as chips. Of all the components types that have been "threatened" by ICs, the miniature ceramic capacitor has been the least affected—partly because its configuration made it easily adaptable for use in hybrid ICs and partly because screen-printed capacitors are limited in their capability.

Figure 10-9 illustrates the variety of sizes, capacitance range, and performance that is available from multilayer chip capacitors. The versatility and volumetric efficiency of the ceramic capacitor have been major factors in their usefulness in thick film hybrids.

Thin Film Capacitors. Silicon monolithic technology can be used to make tiny chips of silicon supporting an oxide capacitor. Up to 50 pF is available on a 20-mil chip. Mounting is done with conventional eutectic and wire-bonding methods. Small thin film chip capacitors are also available on alumina chips. The low values, high cost, and sometimes high assembly cost keep the film chips out of the category of high usage (and the low usage, in turn, keeps the costs up).

Tantalum Capacitors. High values of capacitance have, until recently, been unavailable in chip configuration. It was usually necessary to mount such capacitors outside the hybrid circuit along with other bulky, nonminiaturizable parts. Recently tantalum manufacturers have begun to offer packages that are compatible with thick film hybrid operations. Sprague has a line of "beam lead" or "flip chip" versions that can be mounted on the thick film circuit much like the multilayer ceramic units. In a 180 by 100 mil

Application Notes:

Ceramic capacitors can exhibit significant changes in electrical parameters under varying conditions of applied voltage, frequency and ambient temperature. ·The character and magnitude of these changes differ widely from one dielectric body to another. The High K dielectrics also exhibit capacitance aging (decrease in capacitance value) during storage life, which is a reversible process. These characteristics should be considered in critical design applications. It is recommended that the factory be consulted for detailed information.

COG CAPACITORS

Extremely stable under varying conditions of temperature, voltage and frequency. Shelf aging negligible. No voltage polarization.

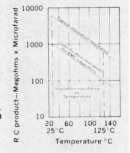

W5P & W5R CAPACITORS

Capacitance and dissipation factor vary with temperature, voltage and frequency. Temporary voltage polarization is characteristic. Shelf aging is typically −1.7% per hour decade of time for W5P and −0.7% per hour decade of time for W5R.

Insulation Resistance for all Electro Materials bodies is rated at 25°C, and is the smaller of 100K Megohm or 1000 Megohm X Microfarad at rated DCWV. COG, W5P and W5R materials are 1/10 of the 25°C values at +125°C, that is 10 K Megohm or 100 Megohm X Microfarad, whichever is less.

X5U CAPACITORS

Exhibit considerable change in capacitance with temperature, voltage and frequency. In a controlled environment, they are excellent where high capacitance is indicated for decoupling, coupling and filtering.

Figure 10-9 Performance data. (Courtesy of Electro Materials Division, ITW.)

COG (NPO) Dielectric

The NPO Ceramic Formulation is a highly stable non-ferroelectric composition which exhibits high Q, and negligible changes in capacitance over a wide range of temperatures, frequencies and bias voltages. Ideally suited for tuned circuits, timing circuits and fast rise time applications.

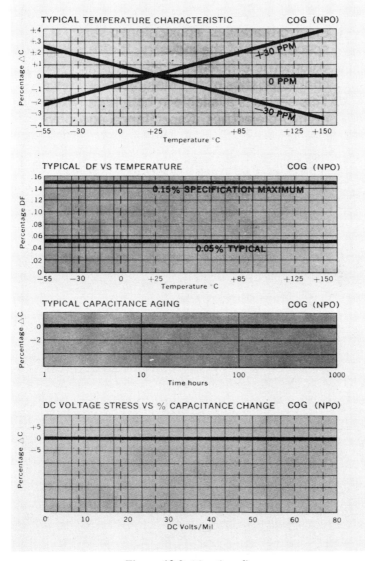

Figure 10-9 *(Continued)*

W5P Dielectric

The W5P material is a ferroelectric dielectric system with a K of approximately 1200 at 25°C. It offers the advantage of approximately 40 times the volumetric efficiency of the NPO material, and exhibits moderate changes in capacitance and D.F. with temperature, frequency and bias voltage. Suited for by-pass, coupling and filtering applications.

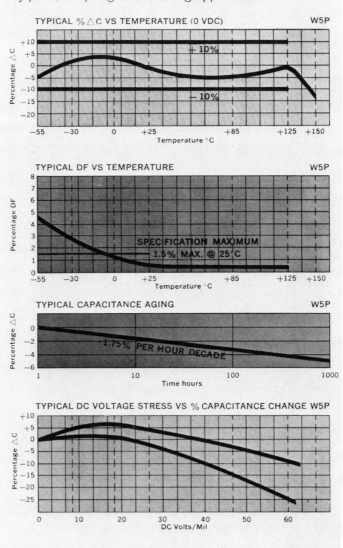

Figure 10-9 (*Continued*)

W5R Dielectric

The W5R material is similar in performance to the W5P material except that it has a higher K and can therefore provide higher capacitance values in a given volume. Suited for by-pass, coupling, and filtering applications where modest changes in capacitance at temperature extremes are acceptable.

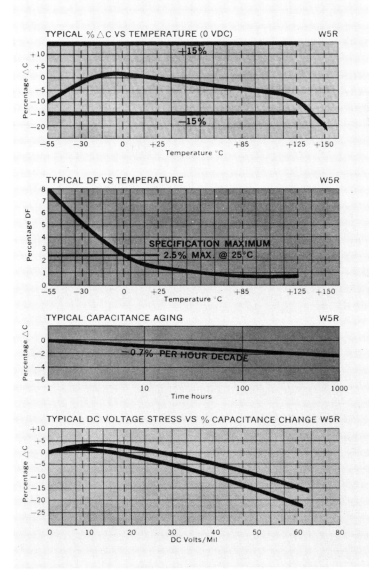

Figure 10-9 (*Continued*)

X5U Dielectric

The X5U material is designed for maximum
capacitance per unit volume. It is a utility body most
suitable for coupling and decoupling where
appreciable changes in capacitance may be tolerated.
A controlled environment will permit use of this

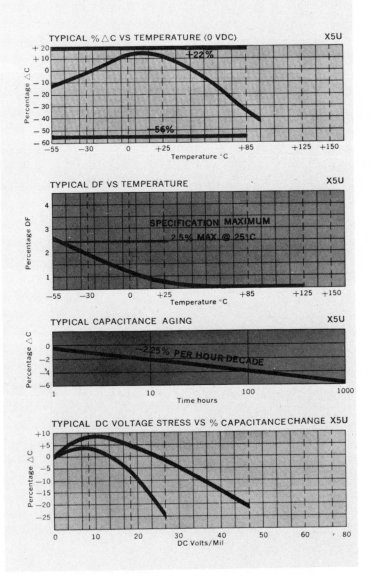

Figure 10-9 (*Continued*)

268

body in applications requiring greater stability. Although short duration exposure to higher temperatures will not degrade X5U, the maximum temperature for long term load life should not exceed 85°C.

The performance characteristics described in these pages and the products defined in this catalog represent the standard Electro Materials' line.

Available upon request is a series of Product Information Bulletins describing the many additional variations to our standard line, as well as performance and application information.

Ceramic dielectric materials can be used for many applications by virtue of our ability to "Tailor" characteristics, whether electrical, environmental, or mechanical.

Our engineering staff is always available to help in your special requirements for dielectrics, metalizations, configurations, or other application problems.

Note: Time is measured from removal of capacitors out of a DE-AGING oven at +150°C for ½ hr.

Figure 10-9 (*Continued*)

COG (NPO) "Chip" Capacitors

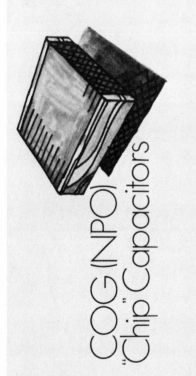

SPECIFICATIONS

Temperature range:
−55°C to +150°C

Test frequency:
100pf and less @ 1MHz, over 100pf @ 1KHz

Temperature coefficient:
0±30ppm/°C (EIA char. COG)

Dissipation factor:
0.15% max. @ 25°C

Insulation resistance:
100K megohms or 1000 ohm-farads, whichever is less @ 25°C

Test voltage:
4x rated WVDC below .012 μf, 2.5x rated WVDC for .012 μf and above

E.I.A. CODE

Capacitance Tolerance	Capacitance Code Examples
10 pf or less:	below 10 pf:
D = ±.5 pf	339 = 3.3 pf
F = ±1.0 pf	"9" digit signifies .1 multiplier
above 10 pf:	10 pf and above:
J = ±5%	101 = 100 pf
K = ±10%	3rd digit signifies number of zeros

DIMENSIONS AND AVAILABILITY

Type No.	0805	0905	1505	1209	1706	1712	2221	3942	Capacitance Code (EIA)
L(±*)	.080"	.095"	.150"	.122"	.170"	.175"	.225"	.390"	
W(±*)	.050"	.050"	.050"	.095"	.065"	.125"	.210"	.425"	
T(max)	.050"	.060"	.060"	.065"	.060"	.065"	.065"	.065"	
MB(±.010")	.015"	.020"	.025"	.020"	.020"	.035"	.035"	.035"	
Capacitance in pf	WVDC 200 100 50	WVDC 200 100 50	WVDC 200 100 50	WVDC 200 100 50	WVDC 200 100 50	WVDC 200 100 50	WVDC 200 100 50	WVDC 200 100 50	
0.47 to 9.1									478 to 919
10									100
12									120
15									150
18									180
22									220
27									270
33									330
39									390
47									470
56									560
68									680
82									820
100									101

Figure 10-9 (*Continued*)

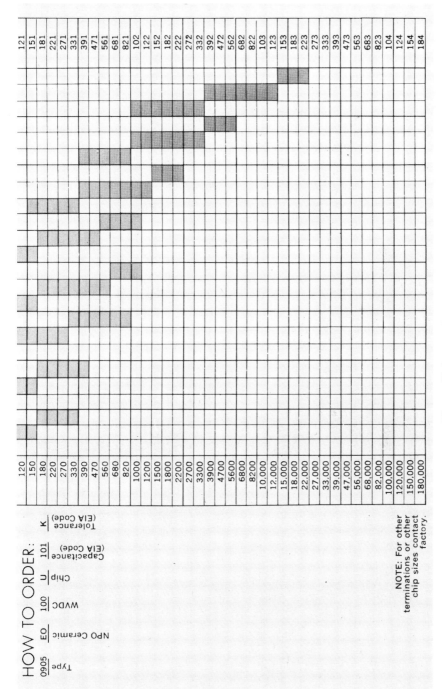

Figure 10-9 (*Continued*)

271

W5P, W5R
"Chip Capacitors"

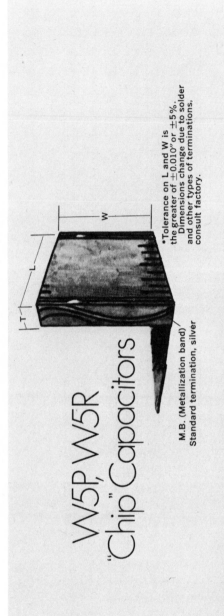

M.B. (Metallization band)
Standard termination, silver

*Tolerance on L and W is the greater of ±0.010" or ±5%. Dimensions change due to solder and other types of terminations, consult factory.

W5P SPECIFICATIONS

Temperature range:
 −55°C to +125°C
Temperature characteristics:
 W5P (±10%)
Dissipation factor:
 W5P: 1.5% max. @ 1KHz, 25°C
Insulation resistance:
 100K megohms or 1000 ohm-farads, whichever is less, @ 25°C
Test voltage:
 4x rated WVDC for values <0.5 µf 2.5x rated WVDC for 0.5 µf and above

DIMENSIONS AND AVAILABILITY

Type No.	0805			0905			1505			1209			1706			1712			2221			3942			Capacitance Code (EIA)
L(±*)	.080"			.095"			.150"			.122"			.170"			.175"			.225"			.390"			
W(±*)	.050"			.050"			.050"			.095"			.065"			.125"			.210"			.425"			
T(max)	.050"			.060"			.060"			.065"			.060"			.065"			.065"			.065"			
MB(±.010")	.015"			.020"			.025"			.020"			.020"			.035"			.035"			.035"			
Capacitance in pf	WVDC 200 100 50			WVDC 200 100 50			WVDC 200 100 50			WVDC 200 100 50			WVDC 200 100 50			WVDC 200 100 50			WVDC 200 100 50			WVDC 200 100 50			Capacitance Code (EIA)
120																									121
150																						W5P			151
180																						W5R			181
220																									221
270																									271
330																									331
390																									391
470																									471
560																									561
680																									681
820																									821

W5P HOW TO ORDER

0905	EL	200	U	102	K
Type	W5P Ceramic	WVDC	Chip	Capacitance (EIA Code)	Tolerance (EIA Code)

Figure 10-9 (*Continued*)

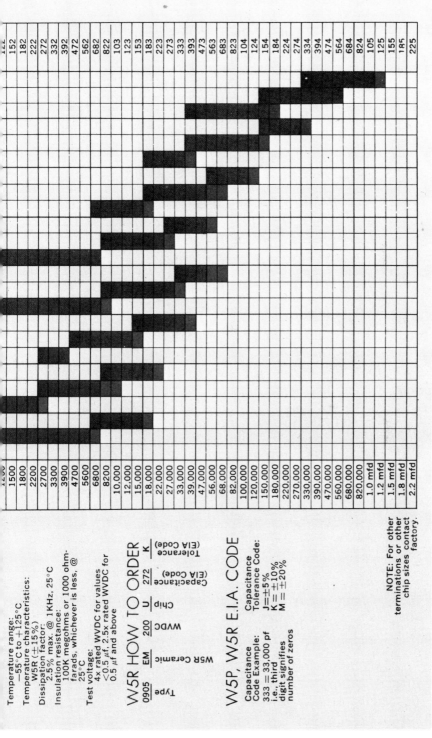

Figure 10-9 (*Continued*)

X5U "Chip" Capacitors

SPECIFICATIONS

Temperature range:
−55 C to +85 C
Temperature characteristics:
X5U (+22%—56%)
Dissipation factor:
2.5% max. @ 1KHz, 25°C
Insulation resistance:
100K megohms or 1000 ohm-farads, whichever is less, @ 25°C
Test voltage:
4x rated WVDC for values <1.0 μf, 2.5x rated WVDC for values 1.0 μf and above. In no case less than 125 VDC

E.I.A. CODE

Capacitance Code Example:
333 = 33,000 pf
i.e., third digit signifies number of zeros

Capacitance Tolerance Code:
M = ±20%

DIMENSIONS AND AVAILABILITY

Type No.	0805		0905		1505		1209		1706		1712		2221		3942		Capacitance Code (EIA)
L(±*)	.080"		.095"		.150"		.122"		.170"		.175"		.225"		.390"		
W(±*)	.050"		.050"		.050"		.095"		.065"		.125"		.210"		.425"		
T(max)	.050"		.060"		.060"		.065"		.060"		.065"		.065"		.065"		
MB(±.010")	.015"		.020"		.025"		.020"		.020"		.035"		.035"		.035"		
Capacitance in pf	WVDC 50	25	WVDC 50	25	WVDC 50	25	WVDC 50	25	WVDC 50	25	WVDC 50	25	WVDC 50	25	WVDC 50	25	
820																	821
1000																	102
1200																	122
1500																	152
1800																	182
2200																	222
2700																	272
3300																	332
3900																	392

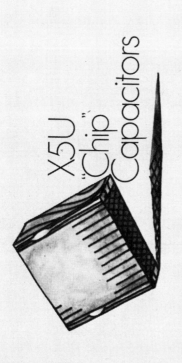

Figure 10-9 (*Continued*)

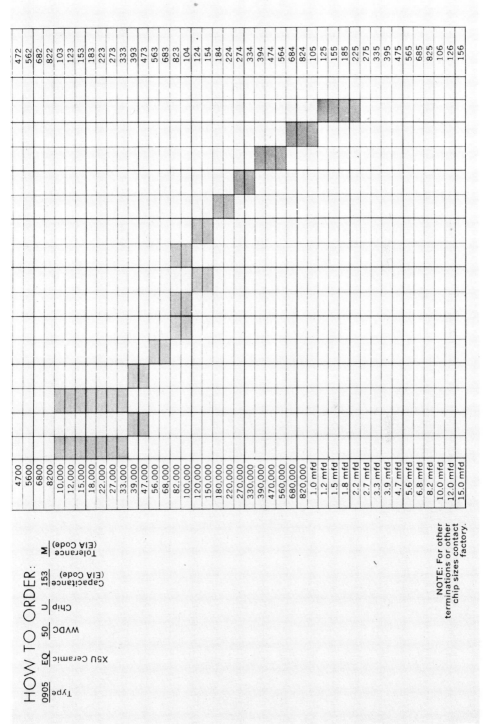

Figure 10-9 (*Continued*)

package, they offer up to 1 μF at 10 V rating. Other manufacturers, such as Components, Inc. and Union Carbide, offer miniature leaded devices (minicomponent configuration) that are small enough to mount on a thick film substrate.

Tantalums are now "somewhat" available in sizes and configurations that are compatible with hybrid needs. The range, volumetric efficiency and availability will no doubt improve in the future.

Other Discrete Components. Easy mounting, compatible, and reasonably priced, discrete passive components available for thick film hybrids are generally limited to resistors and capacitors.

Inductors—Bad News. Not only have inductors resisted miniaturization successfully; but will probably continue to do so. To make high inductance, one still has to resort to many turns of insulated wire around ferromagnetic material. The best efforts to date have produced a variety of minicomponents, but even as minicomponents they cannot be squeezed into many standard packages.

Low-inductance value, low-Q chips are available. Tiny spirals are made using thin film techniques, giving up to 250 nH on an alumina base measuring about 200 mils square. Thin film inductor chips offer enough inductance to be useful in higher frequencies, but they are expensive.

Most circuit designers go to great lengths to avoid use of inductors. When this fails, the best bet for inductance on thick film is the encased miniature toroidal types or some of the small plastic encapsulated minicomponents.

Other Discretes. Other kinds of components are not yet available in form factors specifically designed for thin film, although a variety of minicomponents can be adapted with varying degrees of success. Trimmer capacitors, for instance, are available in sizes below 200 mils in diameter. Miniature potentiometers are available in ever smaller sizes. The smallest of these types of components are usually the most expensive because of the high costs of miniaturization. This high cost limits their use in thick film hybrids. In cases where these components are needed, the thick film hybrid is often unable to operate at an advantage over conventional circuitry. Frequently the best answer in trying to adapt inductors and adjustable components to thick film lies in giving up and mounting them outboard.

Remember that many variable components applications with discrete circuitry can be converted to trimmable thick film capacitor or resistor situations in thick film versions of the circuit.

Chapter 11

PACKAGING

Packaging has often been relegated to the "back seat" in making ICs. One of the reasons for this probably is that the package, since it usually plays no direct electronic role, does not seem to be important. Moreover, other parts of the circuit are much more expensive, hence seem more important. Actually, packaging demands as much consideration as the other parts of an IC. The performance of a circuit can be ruined by the package, and the overall cost of the IC can be greatly affected (because of decreasing costs of the various other circuit parts, the cost of the package looms larger). Thus from both cost and circuit performance standpoints the package becomes critical.

BASIC FUNCTIONS OF IC PACKAGES

The basic functions of a package for thick film ICs are the following:

1. Many individual parts of most integrated circuits need to be protected from the "outside world."
2. The outside world must be protected from the integrated circuit.
3. The integrated circuit must "communicate" (both electrically and physically) with the outside world (in spite of the need for isolation).

The third function of packaging is almost always in basic conflict with the first two. Performing any *one* of the functions is relatively easy—even handling the first two at the same time. But fulfilling the third function, the need for electrical connections and the need to be compatible in a physical way with the "outside," calls for compromises. Minimizing these compromises is what might be called the "art" of packaging. The basic technologies behind this "art" are *sealing* and *encapsulation*.

Function 1—Protecting the Circuit from the Outside World. As far as the average IC is concerned, the outside world is a cruel place, and the individual components need to be protected from a variety of "cruelties."

Heat and Humidity. Circuits must operate at temperatures ranging from well below freezing to well above the boiling point of water—across a range of 200°C. Therefore, packages also must perform their duties under the same conditions. (A package does not "protect" a circuit from heat, but it must operate across the same temperature range as the IC does.)

Humidity as high as 100% can be encountered. Protecting the circuit against humidity is probably the most difficult feat of all. Moisture vapor is able to get through almost anything to some extent, and extremely small amounts can wreak havoc.

Pressure, Vibration, and Shock. The wide variety of places where ICs are needed include some extremely difficult situations—such as under the hood of an automobile and in applications where the circuit will be "shot out of a gun" (fuses, e.g.). Shipment to the user seemingly is every bit as severe.

Abrasion, Corrosion, and Dirt. Without some kind of protection against these kinds of attack, the relatively delicate monolithic circuits would soon fail. A good example of an extreme case in this category again is the under-the-auto-hood environment (and in the immediate user's assembly line).

Electrical. The outside world often has a wire or another component in close proximity that carries a damagingly high voltage or an unwanted RF signal. Thick film hybrid circuits need protection from situations such as this if they are to function properly.

Radiation and Light. The operation of many elements is affected by atomic radiation and light sources. Circuits sensitive to light must use packages that do not transmit light (as would glass or translucent ceramic). Radiation is able to degrade semiconductor performance seriously; and to the extent that it is possible, a package should protect from this type of damage. Most packages are relatively ineffective against the various types of atomic radiation, so that special types of radiation-resistant circuit elements are used.

Function 2—Protecting the Outside World from the Circuit. There are things that go on *inside* an IC that must be kept localized, to avoid damaging any neighboring devices outside the package. Heat generation, high voltage, and RF signal radiation are the major dangers. This function is easy to fulfill in most cases because meeting other needs often automatically satisfies these demands as well. (Heat generation can be an exception.)

Function 3—Allowing Inside-Outside "Connections" (Communication). This function presents difficulties. Leads must pass through the walls of the package without damaging the protective ability of these barriers. In addition to the need for electrical signal passage, other requirements also exist.

Heat. Heat generated inside the package must be channeled to the outside world in acceptable ways—before it can damage the circuit in the package. Heat can be dumped through the leads, the base, or the lid of the package. It is often necessary to keep different parts in a circuit at uniform temperatures so that circuit performance is maintained at an optimized level. The study of temperature profiles and heat transmission has had to become considerably more sophisticated with ICs because of highly concentrated heat generation spots and close proximity of these to heat-sensitive elements.

Lead Solderability and Bondability. The electrical connections must be in a configuration that allows a bond of the desired type to be made to the connection on the outside. This puts certain restraints on a package and causes numerous complications. For example, the metal needed for thermal expansion matching is not the best for soldering. This leads to complex plating operations.

Strength. A package and its leads must be strong enough and tough enough to survive considerable mistreatment during assembly. The leads will be bent back and forth, placing still another requirement on the electrical connections. The package also has to survive shipment to the final user. If a circuit package can withstand assembly and shipping, it is often strong enough to take anything that comes along in final use, although final use must of course be considered.

Physical Considerations. "Physical communication" places many mechanical and geometric requirements on a package. It can be only so high and so wide; the wires must be of such and such a size and be placed in certain spacing. The package must fit its mounting site.

Electrical Requirements. The signals must be gotten from the inside to the outside in such a way that any possible degradation is minimized. The conductivity of the leads and the nature of the bond will have an effect on such things as voltage drop. Lead shape and length will affect inductance. Lead spacing and the insulation materials used in the package walls will control the capacitance between the leads. The nature of the packaging material will affect shielding. All of these items must be considered because they can seriously affect overall circuit performance. They are all relatively controllable, however.

PACKAGE CONFIGURATIONS

So wide a variety of outside-world and inside-the-package conditions must be handled that, not surprisingly, a wide variety of packaging schemes have sprung up. In addition, the variety of components used in a hybrid IC demand a wide range in the degree of protection needed. A circuit operating in a clean, dry area at a constant temperature certainly can get by with a much less capable package than would one operating under an automobile hood or one being dropped out of an airplane into the ocean. A circuit consisting of thick film only needs much less protection than one containing more delicate components (wire bonded monolithics, e.g.). As might be expected, extra protection costs money, so that economics can be a strong factor.

The basic configurations of integrated circuit packages have to do with their physical mating with the immediate outside world—that is, what they will be hooked up to and the manner in which the hooking-up is to be accomplished. There are four basic configurations: (1) flat packs, (2) dual in-line packages (DIPs), (3) TO types, and (4) nonstandards. Figure 11-1 shows these basic configurations.

Flat Pack. The flat pack usually has leads coming out of two sides, but four-sided egress is becoming more common with the advent of more complex circuits. The leads are uniformly spaced metal ribbons. The usual spacing is 50 mils. The ribbon leads (4 $\times$ 16 mils) are easily bent. Bending

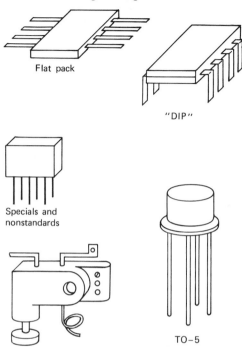

Figure 11-1 IC package configuratons.

is avoided during assembly because the leads are attached to a frame of metal around the perimeter. Special shipping containers can maintain lead straightness after the frame is cut off for testing. (Figure 11-2.)

Flat packs are almost the only packages that allow high numbers of leads (over 80) in a relatively small space. The 50-mil lead spacing and the low profile make the flat pack the most compact of the various packaging schemes. Many materials and constructions are available in the flat pack configuration.

The leads from a flat pack IC are attached to printed circuit boards by soldering or welding. The flat pack cover can be sealed by welding, by brazing, or with soft glass.

Advantages of the flat rock configuration are that: (1) it is lightweight and compact, (2) the area available inside the package for mounting is large compared to the overall package area, and (3) it allows many leads, hence can be used for complex circuits. Disadvantages of the flat pack are that (1) it tends to be expensive (ranging from 25¢ for small flat packs purchased in high volume to more than $5.00 each for larger, more complex packages) and (2) the leads are easily bent and damaged. (Flexing

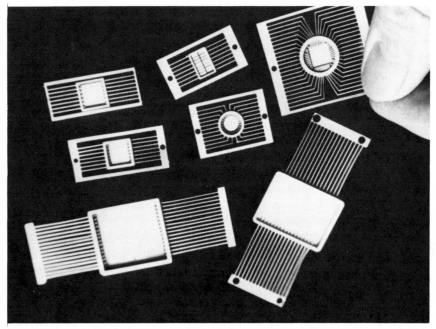

Figure 11-2   Flat packs. (Packages from Tekform and Alloys Unlimited; photograph by State of the Art, Inc.)

of leads can cause seal damage and loss of hermaticity.) Carriers and special jigs are used to cut down on lead damage, but these add even more to the cost.

The package specifications of Figure 11-3 give additional dimensional detail on flat packs as well as the DIPs and TO types.

The Dual In-Line Package. The DIP is designed for insertion into holes in a printed circuit board or into a special connector mounted on the PC board, where the flat pack has its leads attached to the PC board metallization without resorting to holes or connectors. The DIP consists of a ceramic substrate on which stamped metal leads are attached at 100-mil intervals. The leads leave the substrate on a horizontal plane, but they are bent 90° so that they are orthogonal to the plane of package. The leads are much more sturdy than flat pack ribbon leads. This sturdiness allows damage-free shipping and automatic insertion into printed circuit boards. The DIP package is less expensive than the flat pack and is available in either plastic or ceramic construction. (The flat pack is available in plastic and ceramic construction; as well as in metal and glass.) Although less compact,

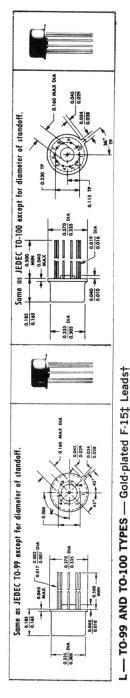

L — TO-99 AND TO-100 TYPES — Gold-plated F-15‡ Leads†

Figure 11-3 Dimensional details of some common standard packages. (Reprinted from *1970 Texas Instruments Catalog*, by permission of Texas Instruments.)

283

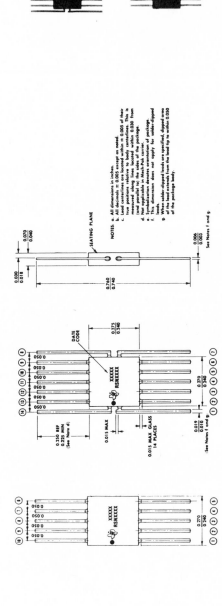

NOTES: a. All dimensions in inches.
b. All decimals ± 0.005 except as noted.
c. Lead centerlines are located within ± 0.005 of their true positions relative to body centerlines. This is measured along lines located within 0.030 from (and parallel to) the sides of the package.
d. Not applicable in Mesh-Pak corner.
e. Symbolization denotes orientation of package.
f. This dimension does not apply for solder-dipped leads.
g. When solder-dipped leads are specified, dipped area of the lead extends from the lead tip to within 0.050 of the package body.

H—CERAMIC FLAT PACKAGES—Gold-Plated F-15‡ Glass-sealing Alloy — 10 or 14 LONG Leads

Figure 11-3 (*Continued*)

284

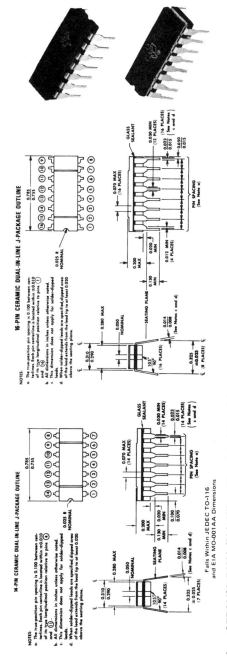

J — CERAMIC DUAL-IN-LINE — Tin-plated Leads†

‡F-15 is the ASTM designation for an iron-nickel-cobalt alloy containing nominally 53% iron, 29% nickel, and 17% cobalt.

†For leads as described add suffix —00. For solder-dipped leads add suffix —10.

Figure 11-3 (*Continued*)

and limited in the possible number of leads, the DIP finds very wide use, especially in high-volume situations. (Figures 11-4 and 11-3.)

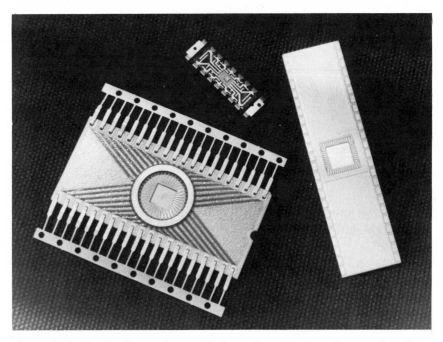

Figure 11-4 Dual-in-line packages. (Packages from American Lava and DuPont; photograph by State of the Art, Inc.)

Probably the biggest disadvantage of DIPs is the low ratio between overall size to available chip mounting area. A standard 14-lead DIP with 100-mil-spaced leads along each side in two rows 300 mils apart has only about a 150-mil-wide strip usable for thick film circuits and components. There is room for *one* relatively large IC chip or only a few thick film resistors and discrete components. Multichip ICs and most hybrids ICs are usually forced to use another package type offering more real estate. Double sized (0.600-mil row spacing) DIPs also are available if more room is needed. The recently developed DuPont DIPs offer a real estate advantage in that both sides are available. (The leads make contact to *both* sides.) (Figure 11-5.)

The major advantages of the DIP are (1) the increased ruggedness as compared with the flat pack and (2) the low cost. The 14-lead ceramic DIP ("C-DIP") costs 10 to 15¢ each in volume, and a plastic DIP can

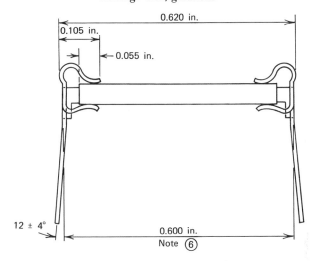

Right side view — 4 X full

Figure 11-5 Cross section of DuPont Multilox^R DIP design, showing double-sided contact made by leads. The leads are not attached unitl the circuit is finished.

be well below 10¢. Although the larger DIPs which can accommodate up to forty leads are more expensive, their general ruggedness is making them a favored package for LSI chips. The larger DIPs remain inexpensive compared to flat packs.

TO-Type Packages. These hat-shaped metal packages were originally popular as highly reliable transistor packages. They have adapted successfully to popular use in ICs. They are available in a variety of sizes and number of leads, including designs that have high heat-dumping capabilities. The height available inside the package allows multilevel hybrids to be made. The leads act as risers to make connections between levels. Where multilevel circuitry is not needed, the height is a disadvantage over flat packs and DIPs. The sealed TO package has excellent hermaticity. (Figures 11-6 and 11-3.)

Although inexpensive itself (because of high-volume transistor usage), the TO configuration is not particularly economical for assembly and is limited in the complexity of the circuit that can be assembled inside. The ready availability of the packages in small volume at reasonable prices have led to wide acceptance of this packaging configuration in spite of disadvantages in cost effectiveness in assembly.

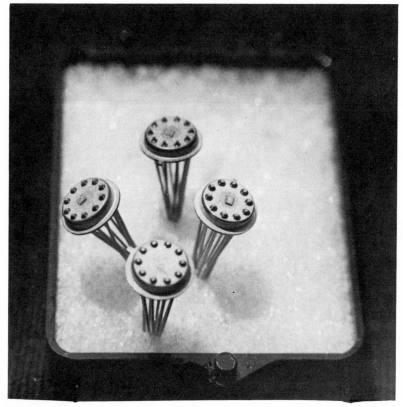

Figure 11-6 TO-5 package. (Prior to adding cover.) (Photograph by State of the Art, Inc.)

The major advantages of the TO series packages is their extreme ruggedness and low cost. A 10 lead TO-5 costs about 15¢. The main disadvantages are the low useful area to overall size ratio and limited number of leads available (12 only for the TO-5). They are not easy to handle in production; the leads get tangled and bent.

Nonstandard Packages (Including Multilayer Substrates). Monolithic integrated circuit makers usually stick with the standard packages, but hybrid makers tend to use nonstandard packages that fit special needs. One of the most popular materials used in special designs (usually in-house-manufactured) is the plastic package. Special packages are used also when special mounting is needed, such as the Delco voltage regulator illustrated in Figure 11-7.

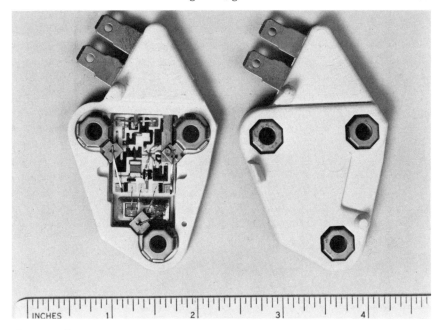

Figure 11-7 Special package design for automotive voltage regulator. (Photograph courtesy of Delco Division, General Motors.)

Another type of package that can be classified as "nonstandard" is one that is designed for extremely complex ICs where many crossovers are needed. When several IC chips are combined on a single substrate, the crossovers must also be handled on the substrate (within the package). Figure 11-8a shows an early (1968) version of a multichip circuit with many crossovers. Figure 11-8b shows a "modern" (1970) version which has many more crossovers. A continuous dielectric layer is used in the latter instead of individual crossover areas.

There are two approaches to multilevel circuits. The first is for the hybrid circuit maker to make his own multilayer circuit by screen printing and firing alternate layers of thick film conductors and thick film insulators as illustrated above. The second is to buy a substrate or a package that has the wiring structure built into the substrate. This is done by printing the wiring pattern on the thin alumina sheets prior to firing. The unfired sheets are laminated together, and the entire assembly is then fired. The result is a substrate with the crossovers *inside* the substrate. This approach, while considerably more costly than the do-it-yourself screen-printed multilevel approach, gives superior electrical isolation and is attractive in high-speed circuits.

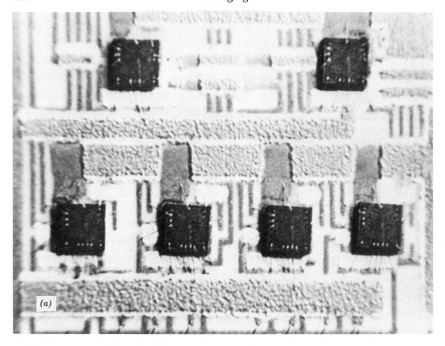

Figure 11-8 (*a*) Simple crossovers in a multichip circuit. (Photograph courtesy of Fairchild.) (*b*) Multichip IC requiring multilayer screen-printing techniques to make the necessary interconnections. (A 12-bit D/A converter containing 6 dual flip-flops, 6 ladder switches, 3 op-amps, 2 clock reset and drive chips, 6 transistors and diodes, 5 tantalum nitride adjustment resistor chips, and 3 tantalum nitride ladder networks.) (Photograph courtesy of Unisem Corporation.)

TYPES OF PACKAGES

Classified by the primary material used in construction, there are four basic types of packages: (1) metal, (2) glass, (3) ceramic, and (4) plastic.

Metal Packages. Metal packages have been used in electronics for many years, and it was natural to continue using this proven technology with ICs. The technology employed to seal transistors and crystals in metal packages transferred easily to ICs. The ruggedness and the reliability that can be built into the metal package make it logical for high reliability IC uses. Metal packages also offer, automatically, good shielding. (Other package types must have shielding built-in if it is needed.) Metal packages as a class are rather expensive unless used in extremely high volume, such as in the TO-5.

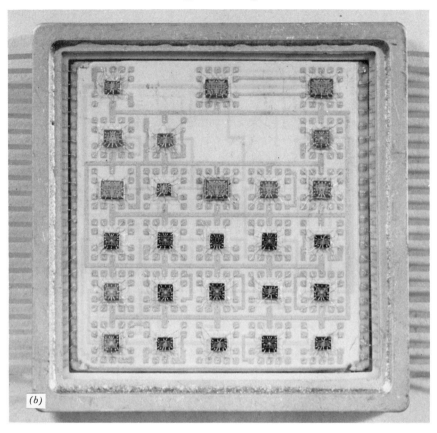

Figure 11-8 *(Continued)*

The TO type is primarily a metal package, and many flat packs also are metal. Metal construction is only occasionally used in the special configuration and rarely in DIPs.

Metal packages have leads passing through holes in the metal, insulated by glass seals. The glass-to-metal seal is an excellent hermetic seal although it is inherently expensive. To keep the seal intact through a wide temperature range, it is necessary that the glass and the metal have roughly equal thermal coefficients of expansion. This requires special metal; Kovar (a cobalt-nickel-iron alloy) is the prime material used. To maintain bondability, solderability, and so on, the Kovar is usually gold plated. Although ICs can be attached directly to a metal package's base, it is more common to use an insulating substrate which is attached to the metal base. Solders

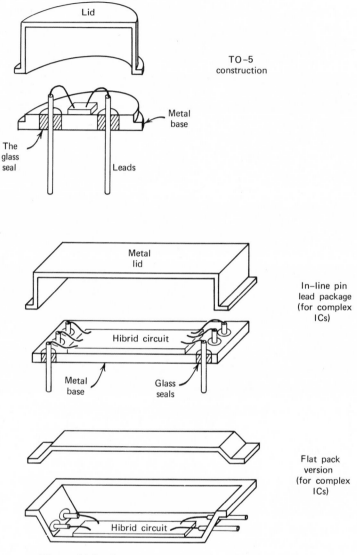

Figure 11-9 Some common metal package configurations.

must be metallized, which adds to expense. Epoxy is used for substrate/package bonding to avoid the need for substrate metallization. For good thermal transfer, care must be taken to ensure the flatness of the substrate; otherwise, voids in the solder (or epoxy) can form, producing areas on the substrate where thermal resistance is high.

The metal package consists of two parts: (1) the metal base, with the leads insulated from the base by glass feedthroughs, and (2) a metal lid. (Figures 11-9 and 11-10.)

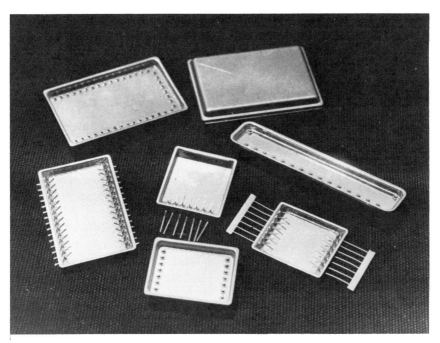

Figure 11-10 Metal packages. (Packages from Techform; photograph by State of the Art, Inc.)

After the IC is mounted and hooked up to the package's leads, the lid must be attached. Several methods are available. One popular sealing approach is brazing with an 80% gold, 20% tin eutectic alloy. The gold-tin eutectic alloy is available as a preform. The 300°C temperature required for the seal presents few problems to monolithic circuits, although in hybrid circuits where there is need to solder discrete devices prior to sealing, 300°C is too high. If this is the case, soft solders can be used. When solders are used to seal the lid, cooling often creates a break in the seal due to the drop in pressure inside the package. To avoid this, a small hole in the lid can be left open; it is sealed in a separate operation later. Flux removal can be a problem, as can the formation of small balls of solder inside the can.

Resistance welding and compression welding are also often used in sealing metal packages. If necessary, the base of the package can be held at low temperatures by heat sinking during the brief welding cycle. Epoxy seals are also used (preforms are available). Curing is done while the lid is held to the base under pressure.

To avoid damage to the components during and after the sealing operation, the process is usually carried out in a neutral atmosphere.

Metal packages are rather expensive, but are very rugged, offer excellent sealing, and give automatic RF shielding.

Ceramic Packages. Ceramic packages are made from alumina (sometimes beryllia) bases and lids with Kovar leads passing through the sides. Glass is used to make a seal between the Kovar and the ceramic. While the metal packages have individual seals for each wire, the seal of the ceramic package is continuous. Ceramic package technology allows a wide variety of construction approaches. Some are illustrated in Figure 11-11.

Ceramic packages (along with glass) have an advantage over metal packages in that they offer automatic electrical isolation; the ceramic is an insulator. In cases where more than one chip is to be mounted and isolation is needed, an insulating package base is advantageous. The metallization pattern for the silicon chip and the wire-bonding pads to receive leads going outside is screen-printed on the package base as the package is built. This can be done with molymanganese and then plated up, or with thick film compositions.

Some ceramic packages—as illustrated in Figure 11-11c—have outside leads that do not go through the seal into the inside of the package. This construction offers high reliability in that flexing of the lead is not likely to break the seal. To increase the ruggedness of the seal, its length between the outside and inside is increased. Figure 11-11c shows package walls as being quite narrow, but they can be made (and often are) considerably thicker so that the seal path is longer. Twenty to forty lead LSI DIPs use this construction extensively. (Figure 11-4.)

Figure 11-11c illustrates an attractive ceramic package approach that is advantageously used in a hybrid circuit operation. The substrate on which the hybrid circuit is built also serves as the base of the package. When the circuit has been built and checked out, a glass seal is screen-printed over the outer periphery of the substrate, and the lid is then attached by glass sealing. This represents a partly homemade package and offers cost reduction possibilities to hybrid manufacturers in addition to added flexibility. DuPont announced a package design in early 1971 that offers essentially this approach.

The ceramic DIP (C-DIP) is a very rugged package that is used extensively for high-volume single-chip ICs (Figure 11-11d). The base of the package has gold screen-printed in a recession to receive the IC chip. The

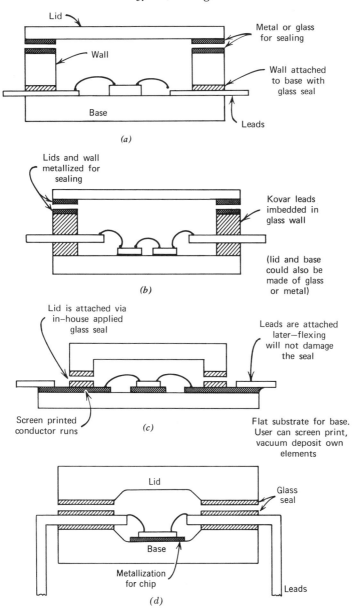

Figure 11-11 Some common ceramic package constructions. (*a*) Leads passing through to inside of package (common with flat packs or DIPs). (*b*) Composite ceramic package—ceramic and glass combination (common with flat packs). (*c*) Alternate design, offering (1) improved seal and (2) extra processing freedoms. (*d*) Ceramic **DIP.**

base has a glass coating covering the remaining surface. The lead frame is attached to the substrate by heating the base until the glass softens. The lead frame is then pressed into the molten glass. Equipment is available that will attach both the chip and leads at the same time. A ceramic lid with glass seal material screen-printed on it is attached later by heating until the glass softens. (A similar version can be plastic-encapsulated; see Figure 11-12.) The major attraction of the C-DIP is its low cost.

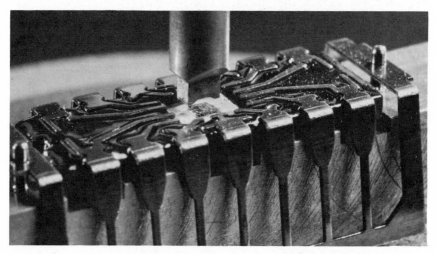

Figure 11-12 Close-up of "C-dip" package during simultaneous attachment of the lead frame (glass bonded to ceramic) and the silicon chip (gold-silicon eutectic bond). (Photograph courtesy of Unitek Corporation.)

Glass Packages. Glass packages, being insulators, have the same advantage over metal as do the ceramic packages in that they offer electrical isolation for separate chips. Glass construction is similar to the ceramic illustrated in Figure 11-11*a,b* except that glass is used instead of ceramic. Glass is weaker, hence is not used in larger packages. Small flat packs are the most likely place to find all-glass packages.

The advantages of glass are low cost and electrical isolation. The disadvantages are poor strength and poor heat conduction. Lower costs of ceramic packages have allowed them to replace glass as a basic package material; but glass, of course, plays a key role in sealing both metal and ceramic packages. Glass-constructed packages are not a factor in thick film circuits.

Some packages are currently being offered made of a mixture of ceramic and glass. Their characteristics are in-between the two. These glass-ceramic combinations are less expensive than the 100% ceramic package.

Plastic Packages. There are three basic types of plastic packages: (1) potted, where a fluid plastic is poured into either a prepared thin-walled plastic case or into a mold that will be stripped after curing; (2) molded, where hot molten plastic is forced around the circuit by pressure; and (3) conformal coatings, where the circuit is dipped into a fluid. The adhering plastic is then dried and cured.

Plastic packages are used because of their great design flexibility and economy. They are generally limited to less demanding applications. No true hermetic seal is available in plastic packaging, although a well-designed and produced system can stand up to all but the most extreme requirements. (The problem here is to get the right materals and to process them properly—a difficult and demanding task requiring much development and control.) Plastic packages are used little in monolithic ICs except for high-volume single-chip circuits. They are much more likely to be used in hybrid applications, especially thick film.

The potted packages are perhaps the easiest to handle. Tooling costs are at a minimum; and, in the case of the preformed cases, softer encapsulating materials can be used that are not so hard on the encapsulated circuit. Figure 11-13 illustrates potting and other plastic package configurations.

Molded packages (usually injection molded) have high tooling costs, but the unit cost can be very low. The low unit cost is attractive for high-volume operations. A common example of this type of plastic package is the plastic molded DIP. Injection molding is a *very* rough process and should be approached with extreme caution.

Conformal coatings (not illustrated) offer extremely low tooling costs and simplicity. Compared to molded plastics, they are very gentle and easy on the circuit. However, they are somewhat ugly which bothers many people. Except for poor edge coverage, they stand up in quality very well in comparison to other plastic packages.

Epoxies are by far the most popular plastic packaging material. Because of the thermal mismatch between the epoxy and the substrate, most components have to be protected from the epoxy with a flexible undercoat. Silicones are also used, both for undercoats and as potting material.

The plastic systems, usually requiring heavy involvement in internal processing, are "difficult" to keep under control. It must be kept in mind that when manipulating plastic systems, one is dealing with very complex chemistry and processes. It is easy to get into situations where, for one reason or another, the plastic encapsulation is not giving the protection it is supposed to give. A common fault is a tendency of the user to oversimplify the process and its problems. Plastic packages should be handled with care and caution—if you don't, they can "turn on you."

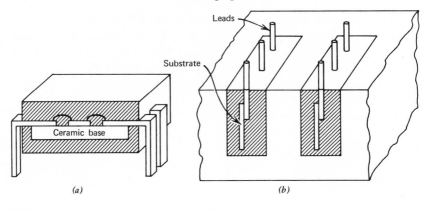

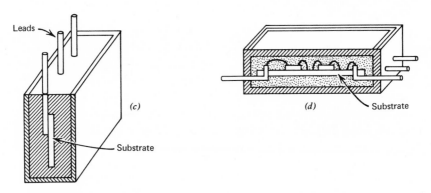

Figure 11-13 Plastic package constructions. (*a*) Molded (DIP). (*b*) Potted in "RTV" molds. (*c*) Potted in a plastic case. (*d*) Potted in a plastic flat pack.

Package Sealing. Packages come to the user in two pieces. It is up to the IC maker to attach the lid to the package body when he is ready. This puts an important part of the package making operation into the hands of the IC maker, and responsibility for doing it properly lies with him. Nevertheless, this often leads to problems, because packaging technology tends to get pushed off to one side as being "simple," as being "the problem of the package maker," or as being "not so important as the rest of the IC process." This attitude on the part of some IC producers in unfortunate and expensive. The more informed IC producers treat both packaging and the sealing process with extreme respect and caution.

The main types of sealing in use are (1) the glass/metal seal; (2) the metal/metal braze or solder seal; (3) metal/metal welding; and (4) plastic sealing.

Glass/Ceramic Sealing. A glass whose thermal expansion matches the ceramic is applied to the lid and to the walls of the package by the package manufacturer. The integrated circuit maker, when he is ready to seal his circuit, places the package on a heated stage (often inside a nitrogen atmosphere so that the atmosphere inside the package will not damage the silicon chips). The lid is placed on the package, and the two are heated under pressure until the glass melts and flows together. Upon cooling, a hermetic seal is made. This sealing occurs at temperatures from 300° to 550°C depending on the glass composition. To keep the eutectic-bonded IC chips from coming off, the base of the circuit is kept cool by heat sinking. Even with heat sinking this type of sealing makes too much heat for many applications. This applies especially when many discretes are attached by solder, as in hybrid circuits. The heat can also degrade some semiconductors. If any of this is a problem, packages requiring glass-to-glass sealing are not attractive. Rather than struggle with the problem, getting into elaborate heat sinking or pushing the seal temperature and time down to borderline limits, it is best to use another sealing approach, of which there are many.

Metal-to-Metal Braze or Solder. This is perhaps the simplest approach and is used with great success by many IC makers. The top of the package wall and the bottom of the lid are metallized. When ready to seal, a preform of a low-melting temperature alloy is placed and heated until it melts. A popular sealing alloy is 80% gold-20% tin. It is possible to use the tin-lead solders also. The former is popular when the circuit consists of silicon chips only. The 300°C sealing temperature is neither harmful to the chips nor does it approach the gold-silicon eutectic temperature close enough to make loosening of the chip bond a possibility. Solder sealing is more popular with hybrid circuits where some of the discrete components ars bonded to the substrate inside the package with various solders. A tin-lead eutectic can be used to seal a package that has discretes inside soldered with high lead solders or with gold-tin.

It is possible to keep the substrate below tin-lead soldering temperatures and still use gold-tin through clever heat sinking offered by some of the currently available sealing machines. (Figure 11-14.)

Contraction of the air inside the package upon cooling often causes a "blow hole" to appear somewhere on the seal. To avoid this, a hole can be left open in the package lid, to be sealed later. Flux and molten solder balls inside the circuit can be problems also. Special soldering approaches avoid these blow holes, such as localized heating, progressing around the package circumference so that most of the package seal remains cool and nonmolten. By being very careful about cleaning and maintaining clean

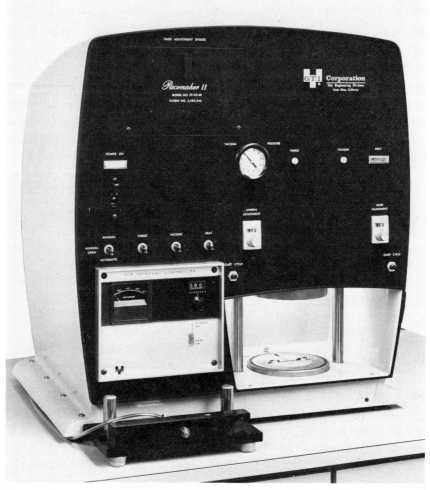

Figure 11-14 A single-station package sealing machine. (Courtesy of Dix Engineering Division, GTI Corporation.)

surfaces, one can make reliable seals without flux, thus avoiding the possibility of sealing flux inside the package.

Metal-to-Metal Welding. Resistance welding is a popular method of sealing metal packages. The heat generated can be kept localized by heat sinks so that the body of the package sees little high temperature. Cold welding is also used for packages designed to accept this method. Metal packages depend on welding to a great extent. Ceramic and glass packages depend more on molten systems.

Plastic Sealing. Suffering to some extent from a reputation of low quality, plastic sealing is nonetheless an excellent approach for many applications and is used with increasing frequency. It has the great advantage of not taking a lot of heat or pressure, one or the other of which is required for *all* of the other sealing methods. It is also inexpensive and can make a good seal. Preforms of thermosetting plastic are usually used. Pressure is applied during the "setting" of the plastic.

Unsealing the Package. After a package has been sealed, a situation often arises with a circuit that is not functioning properly where the circuit maker has to open the package to find out what is wrong, and then possibly make repairs. The alternative is to scrap the circuit. Scrapping may be all right for simple single-chip circuits, but it is not at all attractive for complex circuits into which much time and effort have been put.

If considerable repair is to be done, the sealing scheme and the package design must take this into account. Plastic sealed packages and welded packages are almost totally unrepairable because they are so hard to open. Packages that use molten systems (glass or solder/braze) can be opened up by simple reheating. The metal/metal seals are the easiest to open and repair. Glass seals are not as repairable because they subject the circuit to two more high temperature ordeals—often too much. The glass seal also does not have enough glass to make a good second bond, so a new lid is needed at the very least. With metal seals, a new preform is all that is needed.

Picking the Package. The "best" packages cost the most. The less expensive packages, such as plastic, are quite good—good enough for most applications. With the wide variety of packages available to fit the equally wide variety of possible applications, a choice is not always simple.

There is often a desire for standardization on one type of package within an IC plant. Understandable as this is, it has led to problems in some instances. When a standard in-plant package is picked, certain compromises are made. To cover many applications, a package must be picked that satisfies the toughest conditions. This places an economic burden on the less demanding operations. The opposite choice is to stock *all* types of packages (usually hopelessly expensive and impractical). There is, unfortunately, no simple way to solve this dilemma; both overstandardization and a total lack of standardization are unattractive. Packaging remains an expensive and critical part of the art of building ICs. Enough of the total cost of a circuit is often in packaging to "make or break" a successful design, and a tendency on the part of many to take packaging for granted can be very dangerous.

SUMMARY

A final point about thick film packaging is in order. Thick film is naturally rugged and, of the various types of ICs, requires the least protection. Many thick film circuits operating under fairly rugged circumstances (such as in car radios) use the package mostly for mechanical protection. Modern silicon chips have passivated surfaces that allow them to operate successfully in such nonhermetic packages also. One of the major advantages of thick film is that it holds out promise of integrated circuits that can operate with a minimum of package protection. This ability has strong economic effects.

Author's note. As this manuscript is being prepared, it is becoming obvious that industry is mounting a major attack both on packaging and on eliminating wire bonding. New processes and designs are being announced steadily in early 1971. Three new package configurations that typify the many attempts to reduce cost and increase flexibility that came upon the market in early 1971 are (1) the edge mount ceramic package developed jointly by TI, Coors, and American Microsystems; (2) the Du-Pont package that has do-it-yourself features and can use both sides of the substrate if needed; and (3) the leadless diaphram package offered by Diacon, Inc. Because package cost is looming larger (as other costs are reduced), it will receive increasing attention; other designs, such as the three just mentioned, will surely appear.

The broad subject of packaging had to be covered here in a limited space. For more detail we recommend the August 1970 issue of *Solid State Technology,* which has for several good survey papers on packaging.

Chapter 12

ARTWORK, LAYOUT, AND DESIGN

In this chapter we describe how to get from the original design—a circuit diagram, a breadboard model, or a discrete version that is waiting for conversion—to screen stencils ready to be used in production. Figure 12-1 shows the steps from the early design to the ready-to-print screens.

We delayed discussing this very important part of thick film technology because we feel that it is important for anyone learning about thick film design and layout to have developed a good understanding of the basic technology. As stated earlier, the philosophy of segregation of the design function from the assembly process and from component-making technologies that worked satisfactorily with discrete circuits will not work if applied to IC manufacture.

THE ORIGINAL DESIGN

As shown in Figure 12-1, the original design can start in many forms. It can also start as a combination of several approaches. Probably the most common sequence is to begin with a circuit diagram and then progress to a "prove-out" stage with a breadboard version.

"Breadboard" is a term used in the trade to describe a first-try, crude mock-up of a circuit. Early versions perhaps actually involved use of real

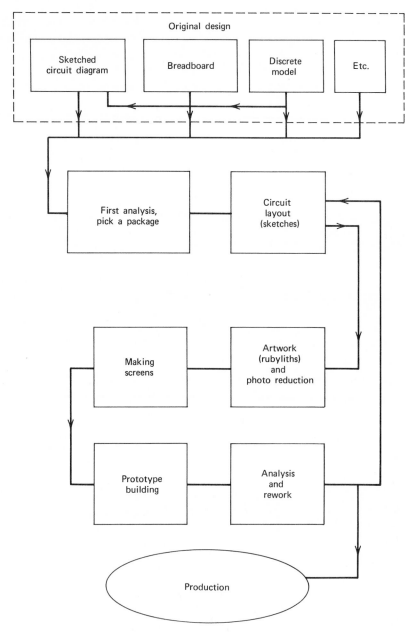

Figure 12-1 The "design" steps in thick film hybrid circuits.

breadboards—or at least pieces of boards through which nails had been driven in columns and rows. Individual discrete components were strung between the columns or rows of nails by soldering or wrapping the leads of the components around the nails. Basic behavior of the circuit was analyzed, and quick adjustments were made by removing one component and replacing it with another of different value. Many circuits were "designed" as much by this cut-and-try approach as by formal mathematical analysis and circuit synthesis. Breadboards today are never slabs of wood, which have been replaced by plastic sheets with a matrix of holes through which mounting posts can be inserted.

Often the basic device to be produced in thick film already exists as a proved design assembled with discrete components. The task of the thick film "designer" here is to design a thick film circuit that will replace the discrete version.

In any case, whether the circuit to be "designed" for thick film is a breadboard model, a circuit diagram, or a discrete model already in existence, the designer of the thick film circuit starts from *something*. It is not the purpose of this book to tell how to get this basic design, but how to convert a basic design into a working thick film circuit.

Differences between Discrete Component Versions and the Final Thick Film Circuit. A problem that sometimes comes up is that a thick film adaptation will not work in the same way as the breadboard model or the original discrete circuit. This is caused by large differences in size, by elements being located closer together, and by the differences between thick film element operating characteristics and those of discrete components. It can almost be *guaranteed,* in fact, that there will be differences. Some of these differences will be "good," some will be "bad." The important thing is to recognize that differences will exist.

Differences do exist between operating characteristics of a breadboard layout and a final discrete component version of a circuit, but these are usually insignificant. The differences between performance of a breadboard layout and the actual thick film circuit are likely to be much more significant. Learning what these differences are, and how to anticipate them, is all part of the process of becoming a skilled thick film circuit "designer."

Attitudes about the differences between performance of breadboard versions and the final thick film circuit vary considerably. Some designers breadboard with carbon composition resistors, because if the breadboard works with this kind of resistor, the final thick film version (with better resistor performance) will *have* to perform better. For other circuit designers the performance to be obtained is more critical, and the breadboard model must be made with components whose performance closely matches the performance of thick film elements (thick film resistor chips are sometimes used in breadboarding for this reason).

Breadboard models of thick film circuits often include small capacitors and resistors to simulate crossover capacitance and resistance of long narrow conductor runs. Parasitic capacitance (such as ground plane capacitance or capacitance of lines running close together) can be simulated by adding discrete capacitors in the breadboard version. Whether or not to include these "phantom" elements depends on how critical the design is.

For some circuits (such as high-frequency designs) a conventional breadboard step is impractical because size and location of the thick film elements are critical. Conventional breadboarding is then eliminated, and the designer goes directly to thick film versions. Several such thick film designs (thick film breadboards) are often necessary before the proper final design is obtained. Considerable prelayout circuit synthesis and analysis is often counted upon to minimize these redesigns.

PICKING THE PACKAGE

Given a ready-to-go circuit design, in the form of a sketch or a breadboard model (which can be also reduced to a sketch), the first task of the thick film "designer" is to pick the package that his circuit will use. The package naturally must be large enough to get all the individual elements into it. It must also be large enough to dissipate heat that will be generated. At the same time, if it is too large, the advantage of compactness will be lost, as well as the advantage of low cost.

Before the designer starts the layout, he or she must know the size and type of the package to be designed for. It is not very practical to start laying out the thick film circuitry for a $1'' \times 1''$ substrate when a round TO-type substrate will be used. It is an equal waste of time to start laying the circuit out to fit a 1-in.^{2} area and find out that only half the area is needed. What is required at this point is some kind of quick prelayout test that will tell the designer what the final circuit size will be.

A package-picking and size-predicting guide of some kind is exactly what most thick film designers develop early in their design experience, to avoid making layouts that do not fit. All of the many guides in use have roughly the same approach—a simple method of assigning a proper area to each component and a method of allowing for each bit of heat generated in the circuit. The method described below is modeled on an article by R. G. Bristol (from CTS) in *The Electronic Engineer*, September 1969.

Area Required for Components. The Bristol article assigned a standard area for each type of component. Table 12-1 gives the specifications for multilayer capacitor chips.

Table 12-1   Area Required for Capacitors

NPO	K1200	K7000	Area to be Assigned
2-500 pF	120 pF-0.02 μF	560 pF-0.056 μF	0.005 in.^{2}
5-1000 pF	180 pF-0.04 μF	560 pF-0.1 μF	0.008 in.^{2}

This assignment was based on two sizes upon which CTS had standardized. The capacitance range listed for the multilayer ceramic chip capacitors represented the range available from their suppliers. As suppliers changed or as they extended their product capability, the range quoted in the table would also change. If sizes other than the CTS standards were to be used, different area assignments would have to be listed. For larger capacitance, the designer would have to resort to supplier literature to see how much space was needed.

For active chips, the areas listed in Table 12-2 were assigned. It can

Table 12-2   Area Required for Active Devices

Small signal silicon transistors	0.0015 in.^{2}
Signal diodes	0.0010 in.^{2}
Integrated circuits	0.0040 in.^{2}
Rectifier diodes	0.0040 in.^{2}
Power transistors	0.0040 in.^{2}

be seen that the area assigned is the approximate *pad* area, not the area of the chip. (A 20 mil square or 20 $\times$ 20 mil transistor is 0.0004 in.^{2}, and the area assignment listed is 0.0015 in.^{2}—approximately 0.040" $\times$ 0.040".)

In the case of screen-printed resistors, the designer should stay above a certain minimum size. He also must check on the power (heat) in each resistor so that the area assigned will not violate a maximum power rating. In the CTS article, a power maximum of 25 W/in.^{2} had been set; the following formula was used to compute area:

$$\text{area} = \frac{0.04 \text{ in.}^2}{\text{W}} \times \text{power dissipation (W)} \tag{1}$$

For avoiding the extremely small resistors that would be indicated for very low power resistors by applying formula (1), a minimum area of 0.001 in.^{2} was set (about 30 $\times$ 30 mils) for all resistors except very high or very low values (above 50,000 Ω or below 10 Ω). The minimum area for these was 0.002 in.^{2}.

If the thick film fabricator used screen-printed capacitors, an allowance would be made in accordance with the capacitance available per unit area for each of the dielectric compositions in use.

By assigning an area to each component, and using the guides above, a tentative total area requirement could be computed. By totaling all of the power dissipation calculations, the total power dissipation in the circuit is calculated. These two figures, total area needed, and the power dissipated, are all that is required to pick a package (along with knowing how many leads will be needed and making sure that the package picked has enough leads).

Area Available in Various Packages. Table 12-3 shows the useable area available in each of several packages. Note that the available area is *not* the total substrate area. The 1×1 in. substrate, for instance, shows only 0.64 in.^{2} available for components. Space must also be allocated to lead pads and for white space between components.

Some TO-5 and TO-8 packages can accommodate two or three substrates, one stacked above the other. When this package type is chosen, not all of the leads will be available for outside connections—some will

Table 12-3   Packages for Hybrid ICs—Area Available and Power Handling Capabilities

Package	Power Dissipation (25°C ambient)	Linear Derating	Area Available
TO-5 0.180 in. maximum height	500 mW	3.3 mW/°C	0.04 in.^{2}
0.250 in. maximum height	500 mW	3.3 mW/°C	0.08 in.^{2}
TO-8 0.150 in. maximum height	1.25 W	0.008 W/°C	0.09 in.^{2}
0.185 in. maximum height	1.25 W	0.008 W/°C	0.18 in.^{2}
0.275 in. maximum height	1.25 W	0.008 W/°C	0.27 in.^{2}
TO-3	4 W	0.02 W/°C	0.25 in.^{2}
$\frac{1}{4} \times \frac{1}{4}$ in.	500 mW	3.3 mW/°C	0.020 in.^{2}
$\frac{1}{4} \times \frac{3}{8}$ in.	500 mW	3.3 mW/°C	0.045 in.^{2}
$\frac{3}{8} \times \frac{3}{8}$ in.	500 mW	3.3 mW/°C	0.055 in.^{2}
$\frac{1}{2} \times \frac{1}{2}$ in.	750 mW	5 mW/°C	0.15 in.^{2}
$\frac{5}{8} \times \frac{5}{8}$ in.	1 W	0.007 W/°C	0.23 in.^{2}
$\frac{3}{4} \times \frac{3}{4}$ in.	1.25 W	0.008 W/°C	0.29 in.^{2}
1×1 in.	1.5 W	0.01 W/°C	0.64 in.^{2}

be needed for interconnections between the substrates. The areas available shown in Table 12-3 represent certain CTS standards having to do with their ideas about proper component spacing, line width, and so on. Other firms using different line spacing and line width standards would arrive at different figures for area available in the various packages. The standards used are dependent on a complex interplay of factors such as internal design standards, cost goals, and reliability standards.

Heat Generation Limitations. A common rule of thumb is that "total heat generated is to be limited to $1\frac{1}{2}$ W/in.²" This applies to a 1×1 substrate, but note (in Table 12-3) that smaller substrates can handle more watts per square inch. The type of mounting to the pc board is also important (see the rating for the TO-3).

The $1\frac{1}{2}$ W/in.² rule of thumb, or the more specific ratings shown in Table 12-3, are for circuits operating at room temperature. A 1-in.² thick film circuit generating $1\frac{1}{2}$ W will run about 25°C above this—or about 50°C. If the ambient is much higher—say 150°C—the circuit will still run about 25°C above the ambient, or 175°C. This would mean that the thick film circuit is in trouble, with soldered leads melting off, plastic encapsulation charring, and individual components running far above their maximum operating temperatures. In fact, trouble can start at lower temperatures. At 125°C ambient, the package is running at 150°C; but individual components near hot spots may be running much hotter—enough to melt solder, for example.

Following the temperature derating column of Table 12-3 helps to avoid extreme overheating. The size of the leads, the length of the leads, the position of the package in relation to air flow, whether or not there is air flow, and many other factors determine what the actual heat dissipation capabilities of a package can be.

The power rating and heat dissipation capabilities given here represent those used by CTS at the time of the Bristol article. Other firms will use somewhat different ratings to satisfy their individual needs. Some firms might, for instance, rate the same resistor compositions up to 50 W/in.²—or use *other* compositions possibly up to 150 W/in.². Power ratings for resistors depend on composition. Power handling capabilities depend on package design and environmental situations. A table with a simple linear derating chart such as Table 12-3 should be taken as no more than a general guide. It should not be stretched too far toward the higher ambient temperatures, because its accuracy is questionable. The subject of heat generation and dissipation is an important part of layout and design. It can be very complex for circuits that are pushing normal design limits. The complexities, however, are far beyond the scope of this book.

Partitioning. If the circuit to be produced is complex, it is likely that the final version will consist of several different thick film circuits—or perhaps of some thick film circuits, some ICs, and some discrete components. Splitting up a circuit into individual subcircuits is called *partitioning*—and this (like the layout of the individual circuit) is a critical process. Ease of assembly, system performance, and final cost are all deeply affected by the way the system is partitioned.

In the days of the all-discrete circuit, partitioning was not particularly critical and was often done by function. (The IF circuit was in one section, the audio amplifier in another, and the RF portions in still another section.) Functional partitioning approaches are not necessarily the proper way to partition thick film circuits. In an article by H. Fenster and F. Gargione (RCA) appearing in the *1969 ISHM Proceedings* (p. 281), "System Partitioning for Hybrid Circuits," the following general guidelines about partitioning were set forth:

1. *"Maintain circuit identity and modular function."* All other things being equal—do this, because it helps to understand how the circuit works. It is also likely to reduce interconnection complexity to the next level of assembly. In addition to being a functional module for one particular circuit, it might also be useful somewhere else. But there are exceptions to this rule. These exceptions make up the rest of the Fenster-Gargione guidelines.

2. *"Do not partition into very small (non complex) units."* Such units are easy to manufacture with high yields, but packaging and testing costs will be high. This approach is not at all economical (if the partitioning goes far enough one is back to individual components). A corollary to this rule is *"do not partition into very large units."* These also tend to be economic disasters. A happy medium must be reached. The proper "happy medium" will be different for different applications, different firms, and different general design approaches.

3. *"Standardize form factor of packages."* Standardization makes for economic purchasing, and for economic handling in assembly. Standardization into a *family* of packages is an attractive goal—for instance, 14 lead DIPs plus 20, 24, 32, and 40 lead versions for more complicated circuits. (Caution: do not carry standardization so far that an economic penalty is encountered. To meet a variety of operating conditions, only the best and most expensive package would always give proper protection. This would place a penalty on applications where a very simple package would suffice. Standardize only when no penalties are encountered.

4. *"Try to redesign circuitry when existing circuits cannot be hybridized because of component limitations."* When a component is needed that does

not lend itself to miniaturization of hybridization, see if it can be designed out of the circuit. This may put a burden on the designer, and complex performance/cost tradeoffs and compromises are often necessary. A serious attempt should be made to design circuits that contain nothing but components that can be hybridized.

5. *"Make use of standard ICs and LSI arrays."* If part of the system can be produced by using a standard monolithic circuit, use it. A hybrid house can seldom beat the costs of a standard circuit produced by a large IC producer.

6. *Last rule: do not be afraid to violate any of the above rules.* Rules should never be followed rigidly. Thus gains in cost and performance can be had by ignoring the rule about "maintaining circuit identity and modular function." A careful study of the entire system might point out ways to combine parts of several different functional modules to make processing much easier. Resistors in similar resistance ranges or performance levels could be grouped so that modules could be made with only one resistor screening per module rather than two or more. Or very sensitive parts could be grouped into a special package. If this is done, advantages outlined in the first guideline will be lost, but compensating reductions in cost may be realized.

We have already mentioned the problems involved in following guideline 3 too closely. Guideline 4, if always followed, would sooner or later result in sublevel performance. It is sometimes best to "give up" and mount the components that resist hybridization outboard.

This last rule was not one of the Fenster-Gargione rules.

MAKING THE THICK FILM CIRCUIT LAYOUT— DESIGN GUIDELINES

Let us say that the package has been picked and the size of the substrate is set. How then does one go about laying out an economic and practical thick film circuit? Later on in this section we list rules and regulations for thick film layout. But none of these rules will really answer the big question: what kind of mental process is involved in making the design? The design rules instruct about the size of the soldering or bonding pads and the width of the conductor runs, but do not specify *where* to put a specific conductor or a bonding pad. The decision about *where* these are to be placed in relationship to each other represents a mental process that does not reduce to simple rules. Attempts to reduce the complex logic of layout geometry to a series of simple rules are always failures. Circuits laid out by use of rigid rules are usually not so good as circuits laid out by a clever layout man. An example is the difficulty in using a computer to help in the design and layout of a thick film circuit. It has been attempted, but to the authors' knowledge has not succeeded as yet. The result has been poorly laid out circuits—more expensive to produce, wasteful of space, and so on.

The circuit layout procedure is critical. The designer is either locking in forever a series of problems that will make the circuit perform poorly or produce expensively (if laid out improperly) or laying out a circuit that performs in a superior way and manufactures economically with a minimum of problems (if done properly). We later introduce a series of simple layout rules, but they no more than hint at what must go through the designer's mind as he transfers the circuit schematic into the thick film layout.

Placement of a transistor too close to a hot running resistor may seriously degrade the transistor's performance, but placing it elsewhere may add considerably to the expense of the circuit. Redesigning the resistor so that it will run cool in turn will crowd the substrate, and unwanted parasitics pop up. A broad and detailed knowledge of the many factors involved, such as the ones just mentioned, is an *absolute necessity* for the layout designer. He will make or break the circuit with his layout. Those who give this job to a draftsman—just because it looks like a draftsman-type job—are asking for trouble, and usually get it.

We make no attempt here to describe the mental process involved in transforming a circuit diagram to a thick film layout. All we can say is that it is a complex mental process, best done by designers who know what they are doing. We can also say that doing it over and over again is very helpful. Experience pays.

Figure 12-2 shows the results of a layout effort on the part of a skilled layout designer. This particular circuit has been chosen because it is simple so that the transition from circuit diagram to layouts of individual thick film conductor patterns and resistor patterns is easily visualized.

There is a tendency to view the thick film layout as a circuit diagram; or to view a circuit diagram as the basic thick film layout pattern. Because of this, the first step in the layout process is to change the original circuit diagram to a topographical layout, such as shown in Figure 12-2, which allows easier visualization as a thick film layout.

Following are a collection of layout "rules" or aids. They summarize experience of other designers, reflect recognition of the limitations of the materials being used, and are the result of application of simple common sense.

1. *Conductors—remember their resistivity.* Thick film conductors can have sufficiently high resistivities so that a significant amount of resistance can be built into the circuit if the layout does not compensate properly. Table 12-4 shows typical resistivities for common types of thick film con-

Table 12-4 Typical Resistivity of Thick Film Conductors

Type	$\Omega/\square$	1 in. long $\times$ 20 mils wide	1 in. long $\times$ 5 mils wide
Palladium silver	0.005	¼ Ω	2 Ω
Palladium gold	0.040	2 Ω	16 Ω
Platinum gold	0.100	5 Ω	40 Ω
Gold	0.100	5 Ω	40 Ω

ductors. The resistivities of a narrow line can build up quite rapidly, as can be seen from the column dealing with the 5-mil-wide line. An adjustment has been made to compensate for the fact that a narrow line will not be as thick as a wider line. This is because printed thickness is dependent on line width (see Figure 8-3) and on the mesh size. Table 12-4 represents the values that would be obtained with a 200-mesh screen, not a fine-mesh screen. Fine lines often are printed with 325-mesh screen (not the more standard 200-mesh screen).

2. *Avoid long conductor runs—especially of narrow lines.* This is a corollary of rule 1. Long runs have high resistance. (It is a good way of making a low-resistance resistor, however.)

3. *Avoid narrow conductor lines when possible—aim for 20-mil-wide lines if possible.* Narrow lines are hard to print and have high resistance. Wider lines are more economical. (Figure 12-3.)

4. *Avoid close spacing.* Long runs of conductors closely spaced promote shorts because of coming together of the conductors. Ten-mil lines with 10-mil spaces are "not too bad" to print, but usually each substrate must be inspected to make sure there are no shorted conductors. Five-mil lines with 5-mil spaces must be *carefully* inspected, and almost invariably there will be a significant yield loss due to shorts or opens. Twenty-mil lines with 20- or 30-mil spacing are to easy to print that not only is the yield very high, but in-process inspection can be eliminated.

There is no economy in narrow lines and close spacing. In high-volume thick film circuits that must be produced with both high reliability and low cost—such as the Delco auto-radio substrates or RCA consumer products circuits—this rule and the two preceding ones are rigidly followed.

5. *Resistor terminations.* Conductor termination pads for resistors should be at least 10 mils larger on each side than the resistor that will be printed over it. This ensures that the resistor makes complete contact—even when one of the setups is off. (Figure 12-4.)

6. *Pad size—active chips.* Pads for active chips could be made with at least a 5-mil border on each side—10 mils if there is room. This allows

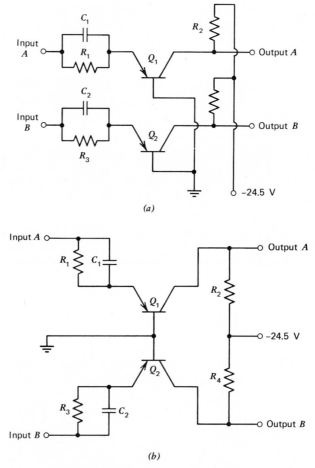

(a)

(b)

Figure 12-2 An example of the thick film layout procedure (a dual MOS driver). (a) Original schematic diagram. (b) Same circuit, rearranged to conform to a thick film layout. (Note that crossovers are eliminated.) (c) (scale 10:1). 1, Composite; hybrid substrate layout. 2, Conductor mask; conductor screens. 3, 10-kΩ/□ mask; resistor screens. 4, 100-kΩ/□ mask; resistor screens. [*Source.* F. Gargione and H. Fenster (RCA), "System Partitioning for Hybrid Circuits," *1969 ISHM Proceedings,* p. 281.]

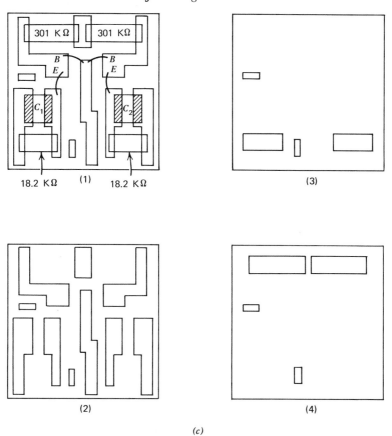

(c)

Figure 12-2 (*Continued*)

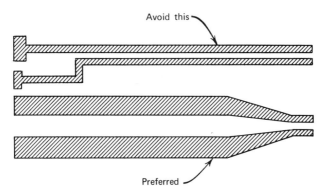

Figure 12-3 Avoid closely spaced long runs of narrow lines.

enough area to "hit the pad" with the chip and makes a good eutectic bond. If there is a possibility that the active chip must be replaced, many designers provide extra space for mounting a second chip. (Figure 12-5.)

7. *Pad size—wire bonding pads.* These should be at least 10 mils square. Smaller ones will slow wire bonding rates.

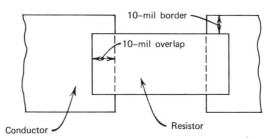

Figure 12-4 Recommended border and overlap minimums for resistor terminations.

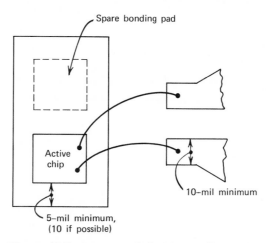

Figure 12-5 Recommended chip bonding and wire bond pad sizes.

8. *Solder bonding pads for wire leads.* These should be three times the wire diameter and 50 mils long (or more). Narrower ones will lack room for a proper solder fillet. Shorter pads will result in leads that peel off easily. (Figure 12-6.)

9. *Bonding pads for soldering discrete components (such as capacitors).* To allow for a proper solder fillet, the pad dimension should be at least

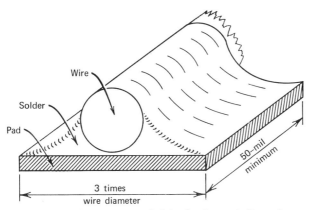

Figure 12-6 Recommended lead wire pad dimensions.

20 mils on each side larger than the chip component being soldered. Some "cheating" on this rule for the smaller chip capacitors is common, but the bond strength may be a bit low. It will be more difficult to tell by visual inspection whether a good solder bond has been made. (Figure 12-7.)

If the circuit will be subjected to wide swings in temperature—especially to extreme cold—a strong bond is essential. Differences in thermal expansion have to be taken up through the ductility of the solder. Before the solder begins to move, considerable shear will be placed on the chip and a small bond area will not be strong enough. (Firing the conductor to maximize substrate adhesion is important here.)

10. *Screen printing over holes.* The conductor area should be at least 10 mils wide (20 mils is preferable). Do not print over the open hole. Otherwise paste will be forced through the hole in the substrate, bleeding onto the reverse side or drying into a plugged hole. A slight overlap (5 mils at the most) is preferable. This will force some ink down the sides of the substrate hole, ensuring a good strong solder bond. (Proper control of the overlap, coupled with two-sided printing can give reliable electrical connection from one side of the substrate to the other.) (Figure 12-7.)

11. *Edges of the substrate.* Keep thick film circuitry at least 20 mils from the edge of the substrate. If the substrate chips during handling, the chip will occur on the edge. If circuitry is close to the edge, chipping will open up the circuit.

12. *Avoid crossovers.* Clever layout can often avoid crossovers (see Figure 12-2).

Some designers get around crossovers by running conductors between the connection pads of a multilayer ceramic capacitor. They sometimes depend on the insulating effect of the ceramic capacitor shell and the fact

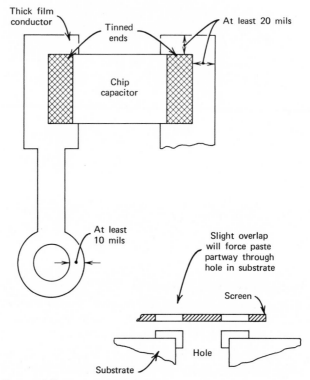

Figure 12-7 Recommended dimensions for pads for soldering discrete chips and for substrate holes.

that the capacitor's end terminations will not extend far along the sides to avoid a short. This dependence is not always justified. It is advisable to give the element passing under the capacitor chip a protective coating. (Figure 12-8a.)

Many crossovers are made by jumping over printed conductors with wire bonding leads in going from the active chip to the various conductor pads. It is necessary to protect the thick film elements over which the lead passes, but this can often be done at no extra cost because a protective coat serves also to protect capacitors, resistors, and so on. (Figure 12-8b.)

It is possible to avoid screen-printed crossovers by using the back side of the substrate. When the substrate has holes for mounting discrete devices, a few extra holes for crossovers do not add significantly to substrate cost. Avoid passing to the other side of the substrate by going around the edge. (Some packaging schemes have leads that attach to both sides of the substrate, offering automatic access to the opposite side.) (Figure 12-8c.)

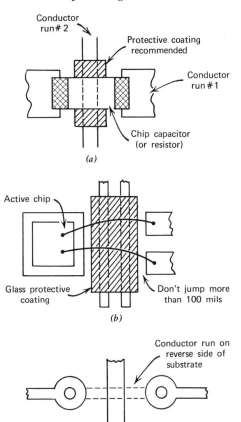

Figure 12-8 Ways of avoiding screen-printed crossovers. (*a*) Going under a chip capacitor. (*b*) Jumping over conductor runs with bonding wire. (*c*) Going through holes to the other side of a substrate.

Figure 12-9 shows a thick film circuit that has used most of the methods just outlined (except two-sided printing) to avoid screen-printed crossovers.

13. *Screen-printed crossovers.* When all else fails, screen-printed crossovers must be used. There is really nothing wrong with this, except that it adds extra screen-printing and firing operations.

One must keep in mind that crossovers have a parasitic capacitance. This capacitance is dependent on the area of crossover and the thickness and dielectric constant of the crossover material. The most stable of the crossover compositions are the recrystallized types. They have K's of at least 14 (as compared with under 10 for pure glass crossovers). The line

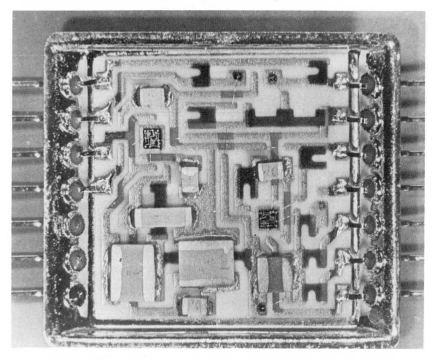

Figure 12-9 A thick film layout that avoids screen-printed crossovers. Note that resistors and conductors are running underneath the chip capacitors. (Photograph courtesy of CTS Corporation.)

width can be reduced to cut down on parasitics, but this will increase the resistance of the conductor. A 400-mil crossover (not that anyone would use one that wide) would have a capacitance of 32 pF if K15 crossover material was used. If the crossover width were 40 mils, the capacitance would be reduced to about 8 pF (not a 90% reduction in capacitance to go with the 90% reduction in area, because of fringing effects). For a 4-mil line, the capacitance would be reduced to 2 to 3 pF, but for such a narrow conductor the resistivity of the conductor would be high.

If parasitics of a few picofards cause circuit problems, one must consider using a *multilayer ceramic circuit board* where the conductors are buried in the ceramic. Parasitics here will be reduced about an order of magnitude, and costs will be increased by a similar amount.

For single crossovers, the dielectric should be wider by at least 10 mils on each side of the conductors than the conductor runs. (Figure 12-10.)

14. *Multilayer screen-printed circuits.* For extremely complex thick film circuits, such as those containing several complex IC chips, dozens and

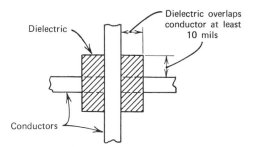

Figure 12-10 Overlap dimensions for screen-printed crossovers.

even hundreds of crossovers are needed. Making a ceramic multilayer "printed circuit board" with thick film techniques is becoming a popular way to produce these complex interconnect circuits. It is accomplished by screening alternate layers of conductor patterns and dielectric patterns. Holes in the dielectric pattern allow interlayer connections.

When the number of thick film layers exceeds three (two conductor planes and one dielectric), the surface will become rather uneven as more and more layers are printed. Precision screen printing over the many discontinuities and ridges becomes difficult, and narrow lines and narrow spacings become impractical. (Figure 11.) (A screen-printed line will spread wider as it is printed over a ridge.) Figure 12-12 shows a method of maintaining a flat surface by printing complimentary layers of dielectric and conductor. This technique is usually necessary if fine line printing is to be maintained past five layers and is sometimes used to maintain flat surfaces for less than five layers.

Multilayer thick film circuits are commonly very crowded and require printing of the narrowest possible lines, but difficulties multiply rapidly when buried lines are printed much less than 10 mils wide. Without compensation techniques, minimum width and spacing must increase with each succeeding layer. Therefore, the designer will often put his most complex level on the bottom and save the simplest for the top. (Note that this was done in the circuit illustrated in Figure 12-11.)

15. *Resistor aspect ratios.* The aspect ratio chosen for a resistor dictates how easily it can be trimmed and how it will perform. The ideal aspect ratio is 1. To print a reasonable range of resistors from a single screen pass, the aspect ratio is extended to a range of about one order of magnitude—say from 0.5 to 5. To make an even wider range of resistors without resorting to an extra screen-printing step, this range is sometimes stretched to two orders of magnitude (i.e., 0.15 to 15). (Figure 12-13.)

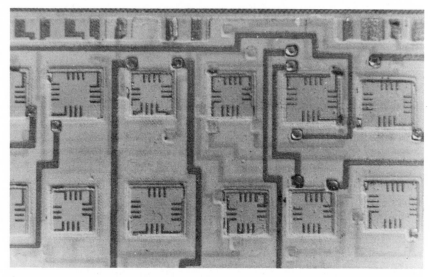

Figure 12-11   Uncompensated multilayer screen-printed circuit. Note the steps made by each succeeding layer and the underlines on the top layer. (Circuit by JW Microelectronics; photograph by State of the Art, Inc.)

If all of the resistors fit into a suitable aspect ratio range except one, using a discrete chip might be a better solution than setting up a separate screen printing of a different resistivity ink.

High aspect ratios are difficult to trim. Once trimmed, they are prone to hot spots. A "top hat" design (see Figure 12-14)) is one way to avoid high aspect ratios.

Meanders in very high aspect ratios are not recommended. A more suitable arrangement would be to use shorting bars (see Figure 12-15). The user should not normally be involved with such high aspect ratios. Designs using meanders are quite rare today in thick film. (They were common in the days before high resistivity inks were available—or useable.)

16. *Resistor size.* The area of a resistor should be kept over 0.005 in.² (approximately 0.070 in.², or 0.050 × 0.100 in.). Figure 12-16 shows how the spread of values increases as resistors are made smaller.

A corollary of this rule is that resistor length should remain over 50 mils. If a resistor is made shorter than this, the interface reaction between the conductor and the resistor plays an increasingly important role. Figure 12-17 shows how interface reactions affect realized values in short resistors.

Another corollary to the minimum area rule is that the resistor width could be kept above 50 mils. As the width goes below 10 mils, control of thickness of the resistor—thence value—becomes more difficult. (See

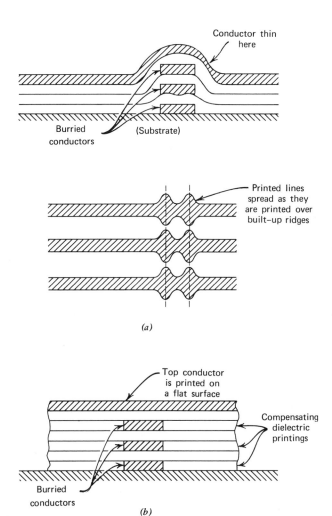

Figure 12-12 Illustrating how compensated (complementary screened) multilevel circuits maintain a flat surface. (*a*) Uncompensated multilayer printing. (*b*) Compensated multilayer printing.

Figure 8-3.) Also, small errors in width play a more significant role.

A third corollary is that the rule is often broken. It would be nice if all resistors could be longer and wider than 50 mils, but the need today for small resistors and increasingly compact circuits simply will not allow this rule to be followed. When it is violated, one can expect to miss targets

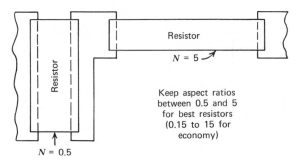

Figure 12-13 Recommended aspect ratio ranges.

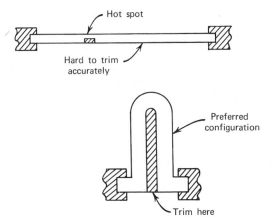

Figure 12-14 The top-hat configuration is easier to trim than a high aspect ratio resistor.

by a wider margin, poorer power handling, poorer TCR and TCR tracking, and wider spreads.

17. *Power ratings for resistors.* There is a maximum power rating, expressed in terms of watts per square inch, for each type of resistor composition and for each thickness and type of substrate. Few firms known enough about the intricacies of heat dumping to be able to have an exact power rating for each of these situations, so they set a conservative rating that they know to be safe and keep all of their designs within this maxium.

A common maximum power rating is 25 W/in.² If more power is generated within the resistor, it will not be able to dump heat into the substrate or into its covering (air, plastic, etc.) fast enough and will overheat. Overheating will (1) exaggerate resistance drift because of the resistor running much hotter than ambient, (2) cause permanent change in resistance, (3)

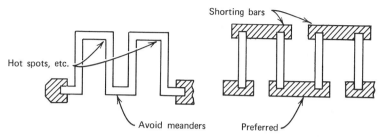

Figure 12-15 Avoid meanders.

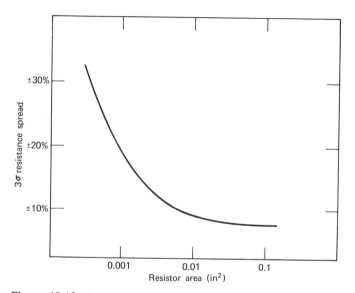

Figure 12-16 Spread in resistors as a function of resistor size. [*Source.* R. C. Headly (DuPont), "Reproducibility of Electrical Properties of Thick Film Resistors," *1967 ISHM Proceedings,* pp. 56–69.]

overheat the surrounding areas of the substrate, perhaps to the point of damaging neighboring components, and (4) damage plastic overcoats or encapsulations.

The 25 W/in.² is a rather conservative rating that has been used with the palladium-palladium oxide-silver resistors. Some firms use less conservative ratings (up to 40 W/in.² of resistor area), perhaps at the risk of increased resistor degradation and drift with time. Some of the newer resistor compositions are much more resistant to heat degradation and can be run at higher power ratings (provided that the package or nearby components are not damaged).

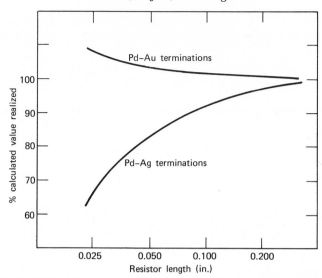

Figure 12-17 Interface reaction effect as a function of resistor length. [*Source.* R. C. Headly (Du Pont), "Reproducibility of Electrical Properties of Thick Film Resistors," *1967 ISHM Proceedings,* pp. 56–69.]

18. *Power ratings for packages and substrates.* A common rule is 1½ W/in.², but different packages have different capabilities of dumping heat. Different environments also play an important role (still air versus moving air, etc.). The 1½ W/in.² rule is a dangerous generalization. More exact ratings are given in Table 12-3.

19. *Voltage limitations.* When resistors are operated in a strong electric field, some resistor characteristics will be changed. If the field is over 1 V/mil, permanent changes can be expected.

Little has been reported on this subject until very recently. As resistors get smaller and smaller, voltage effects will become more important and more will be known about this subject. At present, few resistor composition suppliers report VCR or drift characteristics.

20. *Trimming resistors.* Do not forget to leave room for starting an air-abrasive trim—at least 25 mils. The trim should not begin near another resistor; otherwise trimming of one resistor will change an already trimmed resistor. Try to make all the trims in the same direction, because this facilitates trimming setup. In any case, plan trims in only the X or Y directions. Do not forget the potential hot spots that might be created during trimming. Make power handling calculations on *trimmed* resistor geometry, not on the untrimmed geometry.

21. *Trimming closed loops.* Figure 12-18 shows two closed loops. They cannot be trimmed. (Unless the trimming system is very sophisticated.) If the circuit contains these, trimming must be done with the loop open. The loop can be closed later with a wire jumper—or by using a discrete chip capacitor or resistor or a chip jumper.

22. *Wire bonding.* There is a limit to the length of a wire jumper or of a wire running from a chip to the pad. Keep total length below 100 mils. If the wire passes over conductors or resistors, the elements should be insulated (see Figure 12-8*b*).

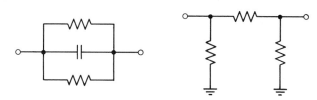

Figure 12-18   Closed loops cannot be trimmed.

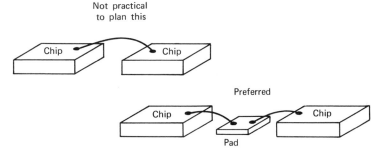

Figure 12-19   Method for chip-to-chip wire bonding.

It is not good practice to connect wires from one chip to another. It is better to drop to a pad from each chip. Most production bonders are programmed to bond from a high bond (the chip) to a low bond (the substrate). Overriding the programmed search heights is normally not possible. However, if one has a bonder that can do this, or is not using preprogrammed search heights on low-volume runs, it is all right to bond from chip to chip. (Figure 12-19.)

ARTWORK—GETTING FROM THE LAYOUT TO THE SCREEN

The Master Sketch. This is the first step on the way to making screen patterns for each individual printing. It is common practice for the layout to be sketched out on coordinate paper, where one square on the coordinate paper is the smallest unit dimension that will be used—commonly 5 or 10 mils. The layout designer will work with a pencil—resorting to lots of erasing as he tries different geometrical approaches.

Once the first layout of the circuit is completed, the next step is to make a final sketch—which is a cleaned-up version of the by now much-erased original. All of the discrete components and thick film compositions that will be used are displayed on this master sketch. Colored pencil or cross hatching will help to keep resistors looking different from conductors and to identify the various other components and patterns.

It is best to have the master sketch made in the same magnification as the artwork will be. For most thick film circuits, the artwork is ten times ($10\times$) the final pattern size. Thus five-squares-to-the-inch coordinate paper can be used for making the original sketches, with one square representing 20 mils in the final pattern. For circuits that are more compact, ten-square-to-the-inch paper is more suitable. If a significant part of the circuit will be made of patterns of under 10 mils—such as metallization for beam lead chips—it is desirable to abandon $10\times$ magnification for something larger.

The Rubylith®. With the $10\times$ sketch finished, the artwork process is ready for the next step—cutting the Rubylith. Rubylith is a trade name for a masking film (Ulano Company). It is so popular that the term is close to becoming generic. Masking film consists of a mylar sheet (3 to 5 mils thick) with a soft layer of transparent red material coating one side. If an area of the red material is scribed, it can be easily stripped from the mylar backing.

After scribing and stripping the red material from a circuit layout pattern, it is placed in front of a light source. Red light will pass through the stripped portion only, and will be absorbed where the red coating remains. A photograph taken of the Rubylith artwork will be exposed only where the stripped-away image passes light. A negative will be black where the red was stripped. If the size of the photographic image is carefully reduced by *exactly* $10\times$ the negative will be an exact reproduction of the desired pattern, $\frac{1}{10}$ the size of the original artwork.

The masking film can be cut and stripped by placing it over the master sketch and having a draftsman carefully cut along the outlined edges of the various patterns—one set for conductors, one for each resistor composition, and so on. Placing the sketch and the transparent masking film over a light box will make it easier to see where to cut. Cutting is done with either a knife or special cutting tools that can be purchased from film suppliers. The latter are somewhat easier to use. A careful draftsman can cut within about 10 mils of where he is aiming, which will permit an accurately dimensioned final negative. A 10-mil error in artwork will reduce to 1 mil. A 20-mil-wide line can be easily held to within ±2 mils. This is accurate enough for many thick film circuits.

For more accuracy—or for someone who cuts lots of artwork and wants to save time and reduce mistakes—a *coordinatograph* is recommended. The coordinatograph is a large light table with a pen mounted on a carrier that is movable in very accurate dimensions in *X-Y* (or rotational) modes. The coordinatograph is screw-driven in each direction. The screw is calibrated. When cutting artwork on the coordinatograph the dimensions are cranked in rather than traced. The original sketch can be placed under the masking film so that one can keep track of where the cutting is—except that to move from one line to the next on the master sketch, the operator will not depend on visual positioning, but instead on the vernier calibration of the pen carriage drive screw. When artwork is cut on a coordinatograph, cutting accuracies of close to 1 mil can be held. When reduced to the final circuit size, the errors are extremely small. (Figure 12-20.)

Coordinatographs are available that have automatic action—the pen (or cutting knife) being driven by numerically controlled tape or a computer.

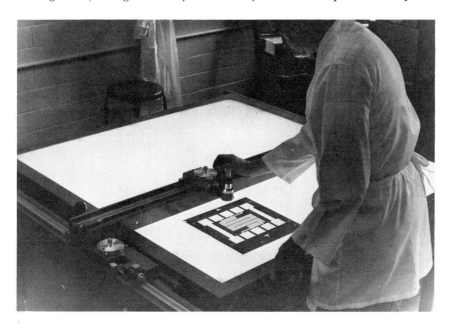

Figure 12-20   A coordinatograph. (Photograph by State of the Art, Inc.)

These are popular for complex monolithic IC artwork, but seldom needed for the average thick film circuit. (Complex multilayer interconnect circuits are an exception).

After the various individual patterns are cut, it is easy to verify that they match the original sketch by placing each sheet of artwork over the original sketch and by laying one piece of artwork over the next. (The designer should put locating marks on each successive piece of artwork—partly to check the artwork by aligning on the marks and partly to make it possible for the screen printer to align successive printings. These marks, commonly small circles, dots, crosses, and so on, are placed in corners of the circuit where they will not be in the way. At least two are needed for proper alignment.)

For complex circuits, the original drawing or sketch is sometimes laid out in several "sections"—one for each of the final patterns, rather than depending on various cross-hatched or colored patterns. If there is to be more than one conductor printing, several resistor printings, glass overcoats, and screen-printed capacitors, a single master sketch is very complicated. It is then difficult to cut Rubylith artwork from it without making mistakes.

Photographic Reduction. A photographic negative is produced by placing the Rubylith over a light source and taking a picture. Special reduction cameras are used where exact reduction ratios can be held. Reduction cameras accurate enough for most thick film circuits are commonly employed by printers and photographic shops. The thick film producer can turn to these sources for his photographic reduction if he wishes to avoid owning such a camera and obtaining the necessary skills for its operation. The camera owner must be convinced, however, that a $10\times$ reduction has to be *exactly* $10\times$, not 9.95, or $10.06\times$.

Screen Making. A screen stencil is made by placing the negative (the master) over an emulsion-coated screen. The emulsion is water-soluble unless exposed to light. When exposed to light (a carbon arc) with the master placed on the screen, the emulsion is rendered insoluble (via a polymerization process, triggered by the light) in all parts except those under the black areas of the master. The unexposed pattern is then washed out (developed), leaving the emulsion-coated screen with the printing pattern in open mesh—an exact reproduction of the master.

Considerable expertise is needed in making good screens, and many thick film producers prefer not to obtain this expertise until their screen demand is high enough to make it worthwhile. The skill of getting the mesh lined up properly, locating the master on the screen, getting the right emulsion thickness, getting an emulsion that does not wear rapidly or deform with use, exposing properly, and many other skills must be mastered in order to make good screens. Qualified screen-making firms offer rapid service at attractive rates and many firms find it advantageous to use these services in varying degrees.

MAKE OR BUY—SCREENS AND ARTWORK

Most screen-making firms offer artwork-generation facilities. They can make a Rubylith from the customer's sketch, reduce it, expose the resulting master to a screen, and ship the developed screen in a matter of days. The hybrid producer can buy into this process at any of several steps.

The most expensive part of the process is cutting the Rubylith, and many thick film producers prefer to cut the artwork in the house, sending it then to the screen maker. This reduces expenses considerably as well as turnaround time.

Some hybrid producers take the process one step further by doing their own photoreductions. The photographic master is sent out. This saves a bit more on cost and reduces delivery time still further.

Larger producers buy frames with screens stretched on them by the screen maker (properly aligned and tensioned) and expose the master themselves. The savings *can* be significant, but the faster turnaround is often more important. Generally speaking, the hybrid producer must be using quite a few screens to make in-house developing profitable (at least five screens a day).

Large firms, and those who are determined do-it-yourselfers, buy screen frames and raw screen and go captive all the way. Smaller firms make their own artwork and screens only for fast turnaround capabilities, readily admitting that savings are not an economic factor.

At what level to enter the artwork screen-making process is often a complex decision and is best made on the basis of the individual firm's special needs. Geographic isolation and a need for fast response will cause a small user to make his own screens, while being next door to a competent screen maker can keep a very large user from going to captive screen making.

Chapter 13

THE ECONOMICS OF THICK FILM HYBRID
MICROCIRCUIT PRODUCTION

We now consider the many economic forces involved in producing thick film hybrid microcircuits. Our approach is to describe step by step the manufacture of an "imaginary" thick film hybrid circuit containing an illustrative variety of components. The components include screened-on capacitors and resistors, discrete capacitors and resistors, transistors, and monolithic ICs. We describe manufacture of the same imaginary circuit in three different thick film facilities: (1) a small prototype facility that builds only 25 circuits, (2) a medium-sized production house, where the production run is 1000 circuits, and (3) a high-volume facilitiy, which makes 50,000 circuits in one production run. The assembly methods and the equipment appropriate to the different production levels are described. Equipment costs and production rates are also covered. A good comparison of relative costs at different production levels results, leading the reader to an understanding of the changing nature of both methods and costs as production levels change.

A good way to illustrate the operation of the many economic forces involved in producing thick film circuits is to investigate in some detail the costs of equipment and labor used to build a specific circuit. While it is necessary to be specific about costs of this particular circuit, generalizations to "average" thick film costs are possible from these specific costs.

THE CIRCUIT TO BE "BUILT"

Components. Our circuit consists of the parts listed in Table 13-1. The makeup of the components has been chosen to illustrate various thick film cost situations. The circuit has no particular function, existing solely for illustrative purposes.

Table 13-1   The Circuit to Be Built—Bill of Materials

12 Resistors	5 Loose tolerance
	5 Precision
	2 Low noise
5 Capacitors	2 High value
	3 Low value (screenable)
3 Transistors	
1 8 lead ICs	

Packaging. The circuit will be built on a 1×1 in. aluminum substrate. It will have six wire leads spaced along one edge of the substrate, attached by soldering. The package will be conformally dipped in an epoxy coating.

ECONOMICS OF DIFFERENT PRODUCTION LEVELS

To give the broadest possible picture, costs will be worked out for three different production levels.

Prototype Production. This is usually a situation where the actual need of the circuit to be designed is very limited, the circuit is being built as a trial design (heavy production to follow), or the design is in-house, but future producton is by an outside firm. Even in a high-production case there are often short trial runs. For every final design production run, there can be several prototype designs leading up to the final design, or several designs that never "graduate" to high production. A production run of 25 circuits has been picked to illustrate prototype-laboratory production levels.

Medium Volume Production. A run of 1000 circuits has been chosen to represent a medium-volume production situation. This would be typical of a firm whose output totals this amount each day. Where the prototype operation visualized above might produce less than 100 parts per day (a few prototypes a week), this medium-sized operation would produce several thousand finished circuits a week with several designs being produced simultaneously.

High-Volume Production. A run of 50,000 has been chosen to illustrate heavy production costs. This would be typical of a shop producing at levels approaching a million circuits per month.

Each of the three levels of production chosen for illustration uses different philosophies of production and experiences different costs. These differences in cost can be illustrated if we work out in detail the cost of producing a circuit at each level.

COSTING GROUND RULES

There are probably as many ways of figuring costs as there are thick film hybrid producers. The method used, of course, influences the final figures. The cost we computed *here* is a "factory" cost. It has little resemblance to final selling prices, or to a total cost.

A labor rate of $6/hr (10¢/min) is used. This allows factory overhead commensurate with the less costly type of firm.

To simplify the presentation, costs are computed at 100% yield. This does not give an accurate picture of the real costs of this fictional circuit; but since it is a fictional circuit, the actual costs are not particularly relevant. Comparisons between specific operations at the three production levels is valid, and so is the comparison of the overall cost between the different production levels. (In actual situations, yields might be somewhat higher for higher production levels. It is worthwhile to strive for yield improvements here because the cost of making the improvements can be spread across more units. The relative costs of the high-volume operation may therefore be overstated.) The actual yields that might be expected in a well-run thick film hybrid shop would range from 70% to the mid- and high-90% levels for a circuit of this complexity. The higher end of this range is the level that would be reached only in experienced, well-established operations that are far down the learning curve.

Design costs are not included in this comparison. It is assumed for comparison purposes that the cost of the design is the same for the different levels. (The same time in making calculations, the same time and care in choosing discretes, the same time in making layouts.) In practice, there is the probability that a high-volume design will be much more carefully done, both because the costs of an error are higher, and because efforts at cost reduction pay off better.

A uniform design has been "forced" here so that comparisons could be made. This is far from a realistic situation. There is every likelihood that a design for high-level production would be different from that for low-level production. For example, a special conformal package may not be chosen for a prototype level because of the trouble involved in controlling the process. A prototype design may use a standard metal package for the sake of easy purchasing, while the higher cost of this package would not be accepted with higher levels.

COST OF TOOLING AND OF PURCHASED MATERIALS AND DEVICES

Tooling—Screens. The only tooling cost that is mentioned here is the cost of the screens. Table 13-2 lists the different screens that will be used,

Table 13-2   Screens Needed

Purpose of Screen	Drafting Time
1. Bottom capacitor electrode	1 hr
2. Capacitor dielectric	1 hr
3. Conductor pattern—soldering	2 hr
4. Conductor pattern—bonding	2 hr
5. Resistor pattern 1	1 hr
6. Resistor pattern 2	1 hr
7. Protection pattern	1 hr
8. Solder paste pattern	1 hr

along with a rough estimate of the drafting time needed to do the artwork. It has been assumed that the three factories all use outside-purchased screens. In each plant a draftsman lays out the circuit from the designer's sketches. He could either work with a "coordinatograph" or by hand, depending on the accuracy needed. The Rubylith artwork goes to the screen maker. The screen maker photo reduces it. Higher-production companies would be likely to do some of this in the house. Also, reduced turnaround time sometimes makes in-house screen-making facilities desirable even though they cannot be economically supported (or at least some in-between step, such as photoreduction and mask reduction, while screen mounting and stretching are done outside.)

The prototype operation and the mid-level operation use small 5×5 screen frames that cost about \$25 each (this breaks down to about \$8

for photoreduction of artwork, $8 for the screen mesh and frame, and
$7 for coating and exposing the screen). The high-volume operation uses
a somewhat different approach. It screens more than one substrate at
once so a bigger screen is needed. It also finds that buying a precision
ground screen frame will give more accuracy and make the screen last
longer. It will thus spend about $40 for each screen, the higher cost being
due to the cost of the precision frame and larger screen. The high-volume
operation uses one metal mask, because in this case the five loose tolerance
resistors will be printed using as much precision as possible so that subsequent trimming can be avoided. The metal mask costs about $140. Because
of the length of the run in the high-volume case, five sets of screens are
needed. These costs are summarized in Table 13-3. (In actual production,
much longer screen life than indicated here has often been reported.)

Table 13-3   Screen Costs

	Prototype (25 pc run)	Medium Volume (1000 pc run)
5 screens $25 each	$125.00	$125.00
7 hr drafting	42.00	42.00
	$167.00	$167.00
Costs prorated	$ 6.68 each	$ 0.167 each
High Volume (50,000 pc run)		
7 Wire screens, $41 each		$ 287.00
1 Metal mesh screen		125.00
		$ 412.00
Need 5 sets (multiply $412 by 5)		2,060.00
Plus 10 hr drafting charge		60.00
		$2,120.00
Prorated cost = 4.2¢ each		

Substrates and Other Materials. Tables 13-4 and 13-5 summarize the costs
of substrates and other materials. The differences in unit costs as volume
purchasing power comes into play are the primary reason for the differences
noted, but some account is also taken of the waste involved in the lower-
volume operations. This is most evident in the cost of the plastic encapsulation material. Limited pot life causes much more plastic to be thrown
away than is actually used.

Table 13-4   Substrate Costs

96% Alumina—1 × 1 × 0.025 in.

Operation	Size of Buy	Cost
25	1,000 pc	15¢ each
1,000	10,000 pc	8¢
50,000	250,000 pc	4¢

Table 13-5   Costs of Other Materials

	25 pc run	1000 pc run	50,000 pc run
Wire	2.0¢	1.5¢	1.0¢
Plastic	8.0¢	3.6¢	1.8¢
Solder	0.5¢	0.5¢	0.4¢

Ink Costs. The area covered by the various thick film compositions can be calculated. Let us say that 30% of the surface of the substrate is covered with conductor ink. An average conductor ink covers about 3 ft²/oz when a 200-mesh screen is used. This means that about 0.007 oz of conductor paste is used per circuit.

A platinum-gold ink is used for the prototype operation so that soldering irons, resoldering, and so on, can be utilized without fear of leaching the conductor. This type of ink costs about $100/oz. The middle-volume operation, while still needing some solder leaching resistance, exercises more care and is able to use a palladium-gold ink costing only $60/oz. The high-volume operation uses a palladium-silver costing only $30/oz because their skills and controls are even more sophisticated. All of the operations use gold ink for mounting pads (for the transistors and the IC).

There are ink losses in setting up and in final clean-up of the screens. These losses are relatively important in the prototype cost structure as illustrated in Table 13-6, but have little importance in the other operations.

About 20% of the surface of the substrate is covered with resistors. Resistors are thicker—160-mesh screens are used—but the specific gravity of the paste is lower, so that the average coverage is about the same as for conductors.

Table 13-6   Ink Costs

Type Paste	Cost	25 pc run	1000 pc run	50,000 pc run
Platinum-gold	$100	7.1¢	—	—
Palladium-gold	60	—	4.0¢	—
Palladium-silver	30	—	—	1.8¢
Gold	75	0.7	.6	0.5
Pd-PdO-Ag resistor	25	1.6	1.6	1.0
Capacitor electrode	30	—	—	1.4
Capacitor dielectric	15	—	—	0.7
Protective glass	10	0.4	0.4	0.3
Screen loss	—	20.0	0.4	0.1
Total cost per circuit		29.8¢	7.0¢	5.8¢

The amount of area covered in our example is rather high. Most hybrid circuits do not utilize this much of the total area. The cost figures generated here could be considered higher than for most circuits.

In the case of screened-on capacitors, used in the high-volume operation (but not the others), about 10% of the substrate area is used for dielectric printing. Two electrode printings are needed, and a double thick dielectric layer will be employed. Coverage is about the same with the dielectrics as with the other inks—3 ft^2/oz—but with the double thickness, this is cut in half.

The costs for the various inks are summarized in Table 13-6.

Purchased Discrete Components. Table 13-7 shows costs of the discrete components. The volume price breaks are important. The prototype opera-

Table 13-7   Purchased Components

Kind of component	25 pc run	1000 pc run	50,000 pc run
3 transistor chips	$1.50	$0.75	$0.65 ⎱ + 20%
1 8-lead IC chip	2.00	1.00	0.85 ⎰
2 .1µF chip Capacitors	1.20	0.60	0.40
1 .01µF chip Capacitor	0.40	0.20	0.16
2 1000-pF chip Capacitors	0.40	0.20	
2 Resistor chips	0.60	0.30	0.25
Face-bonding premium			0.30
Total cost per circuit	$6.10	$3.05	$2.61

tion buys in low volume from a distributor—or at least pays distributor prices even though purchasing from the factory. The middle-level operation buys in 1000- to 10,000-piece lots (or, in other words, pays the "standard" OEM price). The high-volume operation will be "wheeling and dealing," making buys of up to a million pieces. (These costs do not include the internal costs of receiving and inspecting the components, which is normally part of general overhead.)

The 20% premium paid by the high-volume operation for active devices is due to the parts being in beam lead or flip chip configuration. A 20% premium is low today, but could be attainable in time. The important point to keep in mind is the specific sum spent as a premium payment, which will be compared with savings in assembly costs.

Note also that the two 1000-pF capacitors are screened-on in the high-volume operation, but are purchased as chips in the lower-volume operations. The added material costs are (see Table 13-6) 2.2¢ (plus labor for printing); these parts would cost 16¢ if purchased as discretes, however.

Summary of Purchased Parts and Tooling. Spreading of tooling costs over longer production runs and the economy of buying in large lots is illustrated in Table 13-8, which summarizes the cost of purchased parts and materials. (Costs quoted here and elsewhere reject prices of early 1970.)

Table 13-8   Summary of Purchased Parts and Materials

	25 pc run	1000 pc run	50,000 pc run
Tooling	$ 6.680	$0.167	$0.042
Substrates	0.150	0.080	0.040
Inks	0.298	0.070	0.058
Other materials	0.105	0.056	0.032
Components	6.100	3.060	2.61
Total	$13.33	$3.43	$2.78

LABOR RATES AND EQUIPMENT COSTS

In this section we discuss the 21 operations required to produce the circuit, and equipment needed for the different production levels, rates attainable with different equipment, and the setup times.

The 21 operations are:

1. Capacitor and resistor setup.
2. Print capacitor electrodes.
3. Fire capacitor electrode.
4. Print capacitor dielectric (two passes).
5. Print top electrode and conductor pattern.
6. Print bonding pads.
7. Fire conductors and dielectric.
8. Test capacitors and inspect.
9. Print resistor pattern 1.
10. Print resistor pattern 2.
11. Fire resistors.
12. Trim resistors.
13. Print and fire protective coatings.
14. Test and inspect.
15. Attach active devices to substrate.
16. Wire bond.
17. Attach passive devices.
18. Attach lead wires.
19. Encapsulate.
20. Mark.
21. Test.

1. Capacitor and Resistor Setup. In the precision printing of the resistors for the high-volume operation, where it is desired to avoid 100% trimming, a very careful setup is required. This normally involves extra test firings of the ink to determine exactly what resistance will be obtained plus possible additional blending. A test firing may be done on the line to check out screen tension, blade attack angle, and so on, because these also influence the resistance value obtained.

The same setup efforts are required to make capacitors. A setup charge of 120 min has been allowed for this operation, but only for the high-volume plant, since they are the only one attempting precision printing.

Printing and Firing Equipment and Rates. Both the prototype and the low-volume production operation could use a laboratory-type screen printer costing about $5000. In the prototype operation, a rate of about 5 parts/min will be realized. This rate will be doubled—to 10 parts/min—in the 1000-circuit operation because care will be taken with jigging and the operators will be more skilled. Average setup times would be about 20 min for the prototype operation and 15 min for the low-volume operation. The high-volume operation will use an automatic printer that will cost about $15,000 and will print 60 parts/min. Setup time will be 15 min.

For kilns, the prototype operation could use a small metal belt laboratory furnace costing about $5000. Substrates would be hand-loaded onto the belt at the rate of about 10 pieces/min. The middle-volume operation will have a somewhat larger furnace—costing about $8000. It will have a wider belt and longer hot zone. A loading rate of about 30 parts/min can be reached. Again, the parts are hand-loaded. The high-volume operation would require a much larger kiln costing $20,000 or more. Semiautomatic loading methods could be used, allowing kiln loading labor rates of about 150 parts/min. It is practical to go automatically from the screen printer through a dryer into the kiln also, thus reducing firing labor costs even further.

2. Print Capacitor Electrode. This operation is done only on the high-volume line. The smaller operations cannot reduce costs by screen printing their capacitors. Material savings is about $140 per thousand capacitors. Labor costs and tooling must be deducted from this figure to get the actual savings. Design, setup time and screen amortization make use of screened-on capacitors for a thousand-piece run very doubtful from an economic standpoint.

The screening rate for the bottom capacitor electrode in the high-volume operation is 60 (min/0.017 min each).

3. Fire Capacitor Electrode. The high-volume firing operation proceeds at the rate of about 150 substrates/min. The setup time required at the kiln is minimal—only 5 min or so—most of this spent in lot marking, bookkeeping, and so forth. (A 5-min minimum setup time has been assigned to cover such items for each operation to follow.)

4. Print Dielectrics. This operation proceeds at the high-volume screen-printing rate of 60/min. Two passes are required to build up the proper thickness of the dielectric and to reduce the incidence of shorts caused by bubbles or voids. Extremely close monitoring of thickness, paste viscosity, liquid-to-solid ratio, and anything else that might affect the dielectric thickness is required. At present, the screen printing and firing of dielectrics must be considered more difficult than resistors—not because of an inherent difficulty, but because the art is not so well known and is not practiced so widely.

5. Print Conductors. This is the first operation for the lower-volume operations. The prototype operation prints at the rate of 5/min, the middle level at 10/min, and the high-volume operation (with its automated printing operation) at the rate of 60/min. Setup takes a little longer with the prototype operation.

6. Print Gold Bonding Pads. This is likely to be a fine-line printing operation; setup times should probably reflect this, but for the sake of simplification they have not been changed. The printing rates are the same as in Set 5. A 100% inspection of fine-line printing is often necessary. Labor costs for 100% inspection are not included here. If the narrow conductor runs are kept very short, the setup is done carefully, and the equipment is adequate for the task, this inspection is not needed. Avoidance of this type of cost is something to strive for, at least.

7. Fire Dielectrics and Conductors. The conductor patterns and the dielectric are cofired at whatever temperature is required to develop the proper capacitance. If adhesion, conductivity, or solderablity were very critical, the conductors would have to be fired at their own best temperatures. This, however, can usually be avoided, and conductors can be fired at the same time as the dielectrics. The two low-volume operations hand-load substrates onto the smaller furnaces, which are somewhat limited in their capacity; hence the lower rates of 10 or 30/min. The time spent to get the proper peak temperature and overall profile is not included—this either being part of the original setup mentioned earlier or part of the general overhead.

8. Test and Inspect Capacitors. This operation could be performed on an automated turntable-like device (as an example) where the substrates would be hand-loaded into position on an indexing turntable. They would then pass under test probes, where the capacitor would be probed and tested on a go-no-go basis. Such a machine would probably cost $25,000 and would test capacitors at the rate of 60/min. The same type of machine could also test resistors.

The prototype operation, if it were to test capacitors at this point or later when testing discrete components or screened resistors, would use a bridge and a simple fixture—costing about $1000. The middle-volume operation would use some faster device—probably a comparator—which would allow speeds of 20/min, at a cost of about $2000. The prototype operation would test at the rate of 5 elements/min.

9. Print Resistor Pattern 1. The resistance range is such that two different resistivities are needed. The high-volume operation will attempt precision printing so as to avoid having to trim the five loose tolerance resistors.

The cost of this is indicated (perhaps inadequately) in the larger allowances made for extra setup time (operation 1). In the case of two lower-volume operations, the time to be saved in not trimming the five resistors would not justify the extra setup time, more expensive screens, and so on. The prototype operation would need about 20 min for preparation and setup compared to 15 min for the higher-level operations. The printing rates for this printing, like the other printing operations before, are 5, 10, and 60/min.

10. Print Resistor Pattern 2. This is a repeat of operation 9, but with different resistivity paste.

11. Fire Resistors. This operation is similar to operation 7 except that it takes place at a lower temperature with a different profile. Separate kilns are often used because of the extra time needed and the difficulty of obtaining a proper profile.

12. Trim Resistor. The prototype operation will use a simple air-abrasive trimmer. The part is placed in a jig by hand, a button is pushed, and the trimming proceeds automatically to a stop point. Such a system costs about $6500. The rate will be about 3 resistors/min. By adding special fixtures this rate can be increased to between 10 and 20/min. The extra cost of the special fixtures is about $1000. Such a unit would be appropriate for the 1000-unit run.

The 50,000 unit operation would spend from $30,000 to $120,000 for a trimmer that would trim betwen 60 and 250 units/min. High-volume air-abrasive trimmers are available that automatically index the part under successive trimming stations where different resistors or a circuit are trimmed. Laser trimmers are able to shift their beams rapidly, so that with proper indexing control they progress rapidly from one resistor to the next, all resistors in a circuit being trimmed in one pass.

An increasingly attractive approach to trimming is *functional* trimming (dynamic trimming) where resistors are trimmed not to specific values, but to adjust circuit performance to a specific level. Trimmers similar to those described above would do functional trimming if the proper test equipment were added. This type of testing is very complex, and the cost of the electronic testing setup can be very high. Computers are often required to digest all the data and make the proper trimming decisions. The functional trimming step would occur not here, but *after* active devices are attached (operation 17).

With a trimming rate of 3/min in the prototype operation, 3.3 min are required to trim the circuit's ten thick film resistors. The 10/min rate of the middle-level production requires 1 min per circuit. The 60/min rate (or higher) of the high-level operation—as well as the fact that only five are trimmed (the rest being carefully fired to tolerance)—cuts trimming time to less than $\frac{1}{10}$ min per circuit.

With the high trimming rates attainable with the trimmer used in the high-volume operation, why take the extra trouble to fire resistors to tolerance? This is a good question. The reason this approach was chosen here was to illustrate the variety of processing decisions that have to be made. There is every possibility that there would be no net saving—especially when yield is considered. Many real life thick film operations waste time trying to fire to tolerance and avoid trimming.

13. Print and Fire Protective Coating. With a palladium oxide resistor system, a glass coating is needed to protect the resistor from the reduction conditions of the gas blanket used in the bonding operation. If certain other resistor pastes were used (e.g., DuPont's Birox) the resistors would *not* have to be protected. A protective coating over the capacitors usually serves to protect against humidity. Areas on conductors over which wires will bridge are also insulated in this operation. Printing rates here are the same as in the previous printing operations.

Firing the protective coatings is essentially indentical to those in operation 11, except that the temperature will be still lower. The lower temperature will keep the underlying composites from being attacked excessively by the molten protective coating. Also, by staying well under the firing points of the resistor and conductor glasses, reactions *within* those systems will not start again. The greater the temperature difference (generally speaking), the less likelihood there will be of unwanted reactions.

14. Test and Inspect. At this point, a test operation would probably be advisable to make certain that no bad circuits are used to mount relatively expensive components. (Our "theoretical" 100% yield would make this operation a waste of time, but in real life, where yields *are* below 100%, an inspection/test operation here would be advisable.)

Thick Film Summary. Table 13-9 summarizes the time (min) required to perform each of the thick film operations. Setup time is also listed.

15. Attach Active Devices. For this operation the prototype and the middle-production level operations will use the same bonder—a die bonder costing about $3000. Perhaps the middle-level operation would have an extra $500 invested in special jigs to help increase bonding rates. The prototype operation would make only about 1 bond/min. The middle-level

Table 13-9   Summary of Thick Film Operations (Steps 1 to 14)

Operation	25 pc run		1000 pc run		50,000 pc run	
	Time per Piece (min)	Setup Time (min)	Time per Piece (min)	Setup Time (min)	Time per Piece (min)	Setup Time (min)
1 Setup	—	—	—	—	—	120
2 Print capacitor electrode	—	—	—	—	0.017	15
3 Fire	—	—	—	—	0.006	05
4 Print dielectric	—	—	—	—	0.034	15
5 Print Pd conductor	0.200	20	0.100	15	0.017	15
6 Print Au conductor	0.200	20	0.100	15	0.017	15
7 Fire	0.100	15	0.030	15	0.006	05
8 Test	—	—	—	—	0.034	05
9 Print Resistor 1	0.200	20	0.100	15	0.017	15
10 Print Resistor 2	0.200	20	0.100	15	0.017	15
11 Fire	0.100	15	0.030	15	0.006	05
12 Trim Resistors	3.300	20	1.000	15	0.085	15
13 Print coating	0.200	20	0.100	15	0.017	15
13A Fire	0.100	15	0.030	15	0.006	5
14 Test resistors	2.000	10	0.500	10	0.167	15

operation would make about 4 bonds/min, most of the increase coming from operators who have better developed skills. (This is relatively hard to do in a prototype operation.) The longer setup times (see Table 13-10) are needed to get the machines adjusted and operating.

The high-production operation needs a different bonder because beam lead devices will be used. Since beam lead bonders have been available only for a short time, the cost probably will not be very stable—but at present a beam lead bonder capable of bonding 4 chips/min costs about $15,000. When the bond is made, all beams are attached to the substrate pads at one time.

16. Wire Bonding. The wire bonding operation (performed only by the two lower-level operations) uses a wire bonder costing about $4000. Again, better jigging, and so on, may increase the equipment cost of the 1000-piece production operation by another $500. The middle-level operation will average about 17 bonds/min. In our circuit there are three leads to be attached to each transistor (6 bonds), and three transistors make 18 bonds. The

Table 13-10   Summary of Mounting Discretes (Steps 15 to 17)

Operation	25 pc run		1000 pc run		50,000 pc run	
	Rate	Setup Time	Rate	Setup Time	Rate	Setup Time
15 Attach actives	4.000	60	1.000	40	1.000	60
16 Wire bond	5.670	60	2.000	40	—	—
17 Mount passives	3.500	10	1.000	10	0.033	40

integrated circuit with its eight leads has 16 bonds. The grand total is then 34 bonds, and 2 min will be required to make all the bonds on the circuit. In the prototype operation a bonding rate of 6 bonds/min— again mostly because of less developed operator skills—means that 5.7 minutes are required to do all bonding.

17. Mounting Discrete Passives. The simplest possible technique will be used in the prototype operation—a soldering iron. Gold-platinum conductor paste was used to give maximum resistance to solder leaching, so that replacement of devices, hot irons in heavy hands, and so on, can be tolerated. About 2 devices/min will be mounted. With 7 devices to mount, $3\frac{1}{2}$ min will be required. The equipment cost is minimal—less than $50.

The 1000-circuit operation will use solder reflow. Chips can be purchased pretinned, or they can be tinned in-house just prior to mounting. Each substrate is tinned by hand-dipping in solder. Later, a small amount of flux is placed at the various mounting positions. While the flux is still in its sticky/tacky stage, the chips are placed. Putting the substrate (or a group of them) on a hot plate (or in an oven) will remelt the solder. Close control of the time at molten solder temperature is needed partly because the paste used (paladium-gold) does not have quite so much leach resistance as the platinum-gold used in the prototype operation, but mostly because the termination on the chips will be likely to leach rapidly.

Reflow would be equally attractive for the prototype operation. Hand-soldering with an iron was chosen for illustrative purposes, not because it is a better method.

Device mounting in a high-volume operation can be much more sophisticated. For example, solder can be placed on the circuits via screen printing. While the paste is still tacky, the chips are automatically mounted. Reflow is still the basic attachment method, but where $200 would have covered the simple tools used in the 1000-circuit operation, limited to simple jigs to hold the devices in place during reflow—a sum of perhaps $30,000 would be required to handle automatic placement equipment and accessories. The rate of attachment would improve, however, from the 1 circuit/min for the 1000-circuit operation to an automated 30 circuits/min.

18. Attaching Leads. In the prototype operation leads are attached by hand, using a soldering iron. The rate will be only 2 wires/min, or 3 min/circuit; but the equipment cost is zero (covered earlier). The 1000-circuit assembly line will use much the same approach, but will employ simple jigs to hold the wires to the substrates while soldering takes place. The jigging here would be quite elementary, costing no more than $200. The high-volume operation would use wires "made" on a machine which would automatically attach them to strips. Substrates would be held to these wires on the strip, and the entire strip would be soldered at the same time. Equipment cost would be in the area of $5000, but production rates would be increased to 5 or 6 circuits/min.

19. Encapsulate. These operations are very simple. The prototype assembler would prepare a small amount of epoxy (in a paper cup) and hand-dip. The 1000-circuit line would do something very similar, but the length of the run would allow the rate of 1 circuit/min in the prototype to be increased to perhaps 5/min. The high-level production operation would do the dipping while the parts were still attached to the strip holding the leads. The dipping could still be by hand, but 5 or 6 circuits are dipped at one time, so that the rate increases to 25 circuits/min. Jigs, containers, drying racks, and so on, would cost no more than $1000 for the high-volume line—nothing for the other operation. Conformal coating is inexpensive.

A conformal dip coating was chosen for two reasons. The first is to illustrate how inexpensive thick film packaging can be. The second reason was that any other packaging scheme (such as flat packs) would be much more expensive, some to such an extent that the packaging cost could begin to dominate the entire cost and thus mask other costs that should, for illustrative purposes here, be allowed to stand out. In actual situations, while conformal coating could of course be used, it is more likely that another packaging technique would be chosen. Performance standards and user specifications often force more expensive packages.

20. Marking. The trademark, part number, lead numbers, and so on, will be printed on the encapsulated circuit; the prototype and the mid-level operations use hand stamping. The rate difference between the two (3/min versus 10/min) is due only to the higher skills available in the production operation. The high-volume line would stamp all the parts while still on the strip, using an offset printing approach (the ink is transferred to a soft rubber pad, and this transfers to the circuit). The required printing equipment is available for about $5000.

21. Final Testing. Final testing of the circuit might require 5 min using laboratory test gear standard. Special jigs and test circuits could reduce times in the 1000-circuit line to perhaps 3 min/circuit. An automatic testing setup could speed this up tremendously. A $30,000 tester could perhaps handle 10 circuits/min. (More complex test circuits cost much more.) Packaging costs are summarized in Table 13-11.

Table 13-11 Packaging

Operation	25 pc run		1000 pc run		50,000 pc run	
	Rate	Setup Time	Rate	Setup Time	Rate	Setup Time
18 Attach leads	3.000	10	1.500	15	0.200	20
19 Encapsulate	1.000	15	0.200	15	0.040	20
20 Marking	0.333	10	0.100	10	0.040	20
21 Testing	5.000	60	3.000	50	0.100	30

TOTAL COSTS

Table 13-12 summarizes the labor costs involved in making this circuit. The summary is broken down into the three main assembly areas—the thick film operations, the attachment of discretes, and finally the finishing (packaging) operations. Setup costs are prorated across the entire production run. They are not particularly significant in the 1000-piece line, dwindle to almost nothing in the high-volume line, but assume major importance in the prototype operation.

Table 13-13 summarizes the total factory cost—now dollarized. It illustrates the strength of economy of scale—much of which is felt when production gets to the 1000-part level.

This cost structure is one of the important characteristics of thick film— relatively inexpensive production tooling and equipment (mostly laboratory type equipment, simply scaled up a little) allows fairly low production costs at modest production levels. The cost of scaling up to high levels can be considerable, however.

Table 13-12   Summary of Labor Costs

	25 pc run		1000 pc run		50,000 pc run	
	Time per Piece (min)	Setup Time (min)	Time per Piece (min)	Setup Time (min)	Time per Piece (min)	Setup Time (min)
Thick film operations	6.700	165	2.090	145	0.445	280
Attach discretes	13.170	130	4.000	90	1.033	100
Packaging	9.333	95	4.800	90	0.380	90
Total assembly time	29.203	390	10.890	325	1.858	470
Prorated setup time	15.560		0.325		0.009	
Total time per circuit (min)	44.763		11.215		1.867	

Table 13-13   Total Factory Cost*

	25 pc run	1000 pc run	10,000 pc rnn
Materials	$13.33	$3.42	$2.85
Labor	4.47	1.21	0.19
Total	$17.80	$4.65	$3.07

* Not total cost (selling price) but *factory* cost.

Equipment Cost Comparisons. Table 13-14 summarizes and compares equipment costs. This summary is not meant to be a list of *everything* needed to produce at these levels. It is shown only for comparison's sake. Nor does it indicate *how many* pieces of each equipment are needed. Do not make the mistake of totaling each column to see how much capital equipment funding is needed.

Cost Reduction Possibilities. One of the most significant things to be seen in the cost summary (Table 13-13) in the high-volume operation is that almost all of the cost is in purchased materials. The money spent for automatic equipment reduced labor costs drastically, but had no effect on outside-purchased parts. Volume discounts brought material cost down slightly.

Table 13-14 Equipment Costs

	25 pc run	10,000 pc run	50,000 pc run
Printing	$5000	$5000	$ 5,000
Firing	5000	5000	20,000
Test R's and C's	1000	2000	25,000
Adjust R's	6500	6000	30,000
Die bonding	3000	3500	15,000
Wire bonding	4000	4500	—
Soldering	50	200	30,000
Lead attachment	—	200	5,000
Coating	—	—	1,000
Marking	—	—	5,000
Test	5000	6000	30,000

A look at the outside-purchased items (Table 13-8) shows the following costs: tooling—4¢; substrates—4¢; inks—8¢; other material—3¢; and components—$2.61. It is obvious that further attempts to reduce costs must be centered in the area of the purchased components. Any reductions in the other areas will be pennies or less.

A popular way to reduce costs is to go to captive manufacturing such as in-house screen making, in-house substrate making, or in-house ink making. If only pennies per circuit are to be saved, volume must be very high to pay for cost of entry into these new technologies. Other reasons, such as the need for quick turnaround capabilities, may dictate the use of in-house facilities, even though they may not be justified from an economic standpoint.

The breakdown of the components cost (Table 13-7) shows that the transistors cost 78¢, the IC, $1.05, the capacitors, 64¢, and the resistors 25¢ (50,000 level).

There is little the thick film maker can do about changing the cost of the specific active devices used, but *different* devices can be substituted, thus leading to a cost reduction. Costs can also be reduced by using functional testing, where a less expensive version of the same device is purchased and the resulting "looser" performance is tweaked back to desired levels by trimming resistors (perhaps even adding extra resistors for this purpose). There are also other ways of economizing such as combining all the active devices on a single chip, combining the three transistors, or buying active devices in wafer form.

The main point to be made here is that such a large percentage of the circuit's total cost represents a fertile hunting ground for cost reduction efforts. A 20% savings in active device costs is better than getting the thick film inks and the substrates for *nothing*. The former is quite possible, but the latter is not likely.

With the five discrete capacitors and resistors costing 89¢, while all twelve of the thick film capacitors and resistors costing much less, one can see why there is industry pressure to put these chips within the capabilities of thick film. The ink makers are (or should be) aware of this cost structure, and of the rewards that expanding thick film's capabilities could produce. Thick film capacitor characteristics are improving, and resistor inks are now appearing that have characteristics so far available only in discretes or thin film. Future improvements in thick film inks and processing equipment will mean that discrete chips can be replaced by thick film elements at a significant reduction in cost.

Let us look more closely at thick film element costs as compared to costs of similar discrete elements. Without trying to pin down the cost of each separate resistor, we can see by looking back over the cost tables that for the high-volume plant, ten resistors were screen-printed, fired, trimmed and encapsulated at a total cost of about 5.2¢: raw material—1¢; substrate areas—1¢; printing—0.34¢; firing—0.06¢; trimming—0.85¢; encapsulating with protective glass—0.23¢; and final testing—1.67¢. Five of the resistors were trimmed to close tolerance and five were not trimmed. Ten of the cheapest discrete carbon composition resistors would cost about 10¢. Assembly labor and preassembly checking would bring the total cost of using discrete components up to 13¢. It can thus be seen that thick film resistors can be inexpensive enough to compete with *any* kind of resistor (provided that yield is high—and it should be). This points up one of the best reasons for the existence of thick film—inexpensive, high-performance resistors. Any technology that offers good resistors for a half cent a piece is attractive.

Turning to another situation—the incremental cost of extra resistors—it can be seen that more could be added for only the extra material cost, since the labor is already invested. If a new improved resistor ink were available that would allow replacement of our two-chip resistors by thick film resistors, what would the extra cost be? It will be assumed that all the resistors in this example (previously made with Pd-PdO-Ag resistor paste) will be replaced with the new high-performance paste. If the new ink costs $100/oz, it would cost 4.8¢ to shift the ten resistors to the more expensive ink, plus 1.2¢ for the two extra resistors. The extra cost of trimming would be 2¢, and extra final testing would be perhaps 0.5¢. The total added cost would come to 8½¢. These chips cost at least 30¢ when purchased as discrete elements. This example illustrates emphatically the pressure to get improved performance into thick film resistor pastes. It also should serve to illustrate the foolishness of buying one or two chips so that less expensive resistor ink can be used.

Using a similar comparison with capacitors, let us see what the two screen-printed capacitors cost in the high-volume operation. The pastes cost a total of 2.2¢ (1.4¢ for conductor electrodes, 0.7¢ for capacitor, and 0.1¢ for encapsulation material). The cost of labor to print electrodes, to print dielectric, and to test (0.23¢, 0.34¢, and 0.34¢ respectively) is 0.91¢. The total cost to produce the two capacitors was 3.1¢, or just over 1.5¢ each. Although some disk capacitors can be purchased and assembled at such low costs, the smaller chip-type capacitors are much more expensive (usually close to 10¢ each). The economics of thick film capacitors is attractive also.

What would an extra capacitor cost, if it were made of the same basic material? The extra material would be 1.1¢. The extra labor cost would be limited to 0.17¢ for the testing, since no extra screening or firing work is involved. Screen-printed capacitors are inherently more expensive than resistors (because of the cost of the electrodes). Even so, thick film capacitors can compete on a cost basis with almost any type of discrete capacitor as long as the substrate area required is not too high.

Thick Film versus Conventional Circuits. It would be of interest to compare the costs of a conventional circuit to those of its thick film counterpart. Table 13-15 attempts to do this—with the thick film cost levels of the

Table 13-15   Conventional vs. Thick Film

	Conventional	Thick Film
12 resistors: 5—10%	$0.10 ⎫	$0.08
5—1%	0.50 ⎭	
2—film	0.20	0.30
Active devices	2.00	1.80
5 capacitors	1.20	1.10
PC board, solder, etc.	0.30	0.10
Assembly labor	0.20	0.40
Tooling	0.10	0.17
Total	$4.60	$3.95

1000-piece run as a base. As can be seen, most of the savings are due to the low cost of the thick film resistors. This comparison is not really valid in that it assumes a 100% yield; this is all right when comparing two production levels in a similar technology, but not when comparing two different technologies. The conventionally assembled circuit will, in fact, yield almost 100%. The thick film circuit could yield in the high nineties if built by an experienced team, but might also yield only 70% or even less. If the losses occur early in the process, total cost is not heavily affected; in nearly finished items, however, any edge thick film has over conventional circuits can easily disappear as a result of such losses.

MAKE OR BUY

This is a complex question, and a difficult subject to discuss. Reaching a decision would be much easier if it were a matter of costs only, although costs also are sometimes difficult to define. There are, however, many factors other than cost that influence make-or-buy decisions.

A Prototype Facility. In making thick film, the least costly situation is the simplest possible prototype facility. It will help to look at the basic costs here to find an absolute floor for costs. With a minimum figure in mind, we can then look at the various pros and cons of an in-house facility with a somewhat harder eye.

The simplest thick film operation would have the following equipment:

Printer	$5,000
Resistor trimmer	7,000
Kiln	5,000
Bonders	7,000
Test equipment	8,000
Miscellaneous	4,000
Space	5,000
	40,000

Amortized over a four-year period, the annual facility cost is $10,000. Add to this $30,000 per year to cover wages and fringes of an engineer and a single technician $10,000 per year to supply the operation with materials and possible other operating costs, and one finds that $50,000 per year is required to operate a rudimentary thick film prototype facility. Such a facility could turn out one prototype per week of the type we examined earlier in this chapter.

Let us now consider some of the reasons that are often given for establishing in-house facilities.

Fast Turnaround on Prototypes. This is usually a valid need. But with a capability of only one prototype a week, it would be best not to ask for too many designs at one time in the facility we outlined above—otherwise the turnaround is not so fast.

Many job shops claim fast turnaround time capabilities, and no doubt give it if there is promise of a larger order to follow or if they are not busy with other prototypes. The main reason why in-house facilities provide faster turnaround than do outside job shops is that it is easier for management to assign priorities in accordance with their needs. This is more difficult with outside vendors who also have other customers to satisfy.

The question to be answered is: is *limited* fast turnaround capability worth $50,000 per year? ($1000 extra payment to a job shop might speed things up quite a bit—this might be much less expensive than a $1000 per week in-house operation.)

Better Service on Small Runs. Unquestionably better service is available in-house than at job shops, but again this is probably only because the whip can be more easily cracked in-house than with outside suppliers. If one were willing to pay for faster service at job shops, better service would be available.

Makes Outside Purchases More Efficient (Narrows Communications Gap, etc.). There is not much evidence to support this. At best, in-house knowledge may keep an uninformed purchasing agent from paying too high a price. On the other hand, the in-house facility makes the outside supplier wary. He will often figure (and rightly so) that he is being thrown scraps while the in-house facility is getting the gravy. He will thus tend to be more careful in his pricing. The truth is that in-house facilities often tend to *increase* the cost of outside purchases.

Better Control of Quality and Delivery. Delivery, yes; quality, maybe.

A Source of Technical Innovation. The average prototype shop—such as the one described above (with one engineer)—is not about to do much technical innovation. Very few in-house facilities, unless they are the no-holds-barred–cost-is-no-object types one sees in aerospace facilities, can afford to be technical innovators. They are more likely to be concerned with keeping up with the state-of-the-art. The real gain to be made here is the technical innovations that can be made by the circuit designers as they design new systems that utilize thick film's economic or performance advantage. There is often a problem in getting the designers acquainted enough with the new technology to fully take advantage of it.

Less Red Tape. (A student in one of our thick films seminars—from an aerospace firm—caused us to add this one.) At some firms, it is so difficult to go outside for a circuit—quotes, survey teams, quality assurance, drawing up special purchase specifications, and so on— that it is easier in the long run to build inside. Outsiders should have to face no more of these barricades than do inside sources. To the extent that this is a valid reason, it is a rather sad situation.

Proprietary Circuit Protection. History will show that more information is lost by in-house people defecting to start a competing company than through a supplier's thievery.

Maintains Value Added. This is the most important reason for in-house capability. In some situations the reasons given previously are enough to justify in-house facilities, but the prime reason is usually that they are established to maintain value added—that is, to protect (or increase) profits. In-house facilities often represent a way of either increasing profits or, at the very least, *maintaining* profit levels.

There are two general situations in electronics firms today. In one a "system" is being sold and the electronics content is not really very high; say, something sells for $1000 and only a very small portion of it is electronic in nature, most of it being engineering and sales expense. In-house facilities can hardly be expected to reduce costs in such a case. For example, if only $100 out of the $1000 was electronic, cost reduction or increased value added content could have little effect. The reasons a firm would involve itself with in-house facilities here would be not to reduce to $100 part of the total, but to protect the other $900. Capabilities for faster service, shorter new product cycling, and so on, *are* valid reasons here. It is exceedingly difficult to pin down specific dollar savings, and there is a tendency for overoptimism in the effects that are expected—but the need can be very real.

Note that even though the electronics value added share is small, one should not completely *ignore* cost reduction possibilities.

In the second type of situation the product being sold is an *electronic* product (an instrument, a radio, a voltage divider, etc.). Here the rationale for setting up in-house thick film facilities is totally different. It often has to do with *continued existence,* not with cost reduction. Thus in today's automotive voltage regulator business, an independent voltage regulator manufacturer who has no capabilities of producing a solid state IC regulator has little hope of continuing in business as an electronic manufacturer. He might buy the regulator from Motorola and sell it—but this puts him out of the electronics business. The *only* way to stay in the electronic manufacturing business in such a case is to set up in-house manufacturing. The make-or-buy decision for this type of situation, then, has to do with whether one continues to exist as an electronics firm.

The value added factor is of overriding concern to the firm that is primarily an electronics manufacturer. When the day arrives for his product to go IC (if it has not already done so), he *must* go in-house to survive.

CONCLUSIONS

The cost structures show that there are very definite economic reasons for use of thick film hybrid circuits and materials. The low cost of thick film components (compared to discretes used in hybrids) makes extension of the capabilities of thick film materials economically rewarding.

Given high volume and proper expenditure of capital funds, assembly costs of thick film can be very low.

Hope for major cost reductions in the future lies mostly in reducing costs of the purchased discrete components.

The most common reason for starting an in-house thick film facility has to do with maintaining or increasing value added—or with improving the profit picture. Other reasons should be examined carefully.

Note. An early version of this chapter was given as a paper at the 1970 Electronics Components Conference ("The Economics of Thick Film Hybrid Microcircuit Production," by D. W. Hamer, *1970 ECC Proceedings,* p. 576). Another version was presented at the 1970 International Hybrid Microelectronics Symposium (same title, *1970 ISHM Proceedings,* p. 6.1.1). Quoted here with permission from IEEE and ISHM.

Appendix I

THE TECHNOLOGY OF MONOLITHIC
INTEGRATED CIRCUITS AND THIN
FILM INTEGRATED CIRCUITS

The purpose of this section is to discuss the technologies that, together with thick film (introduced in Chapter 2) make up today's IC world. The presentation is deep enough only to allow the reader to develop a simplified understanding of the technology, its advantages, its limitations, and so on. The discussion here of monolithic and thin film technology is similar in scope and depth to the thick film introduction given in Chapter 2. The basic approach is to describe fabrication of the same simple circuit using monolithic or thin film technology as was done in Chapter 2 with thick film techniques.

Monolithic Integrated Circuits

SILICON—THE BASIC RAW MATERIAL

Silicon is the basic material used for making monolithic ICs. Since other material *can* be used, it is more accurate to qualify the term "monolithic IC" by adding the modifier "silicon"—making it silicon monolithic ICs.

The modifier "silicon" is often dropped. We can assume a monolithic IC is silicon unless noted otherwise.

The starting material for a silicon monolithic IC is a single crystal of very pure silicon. As we shall see, both the single crystal structure and the purity are very important.

The starting purity needed is on the order of parts per million, or even parts per billion. Silicon is a material that will pick up impurities of all sorts very readily; high-purity silicon therefore does not exist in nature—it has to be made. High purity is obtained by using a process called *zone refining*. A chunk of silicon metal, as pure as can be had by regular refining, is placed in a container in a tubular furnace that has a hot spot every few inches (Figure A-1). As the container is slowly drawn past the hot

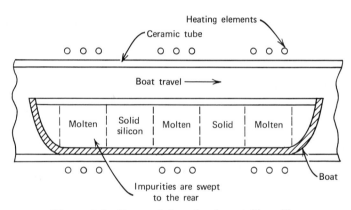

Figure A-1   Zone refining of polycrystalline silicon.

spots, silicon in the region of the hot spot melts. As it travels past each hot zone, the silicon solidifies again.

Impurities tend to stay in the molten zone as the silicon solidifies, since they are more soluble in the molten state than they are in the solid state. The impure silicon, upon freezing, drops out its impurities. The impurities are swept in and by the molten zone to the rear end of the container where they are concentrated.

The pure silicon from the zone refining operation is *polycrystaline* (composed of many crystals). To grow a single crystal, a seed crystal is brought into contact with a crucible of molten purified silicon metal. The crystal is kept at a temperature just below silicon's melting point. As the seed crystal is very slowly removed from the molten metal, the crystal continues to grow at the crystal/molten metal inferface. The crystal is rotated slowly as it is removed from the crucible. The result is a single crystal of silicon in a cylindrical shape. Sizes as large as 3 in. in diameter are available now, although in the past such a large diameter was not practical. (Figure A-2.)

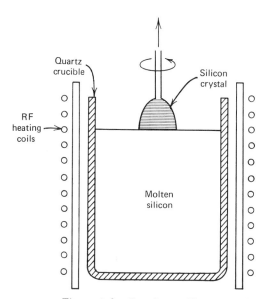

Figure A-2   Growing a silicon crystal.

CONDUCTION IN SILICON

Bulk Resistivity. Silicon in a pure state is a semiconductor, its resistivity (reciprocal conductivity) being between that of insulators and conductors. Figure A-3 shows where silicon is in relation to other relatively well-known materials. The theoretical resistivity for pure silicon is much higher than the value indicated in Figure A-3 for so-called "pure" silicon (such as produced by the zone refining method). This difference is a hint as to what causes a decrease in resistivity—impurities.

Silicon does not conduct electricity well—at least not compared to conductor materials. The molecular structure of a single crystal of very pure silicon is such that the great majority of the four electrons in the outer shell of a silicon atom "belonging" to each atom are shared with the neighboring atom of silicon. This type of bonding (illustrated in Figure A-4) is called covalent bonding. The electrons that are thus tightly held are *not* available for electronic conduction. However, very rarely, certain elec-

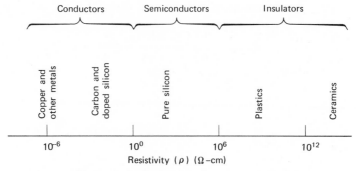

Figure A-3 Resistivity of common materials.

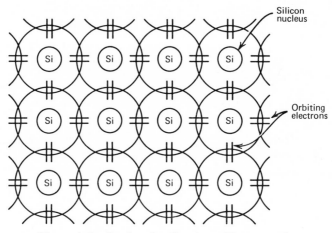

Figure A-4 Covalent bonding in a silicon crystal.

trons somehow get enough energy to break away from the tight covalent bond and become loosely bound. These relatively rare electrons are responsible for what little conductivity silicon has. The holes left where the electron came from can also conduct electricity (hole conduction). The resistivity of theoretically pure silicon is on the order of 10^4 Ω cm.

Pure silicon has 10^{22} silicon atoms per cubic centimeter. With four electrons in each outer shell, there are 4×10^{22} electrons/cc. Of this total, at any one time, about 10^{10} electrons/cc will be energized enough (by temperature, e.g.) to be able to act as a conduction electron. The actual number is large, but the percentage is very low (only one in a billion.)

If small amounts of certain impurities are present, silicon conducts much better however. For example, if an impurity from Group V in the atomic chart (such as phosphorus) is added, conductivity increases markedly. This is because there are 5 electrons in each outer shell of an atom of Group V material. Four of the electrons tie up with the neighboring silicon atoms, leaving 1 electron in an excess position—loosely bound and "available" for conduction. Figure A-5 shows how resistivity goes down as more impurity is added, and Figure A-6 illustrates how holes or conduction electrons are made.

Figure A-5 shows a line for "*p*-type" impurities as well as "*n*-type." The *n*-type refers to silicon containing a Group V impurity such as phos-

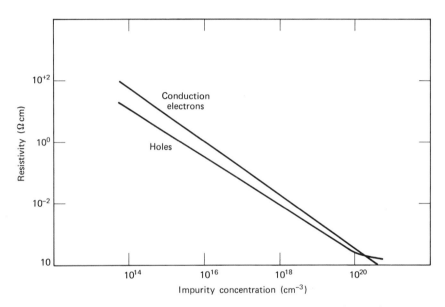

Figure A-5 Resistivity of silicon as a function of impurity levels.

phorus. If a Group III element was added, such as boron, the result would be an impurity site in the silicon crystal matrix that was *short* 1 electron. This would increase the number of holes present and also result in a drop in resistivity (via hole conduction).

Note in Figure A-5 that very small amounts of impurities added to the silicon can result in large decreases in volume resistivity. Keep in mind that 10^{18} impurity atoms in silicon still is only 0.01%, there being 10^{22} silicon atoms/cc.

*p***-Type Silicon and** *n***-type Silicon.** Silicon that has a predominance of *n*-type impurities is called *n*-type silicon (*n* standing for the negative charge

Original structure

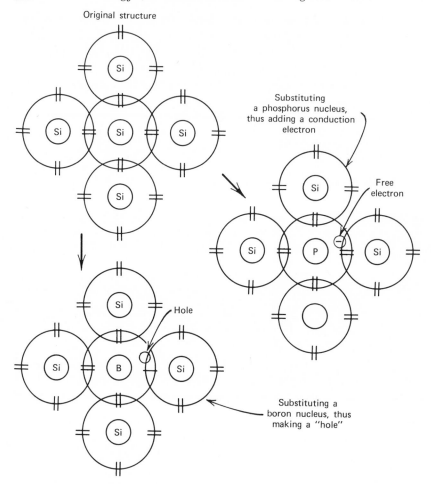

Figure A-6   Making conduction electrons or holes by introducing impurities into the silicon crystal structure.

of the mobile electron). *p*-Type silicon has a predominance of *p*-type impurities (the *p* standing for the positive charge of the mobile hole).

The type designation indicates the *predominant* type of impurity. Silicon of one type can be changed to the other type by adding enough new impurities to overwhelm those already present, since the two types of impurities cancel each other out. The free electrons from one impurity drop into the holes from the other. For instance, silicon that has 10^{18} atoms/cc of *n*-type impurities and 2×10^{18} atoms/cc of *p*-type has a net population of 10^{18}cc *n*-type, the other 10^{18} free electrons/cc having gone to fill up the holes created by the *p*-type doping. This crystal would be *n*-type silicon, because the *net population* is of the *n*-type.

JUNCTIONS

If a situation arises where the impurity type, *n* or *p*, shifts from one to the other in a single piece of silicon, what is known as a *junction* is created at the line where the shift occurs. Besides being a "thin line" where the *n* and *p* populations are equivalent, this junction has special characteristics. Current can flow in only one direction across a junction. If a positive voltage were placed on the *p* side, current would flow easily, but if the same voltage were impressed from the *n* side (polarity reversed, i.e.) very little current would flow.

A junction between *p*-type and *n*-type (a *pn* junction) makes a diode, then (a rectifier). Current will flow only one way. Two of these junctions placed very closely together make a transistor (Figure A-7).

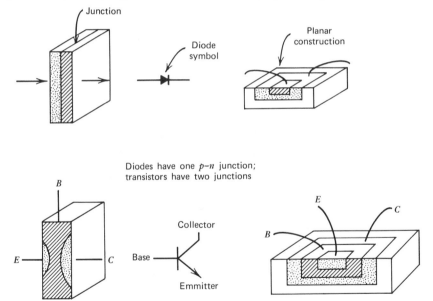

Figure A-7   Basic structure of diodes and transistors.

Two configurations are shown in Figure A-7 for each device. One represents early discrete versions. The planar version is the type that is made via diffusion technology in today's ICs.

The art of making transistors and monolithic ICs can, in many respects, be boiled down to being the art of making junctions between *p*-type and *n*-type silicon. The characteristics and performance of the transistors and other elements so made depend on how accurately the junctions are located and how much of the dopants is introduced. It is a complicated process—but not incomprehensible.

THE MANUFACTURING STEPS IN MAKING A DIFFUSED SILICON TRANSISTOR

The basic principles of making a silicon monolithic IC can be shown by marching through the steps of making a simple circuit. The circuit that we "manufacture" is a very simple amplifier (Figure A-8). The circuit contains one transistor, one resistor, and one capacitor.

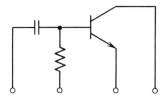

Figure A-8   The circuit to be "produced."

Figure A–9 outlines the basic steps in making a very simple bipolar planar IC via diffusion processes.

Slicing and Lapping—Step 1. The large cylindrical silicon crystal (which can be furnished in either *p*- or *n*-type) is sawed into thin slices about 15-mils thick. The surface of the sawed slices is quite rough. A series of polishing steps are gone through to make a very smooth surface. First the sawed slice is lapped, then polished, and finally etched until its finish is very smooth and mirrorlike. The several steps in the polishing process reduce the thickness to only 5 or 6 mils.

Epitaxial Growth—Step 2. The Random House dictionary defines epitaxis as "an oriented overgrowth of crystalline material upon the surface of another crystal of different chemical composition but similar structure." Epitaxy is a "key" process in making economically practical high performance ICs. It was developed by Bell Laboratories in the late 1950s. In our circuit, we are going to grow a sheet of *n*-type silicon on a polished and etched *p*-type wafer. In doing this, we shall create a *pn* junction. It is the junction so created ("abrupt" and at a uniform depth) that makes the epitaxial process so useful.

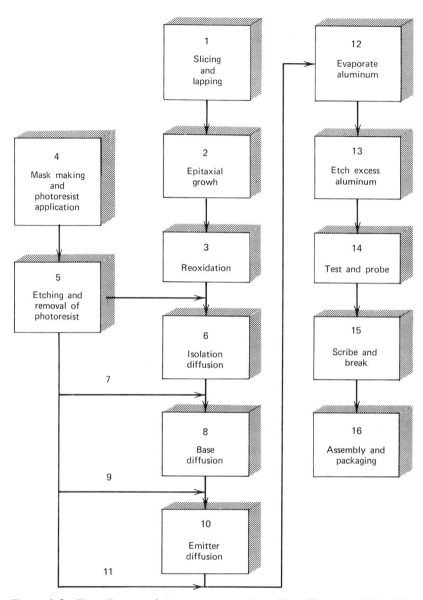

Figure A-9 Flow diagram of the process steps in making silicon monolithic ICs.

Epitaxy starts by heating the silicon wafer in a furnace (an *epi-reactor*) to about 1200°C in an atmosphere of hydrogen (oxygen would oxidize the silicon). When ready to start epitaxial growth, silicon in the form of silicon tetrachloride is introduced with the hydrogen. The hydrogen reduces the SiCl₄, and silicon atoms deposit and grow on the smooth single crystal surface of the wafer. Given a perfect crystalline surface to grow on, the new growth will also be a perfect crystal. Since in the example we are using we wish to grow a layer of *n*-type silicon, an *n*-type dopant gas such as phosphine will be introduced in the proper minute amounts along with the SiCl₄. (Figure A-10.)

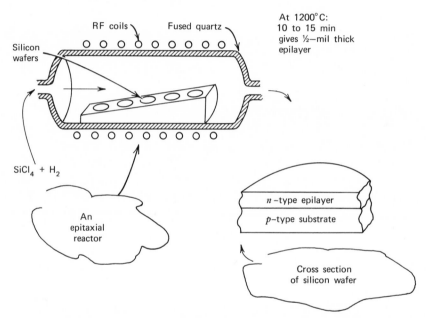

Figure A-10   Step 2: epitaxial growth (cross section of wafer).

The growth takes place slowly, but steadily, at about 1 μ/min. At the end of 10 to 15 mins a layer of 10 to 15 μ ($\frac{1}{2}$ mil) is grown.

Reoxidation—Step 3. The atmosphere in the epireactor is then changed to oxygen (wet). A layer of silicon oxide grows on the silicon slice. (This is listed as a separate step on the flow diagram for clarity, but the two steps are performed together, one immediately after the other). The oxide layer is about 1 μ thick. (Figure A-11.)

The oxide is grown to give certain areas protection from later diffusions. We shall etch windows in this oxide surface in certain areas and reexpose

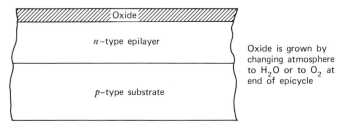

Figure A-11   Step 3: reoxidation of wafer's surface after epitaxial growth.

the wafer to doped atmospheres so that the nature of the silicon immediately under the etched holes can be changed. This reoxidation step is repeated several times in the subsequent operations (at the end of each diffusion) to reseal the exposed surface. In many instances we shall be growing silica layers over already-existing silica layers. This is indicated on the sketches by slightly different thicknesses in different areas. Growth of silica slows as the layer gets thicker, so after a short time it gets thicker very slowly.

Mask Making and Photoresist Application—Step 4. It is necessary to expose certain areas of the silicon oxide layer we just made (in the epitaxial growth step) to acid so that the oxide can be removed. To accomplish this selective etch, we use photolithographic techniques. A thin layer of "photoresist" is applied to each wafer. This is done by placing a drop of the photoresist on the wafer and then spinning it. The centrifugal force throws off the excess, and leaves a thin uniform coating of photoresist.

After the photoresist dries, a *mask* that contains the pattern that is to be etched away is placed over the wafer. (It must be kept in mind that the patterns are very small, and are repeated many times in a single slice of silicon. A 2-in.-diameter wafer can easily have 2000 separate circuits. The patterns to be etched will be smaller than are easily seen with the naked eye.) Light is introduced over the mask and the photoresist coated wafer. Areas touched by light are rendered insoluble by the action of the light, whereas the areas where no light hits remain soluble.

The wafer is washed (developed) to remove the unexposed photoresist. This exposes in selected areas the silicon oxide layer that is to be removed.

Manufacture of the masks begins by making a large drawing of the circuit, many times the final desired size. The size of the original drawing is reduced by photoreduction methods to the proper final size—generally in two or more steps. Since the same pattern is to be repeated all across the face of the silicon wafer, the reduced pattern is repeated by "step and repeat" methods. The mask ends up as a minute circuit pattern repeated accurately hundreds of times in rows and columns across an area the size of a silicon slice. It is in the form of a black photographic emulsion deposited on the surface of a flat piece of glass. Extreme accuracy in the photoreduction is necessary, as are extremely accurately spaced patterns; otherwise misalignment from one mask to the next will create bad circuits.

Etching and Removing Photoresist—Step 5. The silicon slice with windows in the photoresist (where silicon dioxide is exposed) are soaked in buffered hydrofluoric acid where the silica is dissolved. After this has been accomplished the remaining photoresist is removed by use of special solvents.

The wafer now has a many times repeated pattern of "windows" of removed silica, where the *n*-type epitaxial grown silicon is exposed in areas where further processing is desired. The areas where oxide remains will act as diffusion barriers. (Figure A-12.)

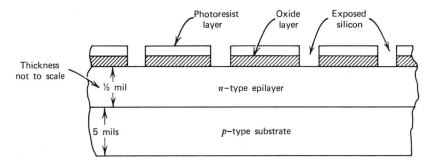

Figure A-12   Step 5: etching the oxide.

Diffusion. Diffusion (along with epitaxy, oxidation, and the photolithographic processes of mask making and exposue of the photoresist) is another of the "key" processes in IC manufacture. Diffusion is the mechanism by which *impurities* (or dopants) are introduced into the silicon wafer. The diffusion phenomenon can be briefly described as one in which matter in regions of high concentration moves to regions of low concentration. Common examples of material movement via diffusion would be (1) perfume spreading through a room and (2) a drop of ink spreading in a glass of water. In the case of ICs, diffusion is the mechanism by which impurities are distributed throughout the thickness of the wafer by introducing a high concentration of the impurity at the surface of the wafer. Time and temperature are the prime determinants of the rate at which diffusion takes place. Close control of both (especially temperature) is needed to ensure accurate control of the amount (level) of the impurity and, even more important, the depth at which a junction is formed.

The role of the oxide on the surface of the wafer is to act as a diffusion barrier. The dopants used will diffuse very slowly—practically not at all—through silicon oxide, but will diffuse at a comparatively brisk rate through silicon in areas where it is exposed to the dopants.

Isolation Diffusion (and Reoxidation)—Step 6. Silicon wafers are loaded into boats and pushed into the hot zone of the diffusion furnace. A diffusion furnace is usually a round quartz tube where temperatures can be controlled with extreme accuracy ($\pm\frac{1}{2}$°C). The ends of the tube are closed or capped so that the atmosphere inside can also be controlled. (Figure A-13.)

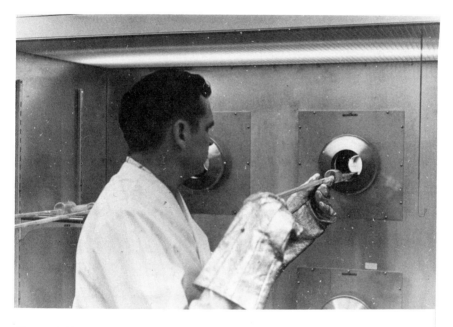

Figure A-13   Loading silicon wafers into a diffusion furnace. (Photograph by State of the Art, Inc.)

The wafers are exposed in the diffusion furnace to a neutral atmosphere (nitrogen). p-Type dopants (boron in the form of BBr_3, e.g.) are introduced in carefully controlled amounts along with the carrier gas. The boron will *diffuse* into the exposed silicon. As more and more boron diffuses into the n-type epitaxially grown layer, the p population eventually gets high enough to shift the silicon to p-type. As time goes by, the p-type layer deepens, and finally after many hours the diffusion converted p-type silicon in the epitaxial layer goes all the way down to the *original* p-type wafer

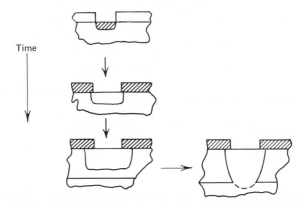

Figure A-14 Conversion of silicon from one type to another as diffusion time increases.

(Figure A-14). The isolation "channels" that are thus formed are in squares; thus the isolation diffusion has created islands of *n*-type silicon surrounded by *p*-type channels—all "floating" on a bed of *p*-type silicon. Each island of *n*-type silicon is isolated from its neighbors by an *np* junction and a *pn* junction. This amounts to two diodes, back to back. No current can flow from one island to the other through back-to-back diodes, so that all the *n*-type islands are electrically isolated from each other. (Figure A-15.)

At the end of the isolation diffusion process, a coating of silicon oxide is grown over the exposed isolation channels in the same manner as outlined in the epitaxial growth operation—by introducing steam and oxygen. This can be done in the diffusion furnace, or in a separate oxidation furnace.

Etch Pattern for Base Diffusion—Step 7. The base pattern is put on the silicon oxide coated wafer in the same manner as was the isolation channel pattern: by coating with photoresist, exposing through a mask so that only the base diffusion pattern is left soluble, then dissolving the soluble portion to expose silicon oxide, and finally etching the exposed silicon oxide away—thereby exposing new areas in the islands of *n*-type epitaxially grown silicon.

While the base diffusion pattern is being made, we can also proceed to make the resistor. Note the meander pattern of the resistor on the middle island of the sketch (Figure A-16). (Most resistors are made with *p*-type base material. Resistivity is in the area of 200 $\Omega/\square$. Low-value resistors can be made during the upcoming emitter diffusion, which produces lower sheet resistivity material.)

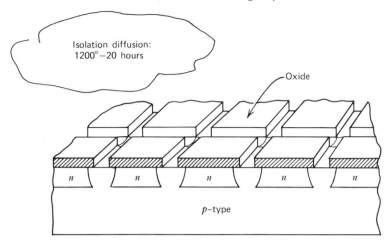

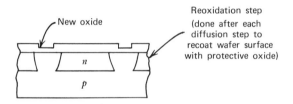

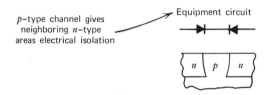

Figure A-15 Step 6: The isolation diffusion.

A plan view of the base diffusion pattern is included in Figure A-16. While the exact orientation of the isolation channel pattern was not very important, the base diffusion pattern must be *very* accurately oriented with respect to the isolation channel pattern and subsequent patterns must also be very accurately located.

The orientation is accomplished at the time the photoresist is exposed. Under a microscope the mask patterns and the oxide steps on the wafer are visible so that alignment of simple patterns is relatively easy. Complex

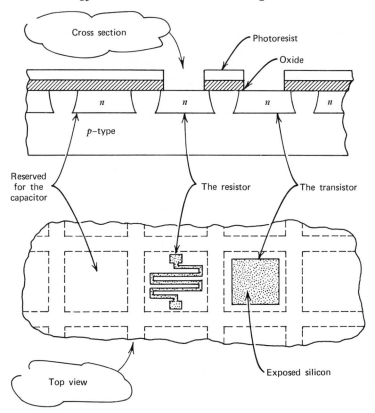

Figure A-16 Step 7: Etch pattern for transistor base (and resistor) patterns.

patterns (common with ICs) cannot be lined up in this manner, however. For complex patterns, alignment *reference marks* are placed on each mask. These are etched into the silicon wafer during diffusion. On the following photoresist exposure, the mask's reference marks are aligned very carefully over the marks in the oxide left by the previous mask. It is possible to manipulate the wafer or the mask very accurately by using the wafer alignment tool's micrometer-style *x, y,* and rotational adjustments. (Figure A-17.)

Base Diffusion—Step 8. This diffusion step will convert some of the areas in the center of the islands of *n*-type silicon to *p*-type in much the same manner as the isolation channel diffusion converted the *n*-type to *p*-type. For this diffusion the junction depth must be controlled *very* precisely.

We reduce the temperature to about 1100°C so that diffusion will proceed

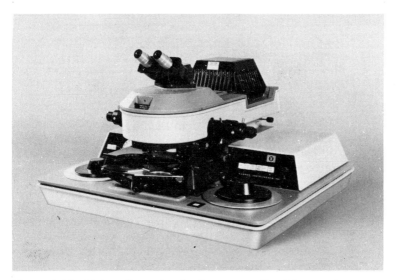

Figure A-17 Wafer aligner (mask alignment tool). (Photograph courtesy of Kasper Instruments, Inc.)

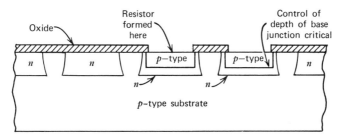

Figure A-18 Step 8: The base diffusion (1100°C, about 1 hour). Often performed in two steps: (1) a "pre-dep" step when all the dopant is introduced on the surface and (2) a "drive-in" diffusion where the impurities are redistributed.

more slowly. Also, at this lower temperature the isolation channel diffusion will change very little. The depth of the junction formed during the base diffusion is only about 3 μ, or only about one-fourth the depth of the epitaxial layer. About 1 hr is required. This diffusion also ends with regrowth of oxide. While the transistor base diffusion is proceeding, we are also diffusing a p-type channel that will form the resistor. One of the attractions of silicon monolithic ICs is that the resistors can be formed at the same time as the transistors are made. No extra processing steps are required. (Figure A-18.)

Expose Emitter Pattern and Etch—Step 9. The emitter region, resting inside the base pattern, is created in the same way as were the isolation channel and base patterns: photoresist application, emitter mask exposure, disolving (developing) unexposed photoresist, and hydrofluric acid (buffered) etch of exposed silica. The bottom electrode of the capacitor is also delineated at this time.

Emitter Diffusion and Reoxidation—Step 10. The diffusion process for the emitter is a reconversion of the already once-converted silicon back to n-type. Again, the depth of the junction is very important. The reason is that the distance between the two junctions (the emitter/base junction and the base/collector junction) is of extreme importance in determining the operating characteristics of the finished transistor. The emitter diffusion temperature is lower by about 50° than the base diffusion temperature (so that the location of the base diffusion junction will not move). Time at temperature is $\frac{1}{2}$ hr or less. The concentration of n-type impurities is much higher here than in the original epilayer, making the conductivity of the silicon in the emitter region much higher. This is to reduce emitter resistance as much as possible and to make a high-conductivity capacitor electrode.

The emitter diffusion step also ends with a reoxidation step. Control of the emitter reoxidation is very important because the thickness of the oxide will determine the capacitance of the capacitor. (Figure A-19.)

Expose Ohmic Connection Pattern and Etch—Step 11. Small windows are etched (in the usual manner—via photoresist, etc.) so that spots on the base, collector, and emitter areas are exposed.

Evaporate Aluminum—Step 12. The wafer is loaded in a vacuum chamber and a vacuum is pulled. Aluminum is melted and vaporized in the vacuum. The aluminum vapor condenses on the entire surface of the silicon wafer. Where there are windows in the oxide, the metal makes physical contact with the exposed silicon of the transistor base, collector, and emitter (and to the resistor and capacitor connections). (Figure A-20.)

Etch Unwanted Conductor Material—Step 13. Aluminum metallization that is not needed is etched away, leaving a pattern of electrical conductors connecting the various elements of the IC. The metallization pattern also furnishes the top electrode to capacitors and is used to make "pads" for wire connections to the package. (Figure A-21.)

Function of the Oxide. We have seen how the first function of the oxide was to act as a diffusion barrier. We now see that it must also serve as an

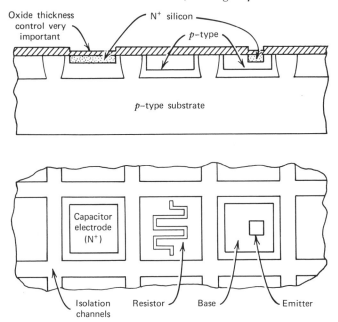

Figure A-19 After step 10: showing emitter diffusion after oxide layer has been grown.

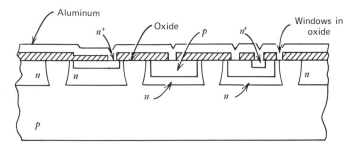

Figure A-20 Steps 11 and 12: cross section of wafer after aluminum metallization.

electrical insulator, keeping the metallization pattern from touching the silicon (except at the windows). Furnishing the dielectric for capacitors, giving *physical* protection to the elements on the surface of the wafer, and acting as surface passivation are some of the other functions.

Making Resistors. Resistors for monolithic ICs are usually made during the base diffusion step. The resistor is made of *p*-type silicon with about 200 $\Omega/\square$ sheet resistance. Each "square" of the resistor channel will have 200-Ω

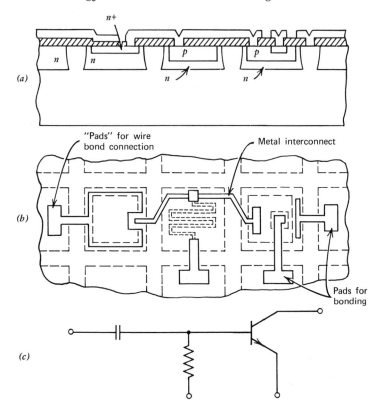

Figure A-21 The finished IC, after step 13. The interconnection etch (*a*) cross section of wafer, (*b*) surface of wafer, and (*c*) the circuit schematic.

resistance. Thus to make a 4000-Ω resistor the channel must be 20 times as long as its width. Photolithographic capabilities make a $\frac{1}{2}$-mil-wide resistor quite practical, so that a 4000-Ω resistor will be only $\frac{1}{2}$-mil wide and 10-mil long. The high-conductivity emitter diffusion is often used to make lower-value resistors. It can be seen that making resistors is quite easy in silicon monolithic technology. No extra steps are needed and very little space is used. This capability is a highly attractive feature of silicon monolithic technology.

Making Capacitors. Capacitors are made on silicon monolithic ICs by using the same silicon oxide (silica) insulation that is used for protection and insulation. The bottom electrode is of high conductivity n^+ silicon—made during the emitter diffusion. The silica layer is grown in the usual manner, except that control must be more exact, since the thickness of the oxide will determine capacitance. The top electrode is evaporated in the same manner and at the same time as the other ohmic contacts are made to the transistors and resistors.

Back-biased *pn* junctions also offer capacitance (very voltage sensitive, however). The *junction capacitor* is one way to make IC capacitors that is *totally* compatible with the rest of the IC process.

A problem that limits the use of capacitors in monolithics is that they take up too much area.

Making Diodes. If a diode is desired, simply use the emitter and the base of the transistor. The collector portion can be ignored.

Testing and Probing—Step 14. Each IC can be checked—at least to some extent—while they are all gathered together on the wafer. Equipment is available to very accurately probe the tiny contact areas of each circuit, moving automatically from one circuit to the next. Every time a bad circuit is found, it is marked with ink for later disposal. (Figure A-22.)

Scribing—Step 15. The silicon wafer is broken up into its individual ICs by scratching or scribing between the circuits. After the scratch is made, pressure will cause the wafer to break at the scribe marks (usually). Laser cutting and abrasive sawing are other methods used to separate the wafer into chips. (Figure A-23.)

Assembly—Step 16. The tested integrated circuits are then mounted to a metallized pad on a ceramic substrate. Alloy bonding is the most common method. Gold and silicon form an allow at about 400°C. The silicon chip is placed on a gold pad on the substrate, which is preheated to over 400°C. The gold and the silicon combine to make a eutectic alloy. Sometimes small preforms of the alloy are used to promote an improved bond.

Once mounted on a substrate, connections between the leads of the package and the pads on the chip are made with very fine gold or aluminum wires. Either of two processes are used to make the bond between the wire and the pad or terminal: thermocompression bonding where pressure and heat are used to make a metallurgical bond between the two metals, or ultrasonic bonding, a process that uses no heat. (Figure A-24.)

After the wire bonding is completed, the package is sealed by a variety of means, ranging from plastic encapsulation to hermetic glass sealing.

The assembly steps just described are common to thick film ICs as well as to thin films. They are described in more detail in Chapter 2. In addition, Chapters 9 and 11 are devoted entirely to bonding and packaging.

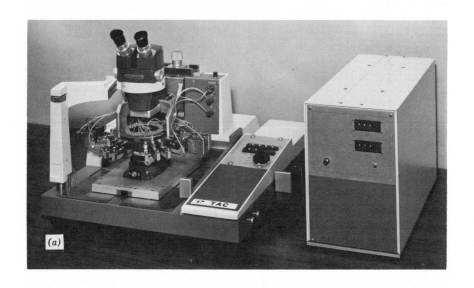

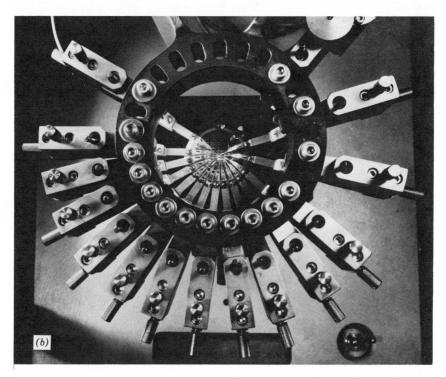

Figure A-22 Wafer prober. (*a*) The entire system. (*b*) The probe assembly. (Photographs courtesy of Teledyne TAC.)

378

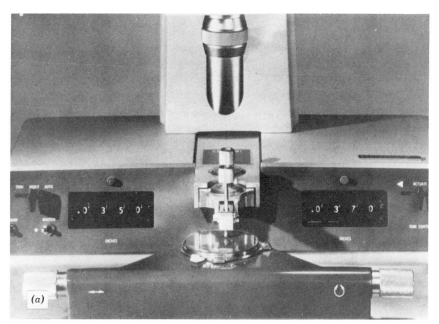

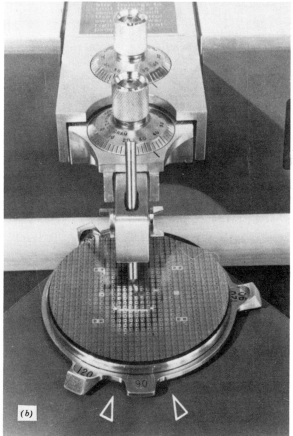

Figure A-23 Wafer scriber. (*a*) The entire scriber. (*b*) Close-up of scribe head. (Photographs courtesy of Tempress Division, Sola Basic.)

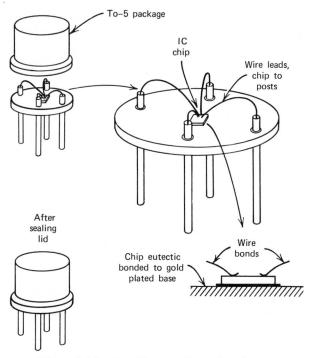

Figure A-24 Step 16: assembly and packaging.

SUMMARY OF THE PROCESS STEPS

We have gone through the steps of making a simple monolithic IC, using diffusion to introduce impurities and control junction depth, conductivity, and other characteristics of the various elements. Photolithographic techniques control *area* geometry. We have also shown how passive components can be made without adding extra processing steps. There has been considerable simplification here, and many of the refinements have been left out. There are, for instance, other diffusion steps that are often, indeed usually, included to improve the characteristics of the transistor. A typical circuit is also much more complex than the one illustrated. Dozens, often hundreds and even thousands of elements are built in a single chip, rather than the three-element IC illustrated here.

We have not discussed many of the problems that go with each step, such as mask misalignment, photoresist that does not always "resist," temperature and time errors in diffusion, damage to the chip in assembly, and a host of other process problems involved in making devices by this process. Each of the many steps in the process must be almost perfect in order to get a visible yield at the end of the process.

The silicon monolithic IC process is very involved, and extreme care must be taken all the way. Any one step is relatively simple, but they all add up to a very complex process. Successful manufacture of monolithic ICs is a technological feat that commands real respect.

RELATIVE ADVANTAGES AND DISADVANTAGES OF SILICON MONOLITHIC ICs

A more detailed comparison is given at the end of Chapter 2. Very briefly, however, silicon monlithics are best, or are most used, where production runs are relatively long, where rather expensive setup and design costs can be amortized. Aside from original design costs, the cost per component (and especially the cost per active component) is extremely low. The silicon monolithic has large volume efficiency. They are most commonly used in digital circuits.

The silicon monolithic IC is at a disadvantage over the thick or thin film ICs, or at times conventionally assembled circuits, in areas such as high voltage, high power, many types of linear circuits, high-precision circuits, low-production runs, and microwave applications.

The various disadvantages of monolithics are being aggressively attacked by the manufacturers, and some inroads into what are now private preserves of thick and thin film can be expected over the years.

Thin Film Microcircuits

In this section the major steps in making a thin film circuit are discussed. Description of the assembly and packaging steps are eliminated. The packaging and assembly techniques used in thick film are essentially the same as used by thin film producers.

In describing the thin film IC process, the fabrication of the same simple amplifier as used for monolithics is described. It consists of one transistor to be added as a *discrete* device—the conductors, the coupling capacitor, and the base biasing resistor to be fabricated using thin film techniques. The order of assembly of the various elements, resistors, conductors, and capacitors that has been chosen is only one of many that might be used. The materials that are chosen for making the resistors and conductors are also only single instances of a large number of materials that could be used. There is little doubt that the materials chosen and the order of assembly is not the best, having been picked to illustrate various processes available rather than the methods that would give the best properties, the least cost, and so on. No one would ever conceivably use this combination of processes in an actual thin film fabrication.

THE BASIC PROCESSES

High vacuum is the environment for manufacturing thin film circuits. The fact that the surroundings are what they are is one of the major objections to thin film. (It is difficult to build a factory inside a vacuum.) High-vacuum equipment is expensive, and to build automated equipment to function inside vacuum chambers is also relatively expensive.

Vacuum Evaporation. Vacuum evaporation is one of the two basic vacuum processes used. As a material is heated in a vacuum, its vapor pressure eventually gets high enough for the material to evaporate. (This, of course, can be said for a nonvacuum situation, but the temperatures needed to evaporate the materials of interest here in air would result in unwanted chemical reactions, primarily oxidation.) When material vaporizes, the individual atoms of the metal travel in a straight line until they bump into something. If what they hit is cool enough, the vaporized material will condense—much like steam condensing on the cool sides of a container of warm water.

The vacuum keeps the vaporized material from oxidizing. The vacuum has to be high enough so that it is very unlikely that the vaporized material will hit an atom of air or nitrogen before it condenses. If it does, it would probably combine and deposit on the circuit as an undesired oxide. Figure A-25 shows a schematic of a vacuum evaporation system.

Sputtering. There are many materials that (1) cannot be heated to a temperature high enough to vaporize without being destroyed by a chemical change or (2) have very high melting points. A technique called *sputtering* is used to vacuum-deposit such materials. Here, since we cannot vaporize the material, we instead strike it with a fast-moving gas ion. The force of the blow can be enough to dislodge the atoms of the "target" material.

To sputter, a high negative voltage is applied to the target (Figure A-26). The voltage causes the small amount of argon in the near vacuum to ionize. The target is negatively charged so that the ions (positive charge) will be attracted to it—accelerating as they approach to the collision point. The dislodged particles of the target material—the material that is to be deposited—go flying off in all directions, until they hit something, at which time they "stick" to whatever they hit.

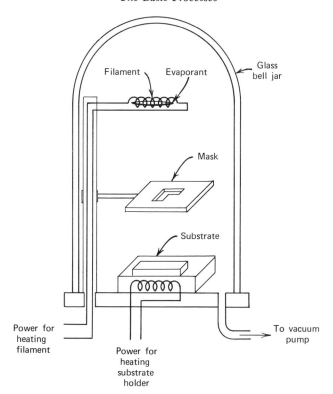

Figure A-25 Schematic showing vacuum evaporation equipment.

For nonconducting materials a space charge builds up near the target, keeping the ions from striking. To get around this, an alternating voltage is applied to the target, which drives off the space charge. On the alternate cycle, some ions strike before a space charge builds up again. This variation is called RF (radio frequency) sputtering.

Pattern Definition. In either sputtering or evaporation, the materials are deposited on the substrate (1) through a mask placed over the substrate so that material is laid down only through open areas in the mask or (2) with no mask, where the completely covered surface will be patterned later by photoresist and etching processes. The latter approach is called "substractive."

Material Thickness. The thickness of the film that is deposited is a function of time. Most thin film depositions are indeed quite thin. Film thickness

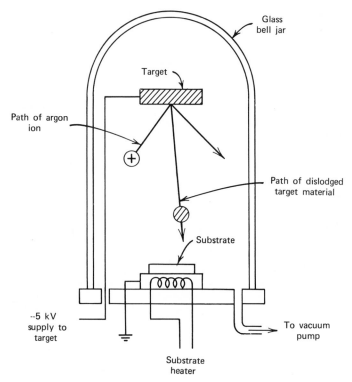

Figure A-26　Vacuum sputtering schematic.

is measured in angstrom units, one angstrom unit (Å) is 10^{-10} meter (1 μ = 10,000 Å, 1 mil = 254,000 Å). Film thicknesses are in the range of several hundred to several thousand angstroms. Deposition rates range from 100 to over 1000 Å/min. Evaporation is faster than sputtering.

MATERIALS USED

Conductors. For conductors, gold tantalum, and aluminum are commonly used. Conductors and resistors *both* can be made of tantalum, the resistor areas being trimmed to desired resistance by anodization.

Resistors. Tantalum is used, as mentioned above, or tantalum nitride. Other commonly employed materials are cermets such as silicon oxide and chromium as well as nickel-chromium mixtures. Tantalum gives the best resistor characteristics and can be trimmed to extremely close tolerance. The cermet systems can give high sheet resistance values.

Sputtering is often used for depositing resistor materials. Combination systems, such as nickel-chromium, are evaporated by utilizing mixtures of small pellets in the proper ratio or sometimes by flash evaporation where the correct proportions are continuously fed onto a hot filament where they are immediately evaporated. The last method maintains exact material ratios better.

Capacitors. Silicon oxide and tantalum oxide are the most commonly used materials, but there are many others that could be used. A high dielectric constant is very desirable, and much work has been done in an effort to employ materials such as titanium oxide and barium titanate. Dielectric strength is also important, and the high dielectric strength of thin films of silica and tantalum oxide makes these materials popular.

Substrate Heating. The substrate is usually heated during deposition. This helps to allow a better film to be deposited. Film density is higher, adhesion is improved, and so on. Characteristics such as sheet resistance and thermal drift of resistors are also influenced by substrate heating.

Summary Materials. Vacuum-deposited films do not usually have the exact properties as the bulk materials. Conductivity of metal films, for instance, can be one or two orders of magnitude higher than that of pure metal. This is because the structure is not continuous, containing voids. Also the material is not always pure, having picked up some oxides or nitrides in its journey from the evaporation source to the substrate.

The Substrate. It is possible to have either active or passive substrates. A circuit of thin film can be built on a silicon substrate—in fact, it is vacuum technology that is used to put the conductors in place on the silicon IC described in the preceding section. Thin film resistors can be deposited over silicon substrates that are protected with a layer of silica (which can be either grown from the wafer or deposited). Such resistors have a great advantage over the resistors made inside the silicon wafer—they have much better characteristics, and capacitance parasitics are greatly reduced. It is possible to do everything on a silicon substrate that can be done on the passive substrates, except that the substrate is quite expensive. For complex circuits requiring large areas for thin film components (such as resistors of high value, and of higher-capacitance capacitors) it is usually preferable to use a passive substrate, adding active devices as discrete chips.

In describing thin film fabrication steps, we use an example utilizing a passive (insulating) substrate. When one refers to thin film ICs one generally is referring to passive substrate circuits. (The discussion in the preceding paragraph was not meant to upset the idea that most thin films are done on passive substrates—just to point out that the thin film process is compatible with the monolithic process and circuits could be built on semiconductor substrates.)

Passive substrates for thin film can be of several materials, the major requirements being that they be good electrical insulators and have a smooth surface. Organic substrates are not used because they cannot take the high temperatures needed for substrate heating and because demands of strength and durability are difficult to meet. The smooth surface is needed because of the thinness of the films. This becomes obvious if one considers the relationship between surface smoothness and the thickness of the films. Figure A-27 illutrates this.

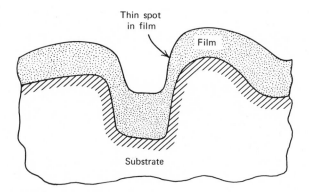

Figure A-27   An 1-microinch surface with a 200-Å film deposited on it.

The nature of the surface in Figure A-27 is one that would not be uncommon on a polished surface, the deep valley being a minor scratch. A vaccum deposition, coming from one direction, comes down somewhat like a snowfall. The vertical sides of the scratch produced a very thin region almost amounting to a disruption. It is easy to see how thin films could lose continuity if the surface were to be rougher.

Surface finishes on the order of 1 μin. are characteristic of glass or of highly polished materials. Glass is a commonly used thin film substrate but is not nearly so popular as glazed alumina has become in recent years. Alumina's strength—heat conductivity characteristics and availability in complex shapes (plus its increasingly economic pricing)—has made it by far the most popular substrate material. Good progress is being made in producing an unglazed alumina of less than 5-μin surface. This is desirable because of the greatly improved capability for conducting heat. Without the development of smooth as-fired surfaces it is necessary to grind and polish the surface. This is quite expensive because of the extreme hardness of alumina. Beryllium oxide (polished) is also used for its extremely high heat conductivity.

In the following description of a thin film manufacturing process, either glass or glazed alumina could be used as a substrate.

THIN FILM MANUFACTURING STEPS

Thin sheets of metal are used as masks where the areas for deposition have been etched away. During evaporation the masks are placed close to the substrate. The closer they are kept to the substrate, the better the edge definition.

The circuit's patterns can also be etched in the same way as in silicon wafer processing—applying photoresists, exposure, and etching (subtractive process). Masks for this are similar to semiconductor masks.

Conductor Evaporation. In our example, conductors will be deposited first. The material can be gold. A charge of gold wire is placed around the heating filament. The substrate or substrates are placed on a heated substrate holder. The vacuum chamber is closed and the vacuum is drawn. It typically takes 15 or 20 min to get the vacuum down to the proper point, about 10^{-5} torr (mm of mercury). Vacuum systems are available that vary greatly in size and complexity. Very fast pumping systems add to the cost considerably. Gold deposition rates are in the order of several thousand angstroms per minute. Only a thousand or so angstroms are needed for many applications, but to keep resistance to a low value in very narrow lines thicker applications are often desired. Thickness can also be built up at a later time by electroplating.

For high-production it is possible to do many plates at one time by either spreading several substates across the bottom of the chamber or by having a manipulatable storage rack where each substrate to receive evaporation is brought out in succession.

Etch Conductor Patterns. The entire surface of the alumina substrate has now been gold coated. The metal areas not needed for conductors, capacitor electrodes, resistor termination pads, or semiconductor chip mountings pads are etched away. The patterns are defined by exposure to photoresist procedures as described in the semiconductor wafer processing portion of this section. (Figure A-28a.)

Sputter Resistor and Capacitor Pattern. After etching the conductor pattern, the substrate is placed again in the vacuum jar. The vacuum needed

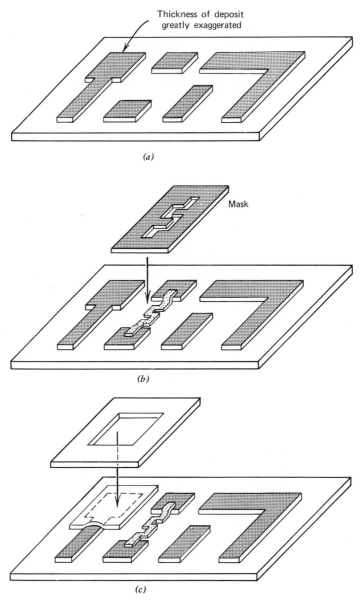

Figure A-28 Fabrication steps for making a thin film IC. (*a*) After etching conductor pattern. (*b*) Sputter tantalum resistor. (*c*) Sputter silica capacitor. (*d*) Evaporate capacitor's top electrode. (*e*) Attach transistor. (*f*) Plastic encapsulated finished thin film hybrid circuit.

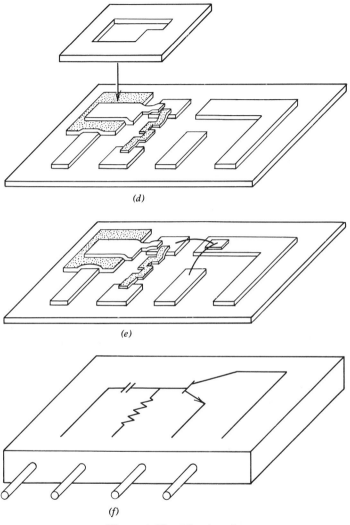

(d)

(e)

(f)

Figure A-28 (*Continued*)

for sputtering is not nearly so high—only about 10^{-2} torr. The atmosphere inside the jar is usually a gas such as argon. With a high voltage between the target and the substrate, the gas atoms ionize. The positive charge of the ionized atoms drives them to the negatively charged target and the energy of impact is often enough to dislodge atoms of the target material. Much of the impact energy results in heat so the target must usually be water cooled. One of the advantages of sputtering lies in the high energy of the atoms leaving the target. They hit the substrates much harder than would evaporated material. This promotes such things as good adhesion and improved electrical characteristics.

Sputtering is slower in its buildup than is evaporation, but a rate of 1000 Å/min is not hard to achieve. Thus in about 2 min we could sputter 2000 Å of tantalum metal for the resistor material. The sputtering is done through a mask which is manipulated into position over the substrate. The refractory nature of tantalum or a need for intimate contact with conductors would be reasons for choosing sputtering. (Figure A-28*b*.)

The capacitor pattern is deposited during the same vacuum by removing the resistor mask and maneuvering a second mask containing the capacitor pattern in its place, and by using a different target.

With film deposition rates of 1000 Å/min, a 1-min deposition of most dielectric materials would produce a capacitor with a dielectric strength of 25 to 50 V. Silica would be a likely capacitor material to put down in this way. (Figure A-28c.)

Control of thickness of the film is very important in resistors and capacitors. The tantalum resistor of our example will be trimmed to exact resistance at a later date so that exact control of thickness in this instance is not quite so important. Thickness can be monitored by various means, such as monitoring conductivity or the resonant frequency changes of a crystal as it picks up weight (because of the deposited material).

Evaporate Capacitor Counterelectrodes. The counterelectrode evaporation can proceed in much the same manner as the deposition of the original conductors, except that in this operation a mask is used to limit the deposition to the area over the silica capacitor material. Precise location of the substrate in relationship to the mask is important in masked deposition steps. (Figure A-28d.)

Adjust Resistors. A need for resistor adjustment is somewhat questionable in the particular circuit chosen for illustration, but for the purpose of illustration we shall adjust anyhow, although it would have been very easy to deposit the resistor to a close enough tolerance for a base biasing resistor.

Tantalum is a material that can be oxidized. As a layer of tantalum metal is oxidized (from the outer surface inward) the resistance of the remaining film is reduced because of reduced thickness. If the resistance is monitored during anodization the resistor can be adjusted to an exact value. Tantalum resistors are trimmed by placing a chemical anodizing solution over the resistor. As electrolytic action proceeds, the tantalum metal cross section is reduced and the resistance increases.

Thin film resistors can also be adjusted by removal of resistor material with air-abrasive systems or with lasers. Tolerances closer than 5% usually require trimming.

Adding Discrete Components and Packaging. A transistor chip is bonded to the pad provided for this purpose. Gold-silicon alloy techniques are used. Wire bonds are made to the proper metallized terminations as shown in Figure A-28e. These processes are common with thick film and are discussed in more detail in the body of the text. Packaging can proceed also by a variety of methods, depending on the final application. (Figure A-28e.)

Thin film, like silicon monolithic technology, is essentially a batch process. Silicon monolithics are inexpensive because it is possible to process many circuits on a wafer. Thin film can also benefit from the same approach. It is quite common to process a rather large substrate—3 or 4 in. on a side. The substrate is broken into individiaul circuits by sawing, scribing, or, lately, laser cutting. The cutting operation, when it is done, occurs after the last vacuum operation. Final assembly operations proceed on a one-at-a-time basis.

Summary. Thin film technology tends to be expensive as far as the cost of producing, but this disadvantage is not felt so much in smaller production runs because initial tooling is less expensive than with silicon monolithics. Great circuit flexibility is available through hybrid approaches. Active devices of almost any complexity can be added. Various active devices with completely different characteristics can be mounted on the same circuit (such as both linear digital IC chips, zeners, and tunnel diodes). Extremely accurate control over line width and geometry makes the thin film IC very good for microwave applications. Excellent resistor characteristics often give thin film ICs advantages over other types. Of the three IC types, the most demanding circuits (where precision geometry and/or values are needed) are done in thin film. (See Chapter 2 for a more thorough comparison between thin film and other types.)

Appendix II

DIGGING DEEPER

This appendix aims to help you to dig deeper into the subject of thick film technology than this introductory textbook can be expected to take you. It is impossible to cover in one book *every* facet of the complicated interplay between materials and processing and between technology and design, marketing, production, or general management. If we have given you a vocabulary sufficient for continued reading and study and have convinced you that an adequate understanding of the materials and processes is necessary for successful application—our time and effort have been well spent. An understanding of the materials is especially important in view of the trend toward more complex materials systems that require even more stringent process controls.

In thick film it is essential to keep up with new developments. This text can only be a start. To aid you in learning more about thick film hybrid technology, we cover here in some detail the following topics: (1) suppliers to the industry, (2) technical and trade journals and government publications, (3) society meetings and symposia, and (4) general references.

Suppliers to the Industry

Materials and equipment suppliers are a very important source of information. Most of them are in a position to provide technical assistance with specific problems in materials and processing. The literature they give out is usually informative and often includes reprints of papers written by their employees. Their sales and technical personnel are usually readily available and can serve as a group of consultants who need not be paid—take advantage of them.

In this compilation of some of the materials and equipment suppliers we have tried to be as thorough as space will allow. Inevitably, some important suppliers will have been left out; for this, we apologize. Only categories that are purely thick film hybrid in nature are included. The list, then, does not include *all* the materials and equipment needed, leaving out categories that people tend to know about or that cover broader areas such as test and measuring equipment, ovens, soldering, and irons.

SUBSTRATES

American Lava Corporation
Chattanooga, Tennessee 37405
615-265-3411
(Alumina, titanate, beryllia, etc.)

Carborundum Company
Box 337
Niagara Falls, New York 14302
(Alumina)

Centralab Division
Globe Union, Inc.
5757 North Green Bay
Milwaukee, Wisconsin 53201
(Alumina, titanate)

Cermetron Corporation
1045 Roselle Street
San Diego, California 92121
714-453-1354
(Short-run alumina)

Coors Porcelain Company
600 9th Street
Golden, Colorado 80401
303-279-6565
(Alumina, beryllia)

Frenchtown/CFI, Inc.
(Subsidiary of The Plessey Co.)
Frenchtown, New Jersey 08825
201-996-2121
(Alumina)

National Beryllia Corporation
Greenwood Avenue
Haskell, New Jersey 07420
201-839-1600
(Beryllia)

Radio Materials Company (RMC)
4242 West Bryn Mawr Avenue
Chicago, Illinois 60646
312-IR8-3600
(Alumina)

Varadyne, Inc.
1805 Colorado
Santa Monica, California 90404
213-394-0271

INKS AND PASTES

Airco Speer Electronics
Box 828
Niagara Falls, New York 14302
716-285-6971
(Resistor, conductor pastes)

Alpha Metals, Inc.
56 Water Street
Jersey City, New Jersey 07034
201-434-6778
(Solder pastes)

* Full line consists of at least five of the following categories: resistors, conductors, capacitor dielectrics crossover dielectrics, encapsulant dielectrics, solder and bonding pastes, and sealing glasses.

INKS AND PASTES

American Components, Inc.
8th Avenue at Harry Street
Conshohocken, Pennsylvania 19478
215-828-6240
(Resistor, dielectrics, conductor)

Cermalloy
Division of Bala Electronics Corporation
14 Fayette Street
Conshohocken, Pennsylvania 19428
215-828-4650
(Resistor, conductors)

Conshom Division
Conshohocken Chemicals, Inc.
Box 224
Flourtown, Pennsylvania 19031
215-835-5700
(Conductors)

DuPont
Electronic Products Division
Wilmington, Delaware 19898
800-441-9442
(Full line*)

Electro-Materials Corporation of
   America (EMCA)
605 Central Avenue
Mamaroneck, New York 10543
914-698-8434
(Full line*)

Electro-Science Labs
1133–35 Arch Street
Philadelphia, Pennsylvania 19107
215-563-2215
(Full line*)

Engelhard Industries
Electronic Products Division
421 Delancy Street
Newark, New Jersey
(Conductors)

Methode Development Company
7447 West Wilson
Chicago, Illinois 60056
312-867-9600
(Resistors, conductors)

Owens-Illinois
Box 1035
Toledo, Ohio 43601
419-242-6543
(Conductors, dielectrics)

Sel-Rex Corporation
Electronic Materials Division
75 River Road
Nutley, New Jersey 07110
201-667-5200
(Conductors, resistors)

The Plessy Co.
Electronic Materials Division
320 Long Island Expressway South
Melville, Long Island, New York 11746
516-694-7900
(Full line*)

CAPACITORS

Aerovox Corporation
740 Belleville Avenue
New Bedford, Massachusetts 02741
617-994-9661
(Ceramic chips)

American Components, Inc.
8th Avenue at Harry Street
Conshohocken, Pennsylvania 19478
215-828-6240
(Ceramic chips)

* Full line consists of at least five of the following categories: resistors, conductors, capacitor dielectrics crossover dielectrics, encapsulant dielectrics, solder and bonding pastes, and sealing glasses.

CAPACITORS

American Lava Corporation
Chattanooga, Tennessee 37405
(Ceramic chips)

American Technical Ceramics
1 Norden Lane
Huntington Station, New York 11746
516-271-9600
(Ceramic chips)

CAL-R, Inc.
1601 Olympic Boulevard
Santa Monica, California 90404
213-451-9761
(Ceramic chips)

Centralab Division
Globe Union, Inc.
5757 North Green Bay Avenue
Milwaukee, Wisconsin 53201
(Ceramic chips)

Centre Engineering
Box P-8
State College, Pennsylvania 16801
814-237-0321
(Ceramic chips)

Components, Inc.
Biddeford, Maine 04005
207-284-5956
(Miniature tantalums)

Dickson Electronics Corporation
Box 1390
Scottsdale, Arizona 85212
602-969-8111
(Miniature tantalums)

Electro Materials Division, ITW
11620 Sorrento Valley Road
San Diego, California 92121
714-459-4355
(Ceramic chips)

Erie Technological Products, Inc.
644 West 12th
Erie, Pennsylvania 16512
814-456-8592
(Ceramic chips)

JFD Electronics
15th Avenue at 62nd Street
Brooklyn, New York 11219
212-331-1000
(Ceramic chips)

Kemet (Union Carbide)
Box 5928
Greenville, South Carolina 29606
803-963-7421
(Ceramic chips, tantalums)

Monolithic Dielectrics, Inc.
Box 647
Burbank, California 91503
213-848-4465
(Ceramic chips)

Motorola Semiconductor Products
Box 20912
Phoenix, Arizona 85036
602-273-6900
(Thin film chips)

Republic Electronics
176 East 7th Street
Patterson, New Jersey 07124
201-279-0300
(Ceramic chips)

San Fernando Electric Manufacturing
Company
1501 First Street
San Fernando, California 91341
213-365-9411
(Ceramic chips)

Sprague Electric Company
North Adams, Massachusetts 01247
(Ceramic and tantalum chips)

United Aircraft
Electronic Components Division
Trevose, Pennsylvania 19047
215-355-5000
(Thin film chips)

U.S. Capacitor Company
2151 North Lincoln
Burbank, California 91504
213-843-4222
(Ceramic chips)

CAPACITORS

Varadyne, Inc.
1805 Colorado Avenue
Santa Monica, California 90404
213-394-0271
(Ceramic chips)

Vitramon, Inc.
Box 544
Bridgeport, Connecticut 06601
203-268-6261
(Ceramic chips)

RESISTORS

Airco Speer Electronics
Venture Product Division
Box 828
Niagara Falls, New York 14302
716-285-6971
(Thick and thin film chips)

American Components, Inc.
8th Avenue at Harry Street
Conshohocken, Pennsylvania 19428
215-828-6250
(Thick film chips)

Angstrom Precision, Inc.
7811 Lemona
Van Nuys, California 91405
213-989-3061
(Thin film chips)

ASC Microelectronics
Division of Acusticon Systems
  Corporation
Danbury, Connecticut 00810
203-744-1900
(Thick film chips)

Caddock Electronics, Inc.
3127 Chicago Avenue
Riverside, California 92507
714-683-3361
(Chips)

Cal-R, Inc.
1601 Olympic Boulevard
Santa Monica, California 90404
213-451-9761
(Ceramic chips)

CTS Microelectronics, Inc.
1201 Cumberland Avenue
West Lafayette, Indiana 47906
(Solid cermet chips)

Dale Electronics, Inc.
Box 609
Columbus, Nebraska 68601
902-564-3131
(Thick film chips)

Dickson Electronics Corporation
Box 1390
Scottsdale, Arizona 85212
602-947-2231
(Thin film chips)

EMC Technology, Inc.
1300 Arch Street
Philadelphia, Pennsylvania 19107
215-516-1340
(Thick film chips)

Kulite Semiconductor Products
1039 Hoyt Avenue
Ridgefield, New Jersey
201-945-3000
(Thick film chips)

Lek Trol, Inc.
Grapevine, Texas 76051
817-268-1101
(Thick film chips)

Minisystems, Inc.
Washington Park
North Attleboro, Massachusetts 02701
617-695-0206
(Thick film chips)

Monolithic Dielectrics
Box 647
Burbank, California 91503
213-848-4465
(Thick film chips)

RESISTORS

Motorola Semiconductor Products
Box 20912
Phoenix, Arizona 85036
602-273-6900
(Thin film chips)

Pyrofilm Corp.
60 South Jefferson Road
Whippany, New Jersey 07981
201-807-8100
(Carbon film pellets)

Sloan Microelectronics Division
Sloan Technology
Box 4608
Santa Barbara, California 93103
805-963-4431
(Thin film chips)

Solid State Scientific, Inc.
Montgomeryville Industrial Center
Montgomeryville, Pennsylvania 18936
215-855-8400
(Thin film chips)

United Aircraft
Electronic Components Division
Trevose, Pennsylvania 19047
215-315-5000
(Thin film chips)

Varadyne
1805 Colorado Avenue
Santa Monica, California 90404
213-394-0271

Vishay Resistor Products Division
Vishay Corporation
63 Lincoln Highway
Malvern, Pennsylvania 19355
215-644-1300
(Thin film chips)

INDUCTORS

Motorola Semiconductor Products
Box 20912
Phoenix, Arizona 85036
602-273-6900
(Thin film chips)

Nytronics, Inc.
150 Springfield Avenue
Berkeley Heights, New Jersey 07922
201-464-9300
(Minicomponents)

ACTIVE DEVICES—CHIPS

Centralab Division
Globe Union, Inc.
4501 North Arden
El Monte, California 91374
(Zeners and diode chips)

Circa Tran, Inc.
Box 832
Wheaton, Illinois 60187
312-858-3727
(LIDS)

Dickson Electronics
Box 1390
Scottsdale, Arizona 85212
602-947-2231
(Zener and transistor chips and lids)

Ferranti Electric, Inc.
East Bethpage Road
Plainview, Long Island, New York
   11803
516-293-8383
(Miniature transistors)

Hughes Aircraft
100 Superior Avenue
Newport Beach, California 92663
(Flip chips)

Microsemiconductor Corporation
11250 Playa Street
Culver City, California 90230
213-391-8271

ACTIVE DEVICES—CHIPS

Motorola Semiconductor Products
Box 20912
Phoenix, Arizona 85036
602-273-6900
(Transistors' diode chips, IC chips)

National Semiconductor
2975 San Ysidro Way
Santa Clara, California 95051
408-245-4320
(IC chips—linear and digital)

Pirgo Electronics (Sprague Affiliate)
130 Central Avenue
Farmingdale, New York 11735
516-694-9880
(Power transistor chips)

Raytheon Company
350 Ellis Street
Mountain View, California 94049
415-968-9211
(Beam leads—ICs and single elements)

Silicon General
7382 Bolsa Avenue
Westminister, California 93683
714-839-6200
(Special IC chips)

Solid State Scientific, Inc.
Montgomeryville Industrial Center
Montgomeryville, Pennsylvania 18936
215-855-8400
(Chips—Single and IC)

Sprague Electric
Semiconductor Division
Pembroke Road
Concord, New Hampshire 03301
(Transistor chips)

Texas Instruments, Inc.
P. O. Box 512
Dallas, Texas 75222
214-238-4801
(Transistor chips, minicomponents, IC chips, beam lead chips)

United Aircraft
Electronic Components Division
Trevose, Pennsylvania 19047
215-355-5000
(Transistor and monolithic IC chips and lids)

SOLDERS, FLUXES

Alpha Metals, Inc.
56 Water Street
Jersey City, New Jersey 07034
201-434-6778
(Full line)

DuPont
Electronic Products Division
Wilmington, Delaware 19898
(Pastes)

Emerson & Cummings, Inc.
Canton, Massachusetts 02021
617-828-3300
(Conductive epoxies)

Epoxy Technology
65 Grove Street
Watertown, Massachusetts 02172
617-926-0136
(Conductive epoxies)

The Plessey Co.
320 Long Island Expressway
Melville, Long Island, New York 11746
516-694-7900
(Preforms and pastes)

PACKAGES

American Lava Corporation
Subsidiary of 3M
Chattanooga, Tennessee 37405
615-265-3411
(Ceramic, buried conductor)

Bendix Corporation
Components Division
Sidney, New York 13838
607-563-9511
(Ceramic)

Centralab Division
Globe Union
5757 North Green Bay
Milwaukee, Wisconsin 53201
414-228-1200
(Ceramic)

Ceramic Metal Systems, Inc.
Box 156
Somerville, New Jersey 08876
201-359-8141
(Ceramic)

Coors Porcelain Company
600 Ninth Street
Golden, Colorado 80401
303-279-6565
(Ceramic)

Dielectric Systems, Inc.
3422 Tripp Court, Sorrento Valley
San Diego, California 92121
714-459-2935
(Burried conductor)

Diacon
4812 Kearny Mesa Road
San Diego, California
714-279-6992
(Ceramic)

DuPont
Electronic Products Division
Wilmington, Delaware 19898
(Burried conductor, ceramic)

Frenchtown/CFI, Inc.
Subsidiary of The Plessey Co.
Frenchtown, New Jersey, 08825
201-996-2121
(Ceramic)

GTE Sylvania
200 Sylvan Road
Bangor, Maine 04401
207-947-8386
(Ceramic)

Interbond Systems, Inc.
1260 Alderwood Avenue
Sunnyvale, California 44086
408-734-3435
(Plastic)

Metalized Ceramics
West River Industrial Park
Providence, Rhode Island 02904
401-331-9800
(Ceramic)

Moldtronics, Inc.
705 Rogers Street
Downers Grove, Illinois 60515
312-968-7000
(Plastic)

Motorola Semiconductor Products
Box 20912
Phoenix, Arizona 85036
602-273-6900
(Ceramic)

National Beryllia Corporation
Greenwood Avenue
Haskell, New Jersey 07420
(Ceramic, beryllia)

Sprague Electric Company
Semiconductor Division
Pembroke Road
Concord, New Hampshire 03301
(Metal, ceramic, glass)

Sylvania (Parts Division)
12 Second Avenue
Warren, Pennsylvania 16305
814-723-2000
(Glass, metal)

Tekform Products Company
2780 Coronada Street
Anaheim, California 92806
714-630-2340
(Metal, glass, ceramic)

PACKAGES

Texas Instruments
Hermetic Seals Department
Dallas, Texas 75222
214-238-2011
(Ceramic, glass)

U.S. Electronic Services Corp.
Holgar Industrial Park
Clifton Heights, Pennsylvania 19018
215-628-5200
(Plastic)

Varadyne
Hanibal Division
1639 East Edinger Street
Santa Ana, California 92705
714-542-4794

Veritron West, Inc.
Subsidiary of Alloys Unlimited
20245 Sunburst Street
Chatsworth, California 91311
(Glass)

SCREENS AND MASKS

Note. Most screen or mask makers have full facilities for artwork, photoreduction, and so on.

A M I
Box 248
Whitehouse, New Jersey 08888
201-534-2103
(Screens)

Aremco Products, Inc.
Box 145
Briarcliffe, New York 10510
914-762-0085
(Screens)

Industrial Reproductions, Inc. (IRI)
Box 888
100 Northeastern Avenue
Nashua, New Hampshire 03060
603-883-5541
(Screens and metal masks)

Microcircuit Eng.
Elm Drive
Medford, New Jersey 08055
609-654-2180
(Screens)

Towne Laboratories
1 U.S. Highway 206
Somerville, New Jersey 08876
201-772-9500
(Etched metal masks)

Ulano
210 East 86th Street
New York, New York 10028
212-MA2-5200
(Rubylith)

SCREEN PRINTERS

A M I (Affiliated Manufacturers, Inc.)
Box 248, U.S. Highway 22
Whitehouse, New Jersey 08888
201-534-2103

Aremco Products, Inc.
Box 145
Briarcliffe Manor, New York 10510
914-762-0685

de Haart, Inc.
12 Wilmington Road
Burlington, Massachusetts 01803
617-272-0794

Precision Systems Company, Inc.
(PRESCO)
U.S. 22, P.O. Box 148
Somerville, New Jersey 08876
201-722-7100

SCREEN PRINTERS

Selrex Corporation
75 River Road
Nutley, N.J. 07110
201-667-5200

Weltek Division
Wells Electronics, Inc.
1701 South Main
South Bend, Indiana 41123
219-288-4657

THICK FILM FURNACES

BTU Engineering Corporation
Bear Hill
Waltham, Massachusetts 02154
617-894-6050

C. I. Hayes, Inc.
800 Wellington Avenue
Cranston, Rhode Island 02910

W. P. Keith Company, Inc.
8323 Loch Lomand Drive
Pico Rivera, California 90660
213-723-1375

Lindberg/Heavy Duty Division
Sola Basic
2450 West Hubbard
Chicago, Illinois 60612

Temtek, Inc.
Box 477
Bartlett, Illinois 60103
312-695-7080

Thermco Products Corporation
1465 North Batavia Street
Orange, California 92668
714-639-2340

Watkins-Johnson Company
Stewart Division
440 Mt. Hermon Road
Scotts Valley, California 95060
408-438-2100

RESISTOR TRIMMERS

Appollo Lasers, Inc.
6365 Arizona Circle
Los Angeles, California 90045
(Lasers)

Arvin Systems, Inc.
1482 Stanley Avenue
Dayton, Ohio 45404
513-222-8279
(Lasers)

Comco, Inc.
1226 West Olive
Burbank, California 91506
213-849-7711
(Air abrasive)

de Haart, Inc.
12 Wilmington Road
Burlington, Massachusetts 01803
617-272-0794
(Air abrasive)

Electroscientific Industries (ESI)
13900 N. W. Science Park Drive
Portland, Oregon 97229
(Laser)

Korad (Union Carbide)
2520 Colorado Avenue
Santa Monica, California 90406
213-393-6737
(Laser)

Micronetics, Inc.
204 Arsenal Street
Watertown, Massachusetts 92172
617-926-2570
(Laser)

MPM Corporation
9 Harvey Street
Cambridge, Massachusetts 02140
617-876-7111
(Air abrasive)

RESISTOR TRIMMERS

Spacerays, Inc.
Northwest Industrial Park
Burlington, Massachusetts 01803
617-272-6220
(Laser)

Teradyne Applied Systems
4034 North Nashville Avenue
Chicago, Illinois 60634
312-725-2011
(Laser)

S. S. White Division
Penwalt Corporation
201 East 42nd Street
New York, New York 10017
212-661-3320
(Air abrasive)

SEMICONDUCTOR BONDING EQUIPMENT

Axion Corporation
6 Commerce Park
Danbury, Connecticut 06810
203-743-9281

Ewald Instruments, Inc.
Route 7E
Kent, Connecticut 06757
203-927-3278

G T I Corporation
1399 Logan Avenue
Costa Mesa, California 92626
714-346-0411

Hughes Aircraft Company
Welder Department
2020 Oceanside Boulevard
Oceanside, California 92054
714-751-1200

Hugle Industries, Inc.
625 North Pastoria Avenue
Sunnyvale, California 94086
408-738-1700

Kasper Instruments, Inc.
983 Shulman Avenue
Santa Clara, California 95050
408-246-2696

Kulicke and Soffa Industries
135 Commerce Drive
Fort Washington, Pennsylvania 19034
215-646-5800

Lindberg/Heavy Duty Division
Sola Basic Company
2450 West Hubbard
Chicago, Illinois 60612
412-921-3778

Mech-El Industries
73 Pine Street
Woburn, Massachusetts 01801
617-935-4750

Micro Tech Manufacturing, Inc.
703 Plantation Street
Worcester, Massachusetts 01605
617-755-5215

Precision Equipment Company, Inc.
(PRECO)
1246 Central Avenue
Hillside, New Jersey 07205
201-351-4442

Sonobond Corporation
310 E. Rosedale Avenue
West Chester, Pennsylvania 19380
215-696-4710

Unitek Corporation
Weldmatic Division
1820 South Myrtle
Monrovia, California 91016
213-359-8367

Wells Electronics
1701 South Main
South Bend, Indiana 41123
219-288-4657

West-Bond, Inc.
2165 North Glassell Street
Orange, California 92667
714-637-2600

MISCELLANEOUS EQUIPMENT

Surface Roughness and Thickness Measurements
Gould/Clevite
4601 North Arden Drive
El Monte, California 91731
213-442-7755

Package Sealing Equipment
Dix Engineering Division
GTI Corporation
1399 Logan Avenue
Costa Mesa, California 92626
714-546-0411

Research Instrument Company
558 Main Street
Westbury, New York 11590
516-333-7440

Substrate Scribers, Paste Rollers
Mechanization Associates
140 South Whisman Road
Mountain View, California
415-967-4262

Chip Handling Equipment
A M I
U.S. Route 22
Whitehouse, New Jersey 08888
201-534-2103

Hugle Industries
625 N. Dastoria Avenue
Sunnyvale, California 94086
408-738-1700

Viscosity Measurement
Brookfield Engineering Laboratories, Inc.
240 Cushin Street
Stoughton, Massachusetts 02072
617-344-4310

Technical and Trade Journals

The increasing interest in thick film technology is evidenced by the number of articles appearing in technical and trade journals. The *State of the Art Digest* reviewed more than 250 articles in both 1969 and 1970, indicating much interest in thick and thin film hybrid technology. Some of the best magazines and journals are listed below. These magazines plus the proceedings of the various technical meetings will give the reader over 90% of what is being published in English today.

*Solid State Technology
Cowan Publishing Company
14 Vanderventer Avenue
Washington, Long Island, New York
   11050
Journal and Bulletin of the American
   Ceramic Society
The American Ceramic Society
4055 North High Street
Columbus, Ohio 43214

Transactions and various *Proceedings of
   the IEEE* plus the *IEEE Spectrum*
Institute of Electrical and Electronic
   Engineers
345 East 47th Street
New York, New York 10017
Electronics
McGraw-Hill Publishing Co.
330 West 42nd Street
New York, New York 10036

* These magazines are aimed more specifically at thick film and publish articles of interest with greater frequency than do the others listed.

Insulation/Circuits
Lake Publishing Company
Box 270
Libertyville, Illinois 60048

*Electronic Packaging and Production
Milton Kiver Publications
222 West Adams Street
Chicago, Illinois 60606

The Electronic Engineer
Chilton Company
Chestnut and 56th Street
Philadelphia, Pennsylvania 19139

Electronic Products
United Technical Publications
Box 465, Ansonia Station
New York, New York 10023

EDN/EEE
Cahners Publishing Company
270 St. Paul
Denver, Colorado 80206

Electronic Design
Hayden Publishing Company, Inc.
850 Third Avenue
New York, New York 10022

Circuits Manufacturing
Benwill Publishing
167 Corey Road
Brookline, Massachusetts 02146

State of the Art Digest
State of the Art, Inc.
1315 South Allen Street
State College, Pennsylvania 16801

Most of these magazines can be obtained by qualified readers at no cost (exceptions: McGraw-Hill's *Electronics,* the Society publications, and *State of the Art Digest*).

Two good English publications are:

Electronic Components
United Trade Press Ltd.
9 Gough Square—Fleet Street
London EC 4
$17.50/year free in the United Kingdom)

Electronic Engineering
Morgan-Grampian, Ltd.
28 Essex
London WC-2
5 £/year

OTHER BOOKS, HANDBOOKS

Government publications are also available. These are listed in "U.S. Government Research and Development Reports," published by the U.S. Department of Commerce, Clearinghouse for Federal Scientific and Technical Information, Springfield, Virginia.

Also of considerable use as a source for information on papers and writings are the compilations of J. T. Milek of the U.S Air Force's Electric Properties Information Center (EPIC) at Hughes Aircraft, Culver City, California, 90230. Milek's various bibliographies and survey papers can be had by writing to EPIC.

Although many of the papers given at the various meetings are eventually published in trade and society journals, some are to be heard only at the meetings or are available only in the transactions of the meeting. The

---

* These magazines are aimed more specifically at thick film and publish articles of interest with greater frequency than do the others listed.

proceedings of ISHM and of the IEEE Component Conferences are particularly valuable as a source of information on thick film hybrids. The NEPCON shows also put out proceedings, but only a considerable time *after* the meeting.

Worthy of mention here is DuPont's *Thick Film Handbook*—available to anyone for $50 (plus yearly updating charges). It has a tremendous amount of general information about thick film and should be obtained by anyone who is seriously interested in thick film hybrids.

State of the Art, Inc. uses in their thick film seminars a text similar to this book (this book is *based* on the thick film seminar text, in fact). It is loose-leaf and is kept up to date through quarterly mailings. The quarterly mailings include much supplemental material beyond the limited scope of this text. The text and one year's quarterly mailings are available for $90. Additional subscriptions are $40/year.

The monthly abstracting service, *State of the Art Digest* has an annual index of articles in the field of hybrid circuits that has published since 1969. The bibliographic references listed below are selected from the *Digest* annual indexes.

Technical Societies and Trade Shows

The following are the most important trade and technical meetings.

The American Ceramic Society. 4055 North High Street, Columbus, Ohio 43214. Annual membership fee: $25 (includes *Journal* and *Bulletin* subscriptions). Annual meeting of the society—in the East in spring each year. Electronics Division Meeting—in the fall of each year, various location. West Coast Regional Meeting—in the fall of each year on the West Coast (no proceedings for these meetings).

The Institute of Electrical and Electronic Engineers, 345 East 47th Street, New York, New York 10017. Annual membership fee: $25 (includes *IEEE Spectrum* subscription; other journals and proceedings extra, but at a substantial discount). Annual meeting—New York City, early spring (questionable value). Parts Materials and Components Group Annual Conference—Washington, D.C., late spring each year; not to be missed. Proceedings available at the time of the meeting.

International Society for Hybrid Microelectronics, 1410 Higgins Road, Park Ridge, Illinois 60668. Annual dues: $15 (includes ISHM journal published in *Solid State Technology*). Annual meeting—various locations each fall; not to be missed. Proceedings available. Many ISHM local section meetings are held several times a year. The sections are extremely active and offer good talks and conversation.

NEPCON (National Electronic Packaging Conference) Given annually in the West and the East, and lately also in the Midwest and in England. All are much alike, although the West Coast meeting is the strongest. Primarily a trade exhibit, but papers are also given. Quite good, although not up to IEEE Components Conference or ISHM meetings. The trade exhibits are excellent—the best place to see what is going on in thick film. Many suppliers show only in these shows. Proceedings are available, although considerably delayed. For information, write Milton K. Kiver Publications, 122 West Adams, Chicago, Illinois 60606.

Bibliography

The references listed below represent the bulk of information published about thick film in the past several years. They are organized by text chapters. Since, inevitably, some articles could fit with more than one chapter, for a particular subject it is probably worthwhile to look under some of the other chapter headings. For instance, an article about resistor processing may fit under Chapter 4 (Thick Film Materials), Chapter 6 (Firing), or Chapter 8 (Trimming). We may have it listed only under one chapter heading. The references include publications through the calendar year 1970.

CHAPTER 1

INTEGRATED CIRCUITS—GENERAL

ABC'S of Monolithic Integrated Circuits. Reprinted by RCA/Electronic Components from International Automotive Engineering Congress Publication, January 1969. M. V. Hoovar (RCA).

Perspective on Integrated Electronics. *IEEE Spectrum,* January 1970, pp. 67–79. J. J. Suran (GE).

Anatomy of Integrated Circuit Technology. *IEEE Spectrum,* February 1970, pp. 56–66. H. Johnson (RCA).

The Art of Building SLI's. *IEEE Spectrum,* September 1969, pp. 29–36. H. T. Hochman (Honeywell).

Large Scale Integration in Electronics. *Scientific American,* February 1970, pp. 22–31. F. G. Heath.

Technological Advances in Large-Scale Integration. *IEEE Spectrum,* May 1970, pp. 50–58. H. T. Hochman and D. L. Hogan (Honeywell).

CHAPTER 2

Comparison of the Use of Thin and Thick Film Resistors and Conductors in Hybrid Integrated Circuits. *ISHM Proceedings,* 1967 (2nd Symposium), pp. 121–125. K. E. G. Pitt, W. J. Pool, and B. Walton (Morganite Research & Development, Ltd.).

Review of the Design and Production of Thick-Film Hybrid Integrated Circuits. *ISHM Proceedings,* 1967 (2nd Symposium), pp. 163–172. D. P. Burks (Sprague Electric).

Hybrid Thick and Thin Film Microcircuits. A Report Bibliography, Interim Report #66, March 11, 1969. J. T. Milek (Hughes Aircraft, Air Force Materials Lab).

An Up-to-Date Look at Thick Films, *EDN,* September 15, 1969, pp. 35–42. J. J. Cox and D. T. DeCoursey (DuPont).

Thick Films or Thin. *IEEE Spectrum,* October 1969, pp. 73–80. R. E. Thum (Raytheon).

Thick Film Integrated Circuits. *Electronic Components (England),* Part I, October 1969, pp. 1121–1176; Part II, November 1969. P. J. Homes and J. R. Corkhill (Royal Aircraft Est.).

Thick Film Materials Capabilities—1969. *Electronic Components,* May 1970, pp. 563–566. J. J. Cox and D. T. DeCoursey (DuPont).

History and Future of Hybrid Microelectronics. *Electronic Engineering,* June 1970, pp. 54–58. D. Boswell (ITT Components Group, Europe).

CHAPTER 4

PROCESSING THICK FILM

Thick Film Production Techniques. *ISHM Proceedings,* 1967 (1st Symposium), pp. 1–10. Also *Electronic Packaging and Production,* February 1967, Special Thick/Thin Film Supplement, TF60-70. H. H. Nester and T. E. Salzer (Microtek).

Practical Production of Thick Film Resistors and Conductors. *ISHM Proceedings,* 1967 (1st Symposium), pp. 12–20. T. M. Place.

Tooling and Part Handling Problems in the Production of Thick Film Microcircuits. *ISHM Proceedings,* 1967 (1st Symposium), pp. 102–13. D. C. Hughes (Precision Systems Co.).

Thick Film Circuit and Substrate Design Considerations for Automation. *ISHM Proceedings,* 1967 (2nd Symposium), pp. 101–105. D. C. Hughes (Precision Systems).

Smoothing the Move into Thick Film Processing. *Insulation/Circuits,* June 1970, pp. 51–56. J. Bowman, E. Stapleton, and J. Turnbaugh (Tektronix).

Recent Advances in Thick Film Resistive Materials. *ISHM Proceedings,* 1967 (1st Symposium), pp. 133–43. S. J. Stein (Electro-Science Labs).

Practical Production of Thick Film Conductors and Resistors. *ISHM Proceedings,* 1967 (1st Symposium), pp. 12–20. T. M. Place.

Controlled Processing for Precision Thick Film Resistors. *Proceedings Electronic Components Conference,* 1967, pp. 229–237. R. W. Ilgenfritz (Raytheon).

Characterization of Thick Film Resistives for Maximum Production Yields. *Proceedings Electronic Components Conference,* 1970, pp. 412–418. W. G. Dryden, R. J. Ost, and R. B. Wolf (Sperry Gyroscope).

Living with a Thick Film Resistor Ink Series. *Proceedings Electronic Components Conference,* 1969, pp. 276–285. H. R. Isaak (McDonnell-Douglas).

Some Practical Considerations in the Fabrication of Printed Glaze Resistors and Circuits. *Proceedings Electronic Components Conference,* 1966, pp. 8–16. S. J. Stein and W. F. Ebling (Electro-Science Labs).

RELIABILITY

Reliability Characteristics of Palladium-Silver Thick Film Resistors. *ISHM Proceedings,* 1967 (2nd Symposium), pp. 143–150.

Achieving Reliable Thick Film Components. *ISHM Proceedings,* 1967 (2nd Symposium), pp. 7–12. H. H. Nester and T. Cocca (Microtek).

Reliability of Screened Metal Film Resistors. *Proceedings Electronic Components Conference,* 1968, pp. 271–277. D. P. Burks, H. Geller, M. Geroulo, J. Herson, and J. P. Maher (Sprague).

Electrical Properties of a Silver Contaminated Borosilicate Glass. *ISHM Proceedings,* 1968, pp. 119–124. A. Hornung (IBM).

Reliability of Hybrid Microelectronic Circuits. *EPIC,* a Report Bibliography, Interim Report No. 65, March 11, 1969. J. T. Milek (Hughes Aircraft, Air Force Materials Lab).

Reliability Improvement Program for Hybrid Circuits. *ISHM Proceedings,* 1969, pp. 23–28. E. M. Cole and D. L. Farr (Litton Systems).

Reliability of Hybrid Microcircuits in Use Today. *Proceedings Electronic Components Conference,* 1970, pp. 16–27. R. J. Straub (GMC Delco Electronics).

Reliability of Thick-Film Circuits in Automobile Environments. *ISHM Proceedings,* 1970, 3.2.1. W. D. Colwell and G. L. Thomas (GMC Delco Radio Div.).

Effect of Soldering Flux on the Reliability of Thick Film Hybrid Microcircuits. *ISHM Proceedings,* 1970, 4.2.1. E. Tsunashima (Wireless Research Labs).

SUBSTRATES

Alumina Substrates for Thick Film Application. *ISHM Proceedings,* 1967 (1st Symposium), pp. 44–48. S. D. Heil (Coors Porcelain).

Design Criteria for Ceramic Substrates. *ISHM Proceedings,* 1968, pp. 405–416. C. E. Nordquist (Coors Porcelain).

Ceramics for Microelectronic Applications. *ISHM Proceedings,* 1968, pp. 387–396. R. D. Dillender (American Lava).

Applications of Laser Systems to Microelectronics and Silicon Wafer Dicing. *Solid State Technology,* April 1970, pp. 63–67. G. A. Hardway (Spacerays).

INDUCTORS

Thick Film Inductors at VHF. *Electronic Components,* June 1970, pp. 611–684. P. Barnwell (Brighton College of Technology).

Properties of Thick Film Inductors. *Electronic Components,* May 1969, p. 593. J. R. Corkhill and D. R. Mullins (Royal Aircraft Establishment).

CONDUCTORS—THICK FILM

Conductor Compositions for Fine Line Printing. *ISHM Proceedings,* 1967 (1st Symposium), pp. 145–155. O. A. Short (DuPont).

Thick Film Conductor Function Inks and Pastes for Microelectronics Applications. Interim Report No. IR-60, Electronic Properties Information Center, c/o Hughes Aircraft, February 1, 1968. J. T. Milek.

Die and Wire Bonding Capabilities of Representative Thick Film Conductors. *ISHM Proceedings,* 1968, pp. 359–371. J. P. Budd (DuPont).

Thick Film Adhesion—Evaluation and Improvement. *ISHM Proceedings,* 1968, pp. 417–423. C. J. Peckinpaugh and R. L. Tuggle (Electronic Communications).

Silver Palladium Fired Electrodes. *Proceedings Electronic Components Conference,* 1968, pp. 52–64. L. F. Miller (IBM).

Study of Surface Oxidation and Solderability on Silver Palladium Thick Film Conductors. *ISHM Proceedings,* 1969, pp. 81–89. T. Kubota and T. Shinmura (Tamura Kaken Co., Japan).

Thick-Film Conductor Adhesion Reliability. *ISHM Proceedings,* 1970, 3.3.1. W. Crossland and L. Hailes (Standard Telecommunication Labs).

Leaching during Solder Immersion—Thick Film Conductors. *NEPCON Proceedings (West),* 1970, pp. 11-1 to 11-6. R. P. Anjard (Delco Division, GMC).

Photoetching and Screen Printing of Conductor Patterns for Face-Down-Bonded Devices. *Proceedings Electronic Components Conference,* 1970, pp. 87–91. L. K. Keys, F. J. Francis, A. J. Russo, and S. Herring (Magnavox).

DIELECTRICS—THICK FILM
(Crossovers, Capacitors, and Encapsulants)

Performance Data on Thick-Film Crossovers. *ISHM Proceedings,* 1967 (2nd Symposium), pp. 39–49. T. Nakayama and L. C. Hoffman (DuPont).

New Dielectric Glazes for Crossover and Multilayer Screened Circuitry. *ISHM Proceedings,* 1967 (2nd Symposium), pp. 151–162. S. J. Stein (Electro-Science Labs).

Screen-Printed Ferroelectric Glass-Ceramic Capacitors. *Proceedings Electronic Components Conference,* 1968, pp. 239–245. J. W. Asher and C. R. Pratt (Corning Glass).

Glass-Ceramic Glazes for Crossover and Multilayer Screened Circuitry. *Proceedings Electronic Components Conference,* 1968, pp. 118–129. S. J. Stein (Electro-Science Labs).

Screen Printed High Q Dielectrics. *Proceedings Electronic Components Conference,* 1968, pp. 246–249. J. J. Cox and L. C. Hoffman (DuPont).

Crystallizable Dielectrics. *ISHM Proceedings,* 1968, pp. 111–118. L. C. Hoffman (DuPont).

Thick Film Glass-Ceramic Capacitors. *Solid State Technology,* May 1970, pp. 63–66. J. V. Biggers, G. L. Marshall, and D. W. Strickler (Erie Tech.).

Multilayer Microelectronic Substrates: A Materials Evaluation. *Electronic Packaging and Production,* October 1969, pp. 41–46. J. E. McCormick and D. W. Calabrese (Rome Air Development Center).

Achieving Multilayer Composite Substrate and Thick Film Materials Compatibility. *Electronic Packaging and Production,* June 1970, pp. 34–38. P. R. Theobald, M. P. Davis, and J. T. Bailey (American Lava).

The Crossover Chip: Multilayer Wiring on a Single Plane. *Electronic Packaging and Production,* May 1970, pp. 39–44. R. P. Moore and G. R. Reid (Burroughs).

Evaluation Testing of a Thick Film Multilayer Interconnect System. *ISHM Proceedings,* 1970, 6.3.1. M. Rossman (Martin Marietta).

Fabrication of Multilayer Thick Film Microelectronic Circuits. *ISHM Proceedings,* 1970, 6.4.1. L. Keys and F. Herring (Magnavox).

RESISTORS—GENERAL

Resistive Metal Glaze and Its Product Applications. *Proceedings Electronic Components Conference,* 1963, pp. 20–24. H. Casey et al.

The Glaze Resistor—Its Structure and Reliability. *IEEE Transactions on Component Parts,* CP-11, No. 2, June 1964, pp. 76–78.

Screened "Thick Film" Resistors. *Proceedings Electronic Components Conference,* 1967, pp. 217–228. D. P. Burks (Sprague).

Thick Film Resistor Functional Inks and Pastes for Microelectronics Applications. Interim Report IR-61, February 1, 1968. J. T. Milek (Hughes Aircraft, Air Force Materials Lab).

Glaze Resistors for Microminiature Hybrid Integrated Circuits. *Proceedings Electronic Components Conference,* 1968, pp. 287–291. R. F. Tramposch (Airco Speer).

Glaze Resistor Paste Preparation. *Proceedings Electronic Components Conference,* 1970, pp. 92–101. L. F. Miller (IBM).

Automation Applied to Establishing Thick Film Resistor Characteristics. *ISHM Proceedings,* 1970, 8.5.1. R. Ost, D. Nash and P. Tramantana (Sperry Gyroscope).

RESISTORS—PERFORMANCE

Precision Glaze Resistors. *American Ceramic Society Bulletin,* **42,** No. 9, September 1963, pp. 490–493. L. C. Hoffman (DuPont).

Properties of Indium Oxide Glaze Resistors. *Proceedings Electronic Components Conference,* 1966, pp. 191–196. M. L. Block and A. H. Mones (IBM).

Thallium Oxide Glaze Resistors. *Proceedings Electronic Components Conference,* 1967, pp. 432–438. F. M. Collins and C. F. Parks (Airco Speer).

The Mechanism of Conduction in Thick-Film Cermet Resistors. *Proceedings Electronic Components Conference,* 1967, pp. 238–246b. L. J. Brady (CTS).

Stability of Palladium Oxide Resistive Glaze Films. *Microelectronics and Reliability,* **6,** 1967, pp. 53–65. E. H. Melan.

Study of the Thick Film Resistor System: Pd-PdO-Ag. Hughes Memo 2741.00/9, September 14, 1967. H. Levin (Hughes Aircraft).

Thallium Oxide Resistive Glazes. *ISHM Proceedings,* 1967 (2nd Symposium), pp. 51–55. F. M. Collins and M. B. Redmount (Speer Carbon Div. of Air Reduction).

Designing with High Reliability Thick Film Resistors. *ISHM Proceedings,* 1967 (2nd Symposium), pp. 57–60. G. D. Lane (Electro Materials Corp.).

Thermal Characteristics of Film Resistor Modules. *Proceedings Electronic Components Conference,* 1968, pp. 69–78. D. Hatzipanagos and J. H. Powers (IBM).

Composition of Thick Film Resistors. *ISHM Proceedings,* 1968; pp. 173–181. D. L. Herbst (Alloys Unlimited).

Thallium Oxide Glaze Resistors on Alumina with Silver Terminations. *ISHM Proceedings,* 1968, pp. 183–187. P. R. Van Loon and C. F. Parks (Airco Speer).

Ruthenium Resistor Glazes for Thick Film Circuits. *ISHM Proceedings,* 1968, pp. 161–171. G. S. Iles (Johnson, Matthey Co.).

Effects of Resistor Geometry on Current Noise in Thick Film Resistors. *ISHM Proceedings,* 1968, pp. 153–160. C. Y. Kuo and H. G. Blank (General Telephone and Electronics Labs).

A Thick Film Resistor Glaze of Precision Properties. *Proceedings Electronic Components Conference,* 1969, pp. 285–288. P. R. Van Loon (Airco Speer).

Thick Film Resistor Pastes for High Performance Use. *ISHM Proceedings,* 1969, pp. 91–110. S. J. Stein, J. B. Garvin, and M. Vail (Electro-Science Labs).

Preliminary Data for a New High Performance Resistor Series. *ISHM Proceedings,* 1969, pp. 111–119. Also *Solid State Technology,* May 1970, pp. 73–76. L. C. Hoffman, M. J. Popowich, K. E. Schubert, and R. J. Bouchard (DuPont).

Tracking Studies in Thallium Oxide Thick Film Resistor Glazes. *ISHM Proceedings,* 1969, pp. 121–127. C. P. Buhsmer (Airco Speer).

Resistor Performance Characteristics in a Liquid Environment. *ISHM Proceedings,* 1969, pp. 233–243. J. H. Powers (IBM).

Voltage Coefficient of Resistance of Thick Film Resistors. *ISHM Proceedings,* 1970, 8.7.1. H. Isaak (McDonnell Douglas).

Variations of Electric Characteristics with Basic Components in Pd/Ag Thick Film Resistors. *ISHM Proceedings,* 1970, 8.6.1. T. Kubota and E. Sugata (Tamura Kaken Co.).

Pd/Ag Thick Film Resistor Stability in Hermetic Packages. *ISHM Proceedings,* 1970, 9.4.1.

Behavior of Thick Film Resistors Deposited on Thick Film Dielectric Layers. *Proceedings Electronic Components Conference,* 1970, pp. 531–535. R. P. Himmel (Hughes Aircraft).

Effects of Particle Size Control in the Metal Powder Systems on the Characteristics of Palladium Silver Thick Film Resistors. *Proceedings Electronic Components Conference,* 1970, pp. 514–519. T. Kubota (Tamura Kaken Co.).

RESISTORS—INTERFACE AND GEOMETRY

The Contact Resistance in Thick-Film Resistors. *ISHM Proceedings,* 1969, pp. 263–269. C. Y. Kuo (Columbia Components).

Termination Anomalies in Thick Film Resistors. *ISHM Proceedings,* 1969, pp. 271–280. J. A. Loughran and R. A. Sigsbee (GE).

Voltage Sensitivity vs. Geometry of Thick Film Resistors. *ISHM Proceedings,* 1969, pp. 345–360. D. L. Herbst and M. Greenfield (Alloys Unlimited).

Termination Resistance in Thick Film Resistors. *EDN,* March 15, 1970, pp. 89–91. C. Y. Kuo (Columbia Components).

The influence of Geometry and Conductive Terminations on Thick Film Resistors. *Proceedings Electronic Components Conference,* 1970, pp. 190–200. J. B. Garvin and S. J. Stein (Electro-Science Labs).

Geometry Dependence of Thick Film Resistors. *Proceedings Electronic Components Conference,* 1970, pp. 209–215. C. F. Jefferson (Tecnetics).

Termination Interface Reaction with Non-Palladium Resistors and Its Effect on Apparent Sheet Resistivity. *Proceedings Electronic Components Conference,* 1970, pp. 520–530. C. J. Peckinpaugh and W. G. Proffitt (Electronic Communications).

Effect of Geometry on the Characteristics of Thick Film Resistors. *Proceedings Electronic Components Conference,* 1970, pp. 102–108. D. E. Riemer (EMR/Weston).

CHAPTER 5

Variables Affecting Uniformity in the Screen Process Printing of Printed and Fired-on Films and the Development of a Squeegee Design for Improving Uniformity. *Proceedings Electronic Components Conference,* 1967, pp. 209–216. D. C. Hughes, Jr. (Precision Systems).

Frame Design and Tension Control for Precise Screen Process Printing of Microcircuits with Mesh Screens and Etched Masks. *ISHM Proceedings,* 1967 (1st Symposium), pp. 21–36. H. L. Coronis (Industrial Reproductions).

Screen Tension and Mesh Alignment for Control of the Off-Contact Printing Process with Direct Emulsion Screens and Indirect Metal Masks. *ISHM Proceedings,* 1967 (2nd Symposium), pp. 127–131. H. L. Coronis (Industrial Reproductions).

Use of Metal Masks to Improve the Printing of Thick Film Geometrics. *ISHM Proceedings,* 1968, pp. 227–232. Also *Proceedings Electronic Components Conference,* 1969, pp. 247–253. W. C. Littell, Jr. (Fairchild).

A Low Cost Master Pattern and Screen Making Technique. *Proceedings Electronic Components Conference,* 1969, pp. 242–246. L. Jacobson (GE).

Paste Transfer in the Screening Process. *Solid State Technology,* June 1969, pp. 46–52. L. F. Miller (IBM).

Thick Film Screen Printing. *Solid State Technology,* June 1969, pp. 53–58. B. M. Austin (AMI).

An Approach to Automatic Screen Printing. *ISHM Proceedings,* 1969, pp. 173–176. E. G. de Haart (de Haart, Inc.).

Indirect and Direct Etched Metal Masks for Deposition Control and Fine Line Printing. *ISHM Proceedings,* 1969, pp. 243–251. L. H. Coronis (Industrial Reproductions).

Repeatability in Screen Printing Hybrid Microcircuits. *ISHM Proceedings,* 1969, pp. 253–262. A. V. Ottaviano (GE).

Fine Line Technologies for Microelectronic Devices. *Proceedings Electronic Components Conference,* 1970, pp. 570–575. C. H. Wang (Fairchild C & I).

Parametric Dependencies in Thick Film Screen Processing. *ISHM Proceedings,* 1970, 5.5.1. D. Kobs and D. Voight (Centralab).

A Storable Emulsion Screen for Thickness Control and Immediate Response. *ISHM Proceedings,* 1970, 5.6.1. L. H. Coronis (Industrial Reproductions).

How Paste Rheology Can Improve Your Fine Line Printing. *ISHM Proceedings,* 1970, 8.4.1. R. Trease and R. L. Dietz (Owens-Illinois).

Process Variables in Thick Film Resistor Fabrication. *Solid State Technology,* July 1970, pp. 58–64 (ISHM Journal I-1). Also *ISHM Proceedings,* 1969, pp. 185–195. J. A. Van Hise (IBM).

Variables in the Thick Film Screen Printing Process and Their Effect on Register Tolerances in Large Scale Production. *Electronic Components,* April 1970, pp. 48–50. J. D. Salisbury (STC).

Controlling the Variables in Thick Film Resistor Fabrication. *Electronic Packaging and Production,* April 1970, pp. 48–50. J. A. Van Hise (IBM).

CHAPTER 6

Some Important Process and Performance Characteristics of "Birox" Thick Film Resistor Compositions. *Proceedings Electronic Components Conference,* 1970, pp. 201–208. Also *Solid State Technology,* January 1971, pp. 33–37. L. C. Hoffman and M. J. Popowich (DuPont).

Firing Characteristics of Palladium-Silver Thick Film Resistors. *Proceedings Electronic Components Conference,* 1967, pp. 389–396. R. C. Headley (DuPont).

Effect of Firing Conditions on Stability and Properties of Glaze Resistors. S. J. Stein.

Reproducibility of Electrical Properties of Thick Film Resistors. *ISHM Proceedings,* 1967 (1st Symposium), pp. 56–69. R. C. Headley (DuPont).

Selection of Furnace Equipment for Thick Film Firing. *ISHM Proceedings,* 1967 (1st Symposium), pp. 37–43. D. J. Spigarelli (Watkins-Johnson Co.).

Firing Thick Film Integrated Circuits. *ISHM Proceedings,* 1967 (1st Symposium), pp. 114–119. J. H. Beck (BTU Eng.).

Note. See listings for Chapters 4, 5, and 7. They contain many references to firing.

CHAPTER 7

See listings for Chapter 4.

CHAPTER 8

Adjusting Depostied Thick Film Resistors in Hybrid Microelectronic Circuits. *ISHM Proceedings,* 1967 (1st Symposium), pp. 178–183. C. Ingulli (S. S. White).

Electric Discharge Trimming of Glaze Resistors. *ISHM Proceedings,* 1968, pp. 145–153. F. J. Pakulski and T. R. Touw (IBM).

Process Information for the Design of Automatic Resistor Trimming Equipment. *ISHM Proceedings,* 1969, pp. 197–200. P. J. Sanders (Microtek).

Resistor Trimming and Micromachining with a Yag Laser. *Solid State Technology,* April 1970, pp. 43–49. R. Waters and M. Weiner-Korad (UCC).

Programmable Continuous Laser Trimming. *Electronic Packaging and Production,* May 1970, pp. 177–186. Also *ISHM Proceedings,* 1969, pp. 177–183. G. B. Stone (Micronetics).

Measuring Techniques for Trimming Thick Film Resistors. *Proceedings Electronic Components Conference,* 1970, pp. 536–546. D. S. Ironside and P. H. Reynolds (James G. Biddle Co.).

Development of Trimming Techniques for Microcircuit Thick Film and Thin Film Resistors. *ISHM Proceedings,* 1970, 3.7.1. S. Caruso and R. Allen (Marshall Space Flight Center).

A Compact Low Cost Thick and Thin Film Laser Resistor Trimmer. *ISHM Proceedings,* 1970, 5.3.1. F. Burns (Apollo).

CHAPTER 9

SOLDERING

Bonding Alloy Placement and Device Attachment by the Use of Metal/Chemical Systems. *ISHM Proceedings,* 1969, pp. 71–79. A. R. Kroehs (Alpha Metals).

Stress Failures and Joining Considerations in Hybrid Circuits. *Proceedings Electronic Components Conference,* 1969, pp. 298–303. S. S. Cole, Jr., and A. R. Kroehs (Alpha Metals).

Selection Parameters for Hybrid Circuit Bonding Alloys. *Proceedings Electronic Components Conference,* 1970, pp. 116–121. A. R. Kroehs (Alpha Metals).

Techniques of Device-to-Substrate Mounting. *Electronic Packaging and Production,* May 1970, pp. 49–56. A. R. Kroehs (Alpha Metals).

Device-Substrate Bonding—Materials and Techniques. *Electronic Packaging and Production,* September 1970, pp. 84–97. A. R. Kroehs (Alpha Metals).

Factors Affecting Solder Welding and Resistance Drift in Thick Film Circuits. *Proceedings Electronic Components Conference,* 1969, pp. 329–333. L. H. Fanelli, W. L. Robinson, and V. J. Leggio (Autonetics).

Formon® Printable Solder and Braze Composition Series. *ISHM Proceedings,* 1970, 8.2.1. R. Amin and J. Conwicke (DuPont).

Noble Metal Scavenging in Hybrid Circuit Bonding Applications. *ISHM Proceedings,* 1970, 8.3.1.

BONDING—GENERAL

Die and Wire Bonding Capabilities of Representative Thick Film Conductors. *ISHM Proceedings,* 1968, pp. 359–371. (See *Handbook,* Section 2.5.1.1.) J. P. Budd (DuPont).

A Survey of Chip Joining Techniques. *Proceedings Electronic Components Conference,* 1969, pp. 60–76. Also (Part I) *Solid State Technology,* August 1969, pp. 47–52, and (Part II) *ibid.,* September 1969, pp. 33–41. L. F. Miller (IBM).

Ultrasonic Bonding of Integrated Circuits to Thick Film Pedestals on Ceramic Substrates. *Proceedings Electronic Components Conference,* 1969, pp. 254–275. (See *Handbook,* Section 2.5.4.) T. J. Matcovich and R. L. Coren (Drexel Inst.); D. G. Kelemen and R. J. Galli (DuPont).

Variables Affecting Weld Quality in Ultrasonic Aluminum Wire Bonding. *Solid State Technology,* August 1969, pp. 72–77. P. M. Uthe (Uthe Technology).

Chip Bonding Promises and Perils. *Electronic Design,* October 25, 1969, pp. 61–79. R. D. Speer (Staff).

Assembly and Repair of Multi-Chip Modules. *Electronic Engineering,* October 1969, pp. 22–24. A. G. Cozens (IBM).

Application of the STD Process to Hybrid Microelectronics. *Proceedings Electronic Components Conference,* 1970, pp. 216–235. R. J. Clark and J. W. Lunden (GE).

Survey of the Major Chip Interconnection Techniques. *NEPCON Proceedings (West),* 1970, pp. 5-1 to 5-11. H. K. Dicken (ICE).

Critique of Chip-Joining Techniques. *Solid State Technology,* April 1970, pp. 50–62. L. F. Miller (IBM).

Spider Bond Packaging. *Electronic Packaging and Production,* May 1970, pp. 296–300. R. Bowman and R. Bond (Motorola).

FACE BONDING

Joining Semiconductor Devices with Ductile Pads. *ISHM Proceedings,* 1968, pp. 333–343. L. F. Miller (IBM).

Handling and Bonding of Beam-Lead Sealed-Junction Integrated Circuits. *ISHM Proceedings,* 1968, pp. 323–332. M. P. Eleftherion (Western Electric).

Flip Chip Microcircuit Bonding Systems. *Proceedings Electronic Components Conference,* 1969, pp. 131–144. T. R. Myers (IIT Res. Inst.).

Optimizing Cyclic Fatigue Life of Controlled Collapse Chip Joints. *Proceedings Electronic Components Conference,* 1969, pp. 404–423. L. S. Goldmann (IBM).

Face Bonding: What Does It Take? *Solid State Technology,* August 1969, pp. 53–57. E. F. Koshinz (Unitek).

Flip Chip Asembly. *Solid State Technology,* August 1969, pp. 62–67. W. Hugle (Hugle Industries).

Screening Materials for Special Chip Joining Procedures. *Electronic Packaging and Production,* September 1969, pp. 82–97. L. F. Miller (IBM).

Compliant Bonding. *Proceedings Electronic Components Conference,* 1970, pp. 380–389. A. Coucoulas (Western Electric).

Mechanical Design of Chip Components for Flip and Short Beam Lead Mounting. *ISHM Proceedings,* 1969, pp. 5–15. D. Boswell (ITT Components Group Europe).

Face Bonded Chips and Thick Film Compatibility. *Electronic Packaging and Production,* May 1970, pp. 87–100. A. F. Khambatta and P. A. Castle (Welwyn Electric).

Installation of a Specialized Manufacturing Facility for the Production of Face-Bonded Chip Semiconductors for Use in Hybrid Thick Film Circuits. *ISHM Proceedings,* 1970, 2.6.1. P. Kirby (Welwyn Electric).

Bonding Conditions and Tests and Fine Line Technology for Attaching Beam-Lead Devices to Hybrid Integrated Circuits. *ISHM Proceedings,* 1970, 7.6.1. L. Keys, F. Francis and A. Russo (Magnavox).

Design Considerations for a Flip-Chip Joining Technique. *Solid State Technology,* July 1970, pp. 48–54. P. Lin, J. Lee and S. Im (IBM).

Rigid and Non-Rigid Beam-Lead Substrates. *Solid State Technology,* August 1970, pp. 62–66. F. J. Bachner, R. A. Cohen, and R. E. McMahon (MIT-Lincoln Lab).

CHAPTER 10

ACTIVE DISCRETES

Factors Involved in Specifying Semiconductor Chips for Hybrid Microelectronics. *ISHM Proceedings,* 1967 (2nd Symposium), pp. 83–89. J. K. Logan and H. B. Bell (Integrated Circuit Eng. Corp.).

Beam Lead Devices—The New Hybrid Circuit Element. *ISHM Proceedings,* 1968, pp. 317–322. W. H. Legat, W. C. Rosvold, and W. Ward (Raytheon).

Supplying Semiconductor Chips to the Microelectronic Industry. *ISHM Proceedings,* 1969, pp. 1–3. G. R. Broussard (Texas Instruments).

Care and Feeding of Semiconductor Chips. *Electronic Products,* July 1970, pp. 32–38. E. W. Callander and L. J. Palmer (Centralab).

Chip Handling Equipment. *NEPCON Proceedings (West),* 1970, pp. 5–21. B. M. Austin (AMI).

INDUCTORS

Adjustable Reactive Components for Direct Mounting on Thick Film Substrates. *Proceedings Electronic Components Conference,* 1968, pp. 191–197. R. L. Weber (Texas Instruments).

RESISTORS

Survey of Chip Resistors. *Electronic Products,* January 18, 1971, pp. 29–32. G. Flynn.

CAPACITORS

Reduced Titanate Capacitor Chips for Thick Film Hybrid IC's. *Proceedings Electronic Components Conference,* 1968, pp. 256–264. D. W. Hamer (State of the Art).

Ceramic Capacitors for Hybrid Integrated Circuits. *ISHM Proceedings,* 1968, pp. 99–109. D. W. Hamer (State of the Art).

Tantalum Chip Capacitors. *ISHM Proceedings,* 1968, pp. 125–135. D. E. Maguire (Union Carbide).

Non-Conventional Applications for Multilayer Ceramic Capacitors. *Proceedings Electronic Components Conference,* 1969, pp. 223–230. D. W. Hamer (State of the Art).

The Multilayer Ceramic Capacitor—A New Industry Approaches Maturity. *Ceramic Industry,* July 1969, pp. 49–56. D. W. Hamer (State of the Art).

Improved Tantalum Chip Capacitors for Hybrid Circuits. *Proceedings Electric Components Conference,* 1969, pp. 211–217. D. E. Maguire (Union Carbide).

Unencapsulated Solid Tantalum Capacitors for Hybrid Circuit Applications. *ISHM Proceedings,* 1970, 4.6.1. R. Lambrecht (Union Carbide).

New End Termination for Ceramic Chip Capacitors. *ISHM Proceedings,* 1970, 6.5.1. H. DeMatos (Union Carbide).

Molded Solid Tantalum Capacitors for Printed Circuit Board and Hybrid Circuit Applications. *Proceedings Electronic Components Conference,* 1970, pp. 437–445. A. Whitman and D. G. Thompson (Sprague Electric).

CHAPTER 11

Laminated Ceramics. *Proceedings Electronic Components Conference,* 1967, pp. 17–26. B. Schwartz and D. L. Wilcox (IBM).

Transmission Line Characteristics of Conductors Buried in Ceramic. *Proceedings Electronic Components Conference,* 1969, pp. 83–86. S. A. Sands and D. L. Wilcox (IBM).

High Density Wiring by the Crossover Chip Technique. *ISHM Proceedings,* 1969, pp. 223–230. R. P. Moore and G. Reid (Burroughs).

Multilayer Composite Substrates for Thick Film Hybrid Microcircuits. *ISHM Proceedings,* 1969, pp. 447–454. P. R. Theobold, M. P. Davis, and J. T. Bailey (American Lava).

Packaging Complex Multi-Chip Systems—Design Considerations and Applications. *ISHM Proceedings,* 1968, pp. 1–10. R. Boggs and E. Kanazawa (Fairchild).

Commercial Application of Thick Film Hybrid Microelectronic Packaging. *Proceedings Electronic Components Conference,* 1969, pp. 231–241. R. C. Abbe (Microtek) and A. P. Mandel (Raytheon).

Metal Problems in Plastic Encapsulated Integrated Circuits. *IEEE Proceedings,* September 1969, pp. 1606–1609.

Encapsulation of Integrated Circuits. *IEEE Proceedings,* September 1969, pp. 1610–1615. M. L. White (Bell Labs).

Study of the Thick Film Resistance Abrupt Change by Resin Packaging. *ISHM Proceedings,* 1969, pp. 51–62. K. Asama, Y. Nishimura, and H. Sasaki (Fujitsu Labs).

The Solution of Parasitic Effects on the Thick Film Hybrid Circuits Resulting from Encapsulation Process. *ISHM Proceedings,* 1969, pp. 63–70. E. Tsunashima and K. Terasaka (Wireless Res. Labs).

Nucleation, Crystallization, and Flow of Sealing Glasses. *ISHM Proceedings,* 1969, pp. 153–158. H. S. Hartmann (Owens-Illinois).

Problems in Hybrid Circuit Packaging. *ISHM Proceedings,* 1969, pp. 217–222. H. T. Groves (Litton Systems).

New Semiconductor Packaging Horizons for BeO. *Electronic Packaging and Production,* December 1969, pp. 64–68. P. S. Hessinger (National Beryllia Corp.).

Plastics Encapsulation of Components. *Electronic Engineering,* January 1970, pp. 50–56. K. A. Pettican (Standard Telecommunication Labs).

IC Packaging: The Variations. *Electronic Packaging and Production,* January 1970, pp. 234–238.

Equipment Designer's Approach to Packaging of Hybrid Microcircuits. *Proceedings Electronic Components Conference,* 1970, pp. 12–15. R. R. Bigler (RCA).

Interconnection and Packaging of Thick Film Microcircuits. *Proceedings Electronic Components Conference,* 1970, pp. 122–126. R. Ilgenfritz and L. Mogey (Raytheon).

Low Cost Packaging of Thick Film Substrates with Ceramic Glass Seals. *NEPCON Proceedings (West),* 1970, pp. 10–40. J. C. Gioia (GE).

Microcircuit Packaging and Assembly—State of the Art. *Solid State Technology,* August 1970, pp. 41–47. G. K. Fehr (Intel).

Resin Systems for Encapsulation of Microelectronic Packages. *Solid State Technology,* August 1970, pp. 48–55. H. Hirsch (IBM).

Hermetic Sealing of Integrated Circuit Packages. *Solid State Technology,* August 1970, pp. 56–61. F. H. Bower (ICE).

Hermetic and Nonhermetic Packaging. *Solid State Technology,* August 1970, pp. 67–70 and 75. A. Postlethwaite (Sylvania).

Hermetic Sealing of Large Ceramic Flat Packages. *ISHM Proceedings,* 1970, 4.3.1. W. Fiedler (Martin Marietta).

Hermetic Packages and Sealing Methods. *ISHM Proceedings,* 1970, 6.2.1. F. Bower (ICE).

CHAPTER 12

APPLICATIONS

Compatible Reactive Components for a Thick-Film Television Video IF Amplifier. *ISHM Proceedings,* 1967 (2nd Symposium), pp. 61–70. R. L. Weber and J. C. Prabhakar (Texas Instruments).

A Hybrid Thick-Film Chroma Demodulator and Color-Difference Amplifier. *ISHM Proceedings,* 1968, pp. 487–496. Also *IEEE Transactions, Parts, Materials & Packaging,* June 1969, pp. 117–123. C. M. Engel, C. F. Hepner, M. L. Kummel, T. O. Melkeraaen, and G. E. Weibel (Zenith Radio).

Thick Film RF Circuitry. *Proceedings Electronic Components Conference,* 1969, pp. 289–297. P. Fosco (Sylvania).

Design Considerations for Power Hybrid Circuits. *ISHM Proceedings,* 1969, pp. 323–344. L. Balents, R. D. Gold, A. W. Kaiser, and W. R. Peterson (RCA).

Hybrid Voltage Regulator for Automotive Applications. *ISHM Proceedings,* 1969, pp. 361–367. G. E. Harland (Delco—GMC).

Merging Technologies—Microelectronics and Microwaves. *EDN,* October 1, 1969, pp. 61–88. J. E. Cunningham and H. F. Cooke (Texas Instruments).

Automotive Microcircuitry. *IEEE Student Journal,* May 1970, pp. 24–29. W. Hugle (Hugle Industries).

.01 MFD. Variable Capacitor. *Proceedings Electronic Components Conference,* 1970, pp. 446–454. J. H. Fabricius and J. Maher (Sprague Electric).

Microelectronics in Consumer Products. *ISHM Proceedings,* 1970, 2.8. W. Liederbach (RCA).

A Thick Film Hybrid, Precision D to A Converter. *ISHM Proceedings,* 1970, 2.4.1. E. Weinberg (AVCO).

Hybrid Components: Development Circuits Capable of Operating at Cryogenic Temperatures. *ISHM Proceedings,* 1970, 3.5.1. C. Turner and H. Blazek (Naval Weapons Center).

DESIGNS

Design Guide for Thick-Film Hybrid Microcircuits. *ISHM Proceedings,* 1967 (2nd Symposium), pp. 91–100. F. Z. Keister and D. Auda (Hughes Aircraft).

Design Guide to Hybrid Package Size. *Electronic Engineer,* September 1969, pp. 45–46. R. C. Bristol (CTS).

System Partitioning for Hybrid Circuits. *ISHM Proceedings,* 1969, pp. 281–288. F. Gargione and H. Fenster (RCA).

Fabrication of Large Scale Hybrid Integrated Circuits by Thick Film Techniques. *ISHM Proceedings,* 1968, pp. 219–225. H. Fenster and P. E. McHale (United Aircraft).

THERMAL CONSIDERATIONS

Thermal Design Critera for Hybrid Microelectronic Modules. *ISHM Proceedings,* 1968, pp. 31–42. A. P. Mandel and P. K. Vahey (Microtek).

Parametric Study of Temperature Distributions in Chips—Joined by Controlled Chip Collapse Techniques. *Proceedings Electronic Components Conference,* 1969, pp. 429–452. S. Oktay (IBM).

Thermal Impedance of Ceramic Packages Using Beam-Lead IC Chips. *IEEE Proceedings,* September 1969, pp. 1616–1620. N. A. Hardwick (Bell Labs).

Designing Hybrid Modules Using Basic Thermal Guidelines. *Electronic Packaging and Production,* July 1969, pp. 112–117. A. P. Mandel (Raytheon).

Thermal Design and Packaging of Hybrid Integrated Circuits. *Electronic Components,* September 1969, pp. 1045–1048. V. T. Guntlow, D. P. Burks, and J. H. Martin (Sprague).

Thermal Analysis of Semiconductor Devices Assembled by Various Packaging Techniques. *ISHM Proceedings,* 1969, pp. 207–216. T. T. Tarone (ITT).

Better High-Power-Density Circuit Cooling through Nucleate Boiling. *Electronic Packaging and Production,* May 1970, pp. 60–72.

Thermal Analysis of Ceramic Based Microcircuits. *Electronic Components,* June 1970, pp. 671–680. J. H. Martin, V. T. Guntlow, and D. P. Burks (Sprague).

Thermal Conductance and Its Effect on Electronic Packaging. *ISHM Proceedings,* 1970, 4.7.1. J. Seely and O. Gupta (IBM).

Thermal Resistance Calculations for Reliability Testing. *ISHM Proceedings,* 1970, 2.5.1. C. Lee and S. Abbas (IBM).

CHAPTER 13

ECONOMICS—THICK FILM

Thick Film Hybrid Economics. *ISHM Proceedings,* 1967 (1st Symposium), pp. 121–132. D. Bailey and G. Doyle (Union Carbide).

In-House Thick Film Facility. *ISHM Proceedings,* 1970, 7.3.1. V. Gundatera (AMF).

Economics of Thick Film Hybrid Microcircuit Production. *ISHM Proceedings,* 1970, 6.1.1. Also *Proceedings Electronic Components Conference,* 1970, pp. 576–584. D. W. Hamer (State of the Art).

Problems in Establishing a Thick Film Microcircuit Facility. *ISHM Proceedings,* 1967 (1st Symposium), pp. 91–101. M. Schneider and D. Auda (Hughes Aircraft).

Experience Curves as a Planning Tool. *IEEE Spectrum,* June 1970, pp. 63–68. P. Conley (Boston Consulting Group).

INDEX

Adhesion (of conductors), 132
Air abrasive trimming, 177; *see also* Trimming
Artwork, 303
  coordinatograph, 329
  the master sketch, 327
  rubylith®, 328
  screen making, 330
  see also Design
Aspect ratio, defined, 71

Beam lead bonding, 226·
Bibliography, 406
Bingham body, 98
Bonding, die (chip), die, 193
  epoxy, 201
  equipment, 197
  eutectic, 195
  introduction to, 44
  see also Face bonding
Bonding, wire, 202
  ball, 207
  equipment, 211
  problems, 215
  stitch, 209
  thermocompression, 203, 213
  ultrasonic, 205, 213
  wedge, 207

Capacitor, chips, use of, 284
  trimming, 185
  see also Dielectric materials; Discrete devices
Captive IC production, 22
Chips, *see* Discrete devices
Conductor materials (inks), adhesion of, 132
  alloy systems, 81
  compatibility, 135
  components of, 74
  functions of, 74
  gold, 80
  inks, 72
  introduction, 31
  line definition, 136
  properties of, 131
  reactions during firing, 119
  resistor interface reactions, 143
  silver, 80
  solderability, 131
Contact Printing, 115
Controlled collapse, 224
Coordinatograph, 329
Costs, conventional versus thick film, 352
  cost reductions, 320
  discrete versus IC, 64
  equipment cost, 310

high volume versus low volume, 333
labor rates for process steps, 339
materials, 336
monolithic cost structure, 56
production, comparisons, 53
startup, facilities, 53
of thick film, 332
thick film versus thin, 65
tooling, 335
Crossovers, *see* Dielectric inks; Multilayer

Definitions, hybrid, 22
microcircuit, 22
microelectronics, 22
MIL STD 280, 22
Design and layout, 303
artwork, 327
design steps, 304
estimating area needed, 307
heat considerations, 309
layout guidelines, 311
partitioning, 310
picking a package, 306
Dielectric constant, 85, 131
Dielectric inks, 84
capacitor, functional materials, 88
crossover, functional materials, 86
properties of, 150
Dielectric materials, introduction to, 33; *see also* Capacitors
Dilatency, 98
Discrete devices, active, face bonded, 251
inspection of, 243
lids, 251
testing, 242
passive, capacitors, 263
configurations, 261
inductors, 276
reason for using, 254
versus screen printed, 254
Dissipation factor, 154
Dual-in line (DIP) packages, 282
Dynamic trimming, *see* Trimming

Economics, *see* Costs
Equipment (thick film); introduction to, 36; *see also* Kilns: Printers
Eutectic bonding, 195

Face bonding, beam leads, 226

flip chips, 222
other approaches, 229
see also Bonding
Firing, conductor reactions during, 117
dielectric reactions during, 122
process, the, 123
reactions, general, 116
resistor reactions during, 119
Flat pack packages, 280
Flip chip bonding, controlled collapse, 224
general, 222
Furnace, 126
introduction to, 41
operation of, 130

Historical developments, electronics in general, 1
integrated circuits, 9
interconnection problems, 8
monolithic ICs, 12
thick film ICs, 15
transistor, 7

Inductors, 276
In-house production of ICs, sales trends, recent years, 22
Inks, conductor, 72
dielectric, 84
making, 89
properties of, 131
resistor, 81
see also Conductor materials; Resistors etc.
Insulation resistance, 155

Kilns, introduction to, 41
operation of, 130
thick film, 126

Laser trimming, 187; *see also* Trimming
Layout, rules for, 311; *see also* Design
LIDs (Leadless Inverted Devices), 251

Make or buy, screens, 331
thick film circuit, 353
Materials, 69
MIL STD 280 (Microelectronics definitions), 26
Minicomponents, 20
Monolithic ICs, comparison to hybrids, 52
processing steps, 364

semiconductor physics, 359
Multilayer, 288, 320

Newtonian fluids, 98
Noise, 141

Overshoot, 178

Packaging, basic functions of, 277
   configurations, 280
      dual-in line (DIP), 282
      flat pack, 280
      nonstandard, 288
      to type, 287
   picking a package type, 301, 306
   sealing, 298
   types, 290
      ceramic, 294
      glass, 296
      metal, 290
      plastic, 297
   unsealing, 301
Partitioning, 310
Plastic, packages, 297
   bonding, 201
Printers, *see* Screen printer
Printing, *see* Screen printing
Process steps in sequence, monolithic, 364
   thick film, 48
   thin film, 387
Pseudoplastic, 98

Resistivity, of conductors, 131
   defined, 71
   sheet, 71, 138
Resistor inks, 81
   blending of, 138
   conductor interface reactions, 144
   firing, effect of, 140
   firing reactions, 119
   functional materials, 83
   introduction to, 32
   materials, 32
   noise, 141
   palladium containing, 83
   properties of, 137
   stability, 146
   TCR, 137
   thallium, 83
   VCR, 141

Resistor processing, controlling spread, 169
   hitting target, 162
   trimming, 173
Resistors, discrete, reasons for using, 256;
      see also Discrete devices
Rheology, 95
   viscosity, 96
Rubylith®, 328

Sales figures, electronics over the years, 2, 5
   electronics, recent figures, 22
   hybrid ICs, recent figures, 22
   ICs over the years, 9
   microelectronics, recent figures, 22
   monolithic ICs, recent figures, 22
   tubes, 4
Screen printers, general, 100
   introduction to, 36
   operation of, 103
Screen printing, contact, 115
   general, 95
   rheology, 95
   squeegees, 111
   theory, 105
   variables, 109
Screens, general, 100
   make or buy decisions, 331
   making, 330
   newer types, 114
Sealing packages, 298
Sheet resistivity, 71
Snap-off, rates, 111
Solderability of conductors, 131
Soldering, alloys, 238
   contamination, 239
   fluxes, 236
   general, 234
   methods, 240
   metallurgy, 238
   reactions, 122
Squeegee, configurations, 112
   introduction to, 41
   materials, 111
Stencils, *see* Screens
Substrates, functions of, 90
   introduction, 30
   making, 93
Suppliers, equipment and materials, 392

Temperature coefficient, of capacitance, 151

of resistance (TCR), 137
Thermocompression wire bonding, 202
Thin film, comparison to thick and, 52
    introduction to, 381
    manufacturing steps, 387
Thixotropic, 98
Trimmers, air abrasive, 177
    introduction to, 42
    laser, 187
Trimming, air abrasive, 177
    capacitor, 185
    functional (or dynamic), 189
    laser, 187
    precision, 179

target values, setting, 177
    techniques, 174

Ultrasonic wire bonding, 205

Value added ratios, ICs compared to dis-
    cretes, 11
    importance of, 355
Viscosity, defined, 96
    measurement, 97
Voltage coefficient, of capacitance, 153
    of resistance, 141

Yields, versus costs, 57

DATE DUE

OCT 1 '86			
SEP 28 '87			
GAYLORD			PRINTED IN U.S.A.